“That’s how we do it…we treat them all the same”

“That’s how we do it…we treat them all the same”: An Exploration of the Experiences of Patients, Lay Carers and Health and Social Care Staff of the Care Received by Older People with Dementia in Acute Hospital Settings

By

Fiona Cowdell

CAMBRIDGE SCHOLARS

PUBLISHING

"That's how we do it…we treat them all the same":
An Exploration of the Experiences of Patients, Lay Carers and Health and Social Care Staff of the Care Received by Older People with Dementia in Acute Hospital Settings,
by Fiona Cowdell

This book first published 2013

Cambridge Scholars Publishing

12 Back Chapman Street, Newcastle upon Tyne, NE6 2XX, UK

British Library Cataloguing in Publication Data
A catalogue record for this book is available from the British Library

ISBN (10): 1-4438-4262-1, ISBN (13): 978-1-4438-4262-4

TABLE OF CONTENTS

ACKNOWLEDGEMENTS

This research was supported by a grant from the Alzheimer's Society.

Grateful thanks are extended to all the participants who gave their time and shared their thoughts so generously, to Professor Kate Galvin and Dr Eloise Carr for their advice and guidance and to Jo Aspland for her editorial support.

Many thanks are also due to KEC and DG who have lived through the production of this work and to RHC for all his encouragement.

INTRODUCTION

'That's how we do it ... we treat them all the same'

This study aimed to explore the experiences of patients, lay carers and health and social care staff of care received by older people with dementia in the acute hospital setting. In view of the ageing population, an increasing prevalence of dementia and the emerging dignity agenda this is a particularly topical subject.

Four elements are included in this book: a literature review, a research study, a practice development project and an integrative review. A literature review sets person-focused research in the context of dementia research as a whole. It also identifies ways in which studies have been conducted in an ethical and meaningful manner.

An ethnographic approach was used in the research study to collect data through observation, conversations and interviews. Findings portray a bleak picture of the care of this vulnerable group. Patients demonstrated, through words and actions, how difficult they found the experience. Lack of communication was an issue as was the obvious distress caused by delivery of personal care. Lay carers were relatively uncritical although this may have been due, in part, to the recruitment process. Staff generally appeared to have good intention. Most stated that they had received little or no preparation or education in dementia care. Many staff functioned almost entirely within the "bed and body" framework. They frequently avoided communication with patients. Staff worked in a deeply embedded habitus, in which they appeared not to really think about what they were doing. They demonstrated a lack of empathy with patients.

The concept that staff were working in a "switched off" mode and lacked empathy called for a practice development project that engaged them on both cognitive and emotional levels. A practice development project based on the philosophies of confluent education and situated learning was implemented. Initial evaluation has demonstrated some tangible changes in practice.

An integrative review draws these elements together into a coherent whole. Potential contributions to the body of knowledge are acknowledged, as are limitations of the work. This study has shown that people with dementia, even those at an advanced stage and with superimposed physical illness, can be engaged in research that is both ethical and meaningful. It has shown that improvements in practice are possible. They need to be underpinned by a belief in the personhood of staff as well as patients. Areas for further research and practice development in this vital subject have been identified.

CHAPTER ONE

LITERATURE REVIEW

Introduction

It is well recognised that the prevalence of dementia in older adults is increasing (Alzheimer's Society 2006). Having worked as a registered nurse in acute hospitals for many years I was aware that some of the care provided for older people with dementia was good and some less so. As the number of people with dementia requiring acute care is ever increasing I felt it was vital to investigate current care and consider much needed developments.

The increase in dementia is reflected by a huge rise in the amount of research into this area. This review addresses the question: is it possible to engage people with dementia in research in a way that is both ethical and meaningful? Three distinct phases in this chapter attempt to answer this question.

Phase one sets person-focused research within the context of dementia research as a whole. This phase considers cumulative reviews of dementia research including systematic reviews, meta-synthesis, meta-analysis, re-analysis and literature reviews. Eight hundred and sixteen papers were identified that met the inclusion criteria. The subject of each of these studies was identified and subjects clustered into ten categories: investigation of disease process, medication, treatment non-pharmacological, diagnostics and assessment, activities of life, care givers, person focused, culture specific, ethics and law and cost. Diagrammatic representation of the categories demonstrates the directions in which dementia research has moved over the last three decades. By far the most work has followed the biomedical model concentrating on investigation of the disease process and the use of medication. There has been a steady rise in studies about the ethics of dementia care, non-pharmacological treatments and techniques for diagnosis and assessment. It is evident that in more recent years there has been a small, but growing, interest in person-focused research studies that seek to understand the experiences and views of people with dementia. Phase one sets person-focused dementia research within the broad landscape of dementia research. Phase two provides an overview of published studies that include people with dementia; forty-five papers met the inclusion criteria. These studies are assessed against a set of criteria that have been developed from existing models for evaluating qualitative research and adapted specifically for use with research involving people with dementia. Studies have been ranked as levels one, two or three according to how closely they met the criteria. Three studies were ranked at level one, meeting the criteria most closely; thirty seven were at level two and five at level three. All studies provided some evidence that it is possible to involve people with dementia in research in a way that is both ethical and meaningful, although the quality of involvement was extremely variable. Reflection on the allocation of studies into the three levels suggested that the way in which decisions had been made was not entirely transparent. It was considered that using a detailed set of criteria may have detracted from reviewing studies from a holistic perspective. This idea generated phase three of the review.

Phase three reconsiders the studies that were categorised at level one. The signal from each of these papers was high. That is, they all appeared to provide an exceptionally valuable contribution to answering a question. However this value was not necessarily fully explicated when using the phase two criteria. The three studies were reviewed again using the fundamental concepts of qualitative research methods and, in particular, the narrative approach. This second analysis allowed a more global review that enabled interpretation beyond that previously achieved and clearly demonstrated the aspects of these papers that identify them as being at the forefront of ethical and meaningful research involving people with dementia.

Background

Dementia is defined by the World Health Organisation as "a syndrome due to disease of the brain, usually of a chronic or progressive nature, in which there is a disturbance of multiple higher cortex functions including memory, thinking, orientation, comprehension, calculation, learning capacity, language and judgment. Consciousness is not impaired" (WHO 1992). The Alzheimer's Society (2003) defines dementia as a "group of symptoms caused by the physical impact of disease or injury on the brain". It is stated that each person will experience it in their own individual way but that most will live through a decline in memory, reasoning and communication skills together with a gradual loss of the skills needed to carry out daily activities.

There are a range of different types of dementia. An estimate of the proportions of people with the different forms of dementia is provided by the Alzheimer's Society (2003). These are: Alzheimer's disease 55%, vascular dementia 20%, dementia with Lewy bodies 15%, fronto-temporal dementia 5% and other dementia 5%.

Diagnosing dementia is not a simple procedure, however early diagnosis is becoming increasingly important as drug therapies for treating different conditions are becoming available. It is also vital in helping the person to plan their future and the early identification of sources of advice and support (Alzheimer's Society 2003). Diagnosis is usually made by excluding other causes of symptoms. Investigations include physical examination, blood tests, computerised tomography or magnetic resonance imaging scans and comprehensive memory testing using one or more validated assessment tools (Brown and Hillam 2004). It is noted that dementia is a complex syndrome to diagnose accurately and it may be that a definite diagnosis is only established after death at post mortem or, in very rare cases, through brain biopsy.

A number of authors have challenged the notion that dementia is wholly a physical disease. Kitwood (1997a) suggests that it is a combination of physical factors and societal attitudes and treatments. Kitwood describes a "new culture" of dementia care in which he suggests that there is a need to move from the traditional view of dementia as a devastating disease of the central nervous system which results in progressive destruction of personality and identity. He argues convincingly that in order to provide high quality care it is necessary to change thinking about dementia towards a view that dementing illness is a form of disability in which care received by the person is crucial to the way in which they are affected by the dementia. Bartlett (2000) investigated the concept of dementia as a disability and suggests that Kitwood's seminal work has enabled a move from thinking about the "dementia sufferer" to a broader view in which the person with dementia is acknowledged to be a person not only with cognitive impairment but also with a variety of social restrictions and barriers.

Kitwood's (1997a) work about dementia care has parallels with the gradual involvement of people with dementia in research. For many years it has been assumed that this group are unable to participate in research and cannot share their views and experiences. It is suggested by Wilkinson (2002) that this attitude does much to reinforce negative stereotypes of this disability. Over the last two decades there has been an increasing call for greater inclusivity in research (for example Cotrell and Schulz 1993, Downs 1997). Such a move has been slow to develop, although there is an increasing body of literature that examines ways in which people with dementia can be included in research. Wilkinson (2002), Barnett (2000) and Sabat (2001) have been particularly influential in this field.

Dementia is acknowledged as being a major issue in the health and social care agenda. Prevalence of dementia is gradually increasing as the population ages. It is estimated that dementia currently effects over 700,000 people in the United Kingdom and that by 2010 this number will have risen to 840,000 (Alzheimer's Society 2006). There is, therefore, a clear need to continue research work into dementia from a variety of perspectives.

Phase One

Phase one provides an overview of dementia research and sets person-focused studies within a wider context. The history of dementia research is long and varied. An extensive review of the literature suggests that McLean's (1987) assertion is accurate in that, for the first half of the twentieth century, mental decline in the elderly generated little interest with cognitive failure being dismissed as an inevitable part of ageing.

A literature search was completed with the objective of identifying the scope and direction of dementia research. In view of the exceptional volume of work on this subject, only review papers were considered. This process produced a trajectory of research over a fixed time period. Databases searched included: Cochrane database of systematic reviews, AMED 1985-12/2004, PsychINFO 1887-12/2004, Medline 1951-12/2004, BNI 1994-12/2004, ASSIA, eLSC and CINAHL 1982-12/2004. Search terms used were dementia, Alzheimer$, literature review, systematic review, meta-analysis, meta-synthesis and re-analysis. Selection criteria were that publications were journal articles, written in the English language, with dementia or Alzheimer$ in the title and have literature review, systematic review, meta-analysis, meta-synthesis or re-analysis as the major descriptor in either the abstract or database information. Studies primarily concerned with people under the age of sixty five were excluded.

It is acknowledged that this strategy would not yield every possible review of dementia research. A total of eight hundred and sixteen papers met the selection criteria. Papers were reviewed and forty one subjects were identified. Subjects were clustered into ten broad categories as shown in table 1-1. A small number of papers included information that could have been categorised in more than one way. In these cases the major subject was identified and used for categorisation.

Category	Subjects Included
Investigation of disease process	Genetics, epidemiology, risk factors, prevention, prediction, reversibility, screening, studies of specific symptoms
Medication	Anti-dementia drugs, other types of medication used for treatment of symptoms of dementia
Treatment non-pharmacological	Reality orientation, validation therapy, Snoezelen, psychosocial interventions, complementary therapies, rehabilitation, behavioural interventions
Diagnostics / assessment	Imaging, biochemical tests, biological markers, assessment techniques used in practice
Activities of life	Respite care, nursing homes, feeding, falls, disclosure of diagnosis, awareness of dementia, nursing roles, environment, pain, sexuality
Care givers	Psychosocial interventions for carers, carer strain, effect of respite care on carers
Person focused	Active involvement of people with dementia in care and research process
Culture specific	Named cultures, nationalities, prisoners
Ethics and law	Ethical and legal considerations in dementia care and research
Cost	Care , medications

Table 1-1: Categories of dementia research

The number of studies in each category was identified and is presented as a graph (figure 1-1).

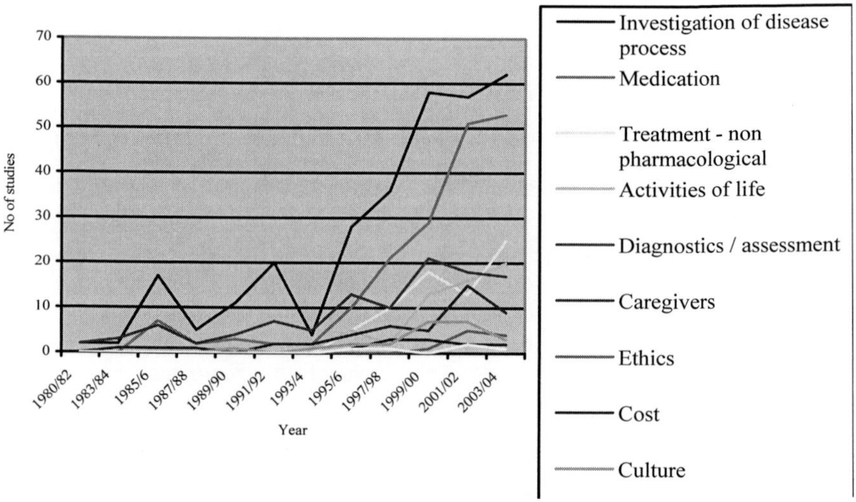

Figure 1-1: Graphic representation of dementia research

Phase one demonstrates clearly how quickly dementia research has developed with the most dramatic rise being in the last decade. This may have been influenced by recognition that the prevalence of dementia is increasing rapidly as the population ages. It has highlighted an ever more urgent need to find ways not only to prevent or cure dementia but also to develop ways in which quality of life for people with dementia can be enhanced.

Greatest areas of growth have been investigation of the disease process and development and use of medication. There is undoubtedly a need to continue biomedical studies that aim to provide a better understanding of the disease process and therefore potential for identifying cause and possibly cure. Research into the use of medication for management of symptoms has continued. However the increase of studies into medication can mainly be attributed to the development in the mid 1990's of anti-dementia drugs that offer some new hope of slowing disease progression.

Whilst biomedical research remains vital, it is equally important that other aspects of dementia research are nurtured to ensure a more holistic picture of the possibilities of dementia care. An increase in studies about the ethics of dementia care and research is noted. This remains an area of much debate for health and social care workers and new thoughts on this aspect of care are being continually generated. There has been a steady rise in studies into non-pharmacological treatments. It can be argued that the move towards more person-centred strategies has been influenced by approaches such as reality orientation, validation therapy, resolution therapy and reminiscence, which have gradually evolved from the 1950's onwards (Kitwood 1997a).

Identification of person focused reviews reveals very clearly that this is a minority area in dementia research at present. The review identified five papers that met the selection criteria; one published in 1996, one in 1997, two in 2002 and one in 2004. Each of these reviews cited a relatively small number of references. Although these papers have been categorised as person-focused their thrust appears to be to provide evidence of a lack of consistent, high quality research that genuinely engages people with dementia. Despite the fact that person-focused dementia research remains comparatively rare, these papers do indicate that there is a growing interest in this field. These papers are briefly reviewed.

In a broadly person-focused literature review, Keady (1996) covers a range of issues concerning dementia care and research in relation to the early experience of dementia and revealing of diagnosis. Keady also considers the impact of dementia on carers and the service demands that it generates. It is noted that much social research has considered the impact of dementia on care givers rather than the person with dementia. Keady (1996) comments that there are a small but increasing number of studies that directly seek the views of people with dementia. Whilst endorsing this growth, he cautions against the tendency to conduct research with people with early stage dementia to the detriment of those with more advanced disease.

An examination of literature relating to three aspects of the person with dementia: a person's sense of self, an individual's rights and the value of seeking the perspectives of the person with dementia was undertaken by Downs (1997). This author provides a concise overview of some of the key work in her consideration of the emergence of the person with dementia in research. She notes that to date the medical model has dominated in this area and even when people with dementia have been involved it has tended to be those in the early stages of the disease that have been included. Downs concludes that current literature increasingly gives value and importance to the person with dementia. She indicates a need to move towards an emphasis on the individual and a distancing from the language of victims and suffering and also suggests that there is a need to embrace people with more severe dementia in the research process.

Nolan et al (2002) take up the issue of involving the person with dementia. Drawing on a wide range of recent literature from health and social care domains these authors identify common themes in dementia care and research. They note that over the last twenty years carer research has been far more in evidence than that which directly involves people with dementia. They identify the paradox that, despite comprehensive literature on this subject, there remains little evidence of the effectiveness of current approaches to care and support. Nolan et al (2002) recognise that there is an aspiration towards including people with dementia in service development and research but that, in reality, the views of this group are rarely sought (Zarit et al 1999, Moriarity and Webb 1997) or may be ignored (Gwyther 1999). Nolan et al (2002) state that there is a need to develop models of research and practice that are more inclusive and empowering and which acknowledge the person with dementia as being "experts in their own experience" (Reid et al 2001). Nolan et al (2002) advocate equality between the person with dementia and the researcher as being a way of promoting effective investigation. They advocate the use of an "exchange" model rather than the more commonly used procedure driven or questioning approach (Qureshi et al 2000).

Ways in which research with people with dementia can be enabled are also considered by Dewing (2002) who critically reviews literature around a competency based approach to informed consent. She argues that a simple extension of this model is not an adequate strategy for people with dementia and may lead to exclusionary ethics. Dewing (2002) describes her work on a theoretical foundation of consent for people with dementia and proposes a model for consent. Dewing (2002:157) suggests that there is a need to adopt a "revisionist, person-centred, inclusionary approach to consent", and goes on to cogently justify and explain this approach.

Traynor et al (2004) discuss inclusion in relation to evaluating effectiveness of drug treatments for dementia. In an extensive literature review, the method of which is clearly described, these authors note the paucity of user involvement in this type of evaluation. Although they acknowledge the constraints placed on researchers, for example the European Agency for the Evaluation of Medicinal Products (1997) defines the areas in which clinical trials of drugs used in the treatment of dementia should provide evidence, they continue to argue convincingly that there is also a need to investigate aspects of quality of life that are important to patients rather than relying wholly on medically defined outcomes.

These reviews offer an insight into the current state of research involving people with dementia. Whilst they view the subject from differing perspectives it can be argued that there are similarities in the key messages that they convey. Keady (1996) and Downs (1997) acknowledge that far more attention has been paid to carers than to people with dementia and that, when people with dementia have been involved in research, it has tended to be those in the earlier stages of the disease process. Nolan et al (2002), Dewing (2002) and Traynor et al (2004) also indicate a lack of involvement. However, the thrust of their arguments appears to be that there is a need to develop new and innovative ways of researching with this group rather than trying to fit approaches to these studies into existing moulds.

It is likely that the gradual emergence of person-focused research has been influenced by a number of factors. A trend towards including service users and carers in research, particularly in health and social care, started in the early 1990s with Government initiatives such as The Health of the Nation (Department of Health 1992). The inclusionary message is clearly restated in more recent documents, for example Patient and Public Involvement in the new NHS (Department of Health 1999b), The NHS Plan (Department of Health 2000) and the National Service Framework for Older People (Department of Health 2001b).

In addition to societal changes there is a gradual but growing movement that supports people with dementia being actively included in research. It is eloquently argued by Bond and Corner (2001) that to understand the meaning of dementia it is vital that we gain the perspectives of people with the condition. These authors are clear that any research must be designed to ensure that the integrity of an individual's personhood is maintained. One powerful proponent of the active involvement of people with dementia is Wilkinson (2002) who, in an innovative text, sets out how such an aim can be achieved. This work is gradually being elaborated on by a range of writers who have considered specific issues in involving people with dementia in research. Examples of these include ethical issues that have been explored by Bartlett and Martin (2002); ways in which user views can be integrated into the evaluation of drug therapies by Traynor et al (2004) and Gibson et al (2004); methods of managing consent by Hubbard et al (2002); the use of focus groups by Bamford and Bruce (2002) and ways in which video recordings can be incorporated into research with people with dementia (Cook 2002). The move towards including people with dementia in research is primarily being driven in the social research arena. There are hints that this approach may be embraced, to some extent, by more traditionally biomedical investigators. For example, one person-focused study has been undertaken by a medical practitioner (Marzanski 2000). There is, to date, little evidence of further person-focused research by medical practitioners.

Phase Two

Phase two involved a literature search for studies that sought the views of people with dementia. In view of the relative scarcity of studies, the search did not follow the precise and linear approach that is advocated for quantitative systematic reviews (Centre for Reviews and Dissemination 2001). A more pragmatic approach was taken. Although the approach is unorthodox, it is transparent, and that is an attribute that Walsh and Downe (2005) consider vital to the integrity of a review. A vast number of studies initially met the search criteria and were judged to be "hits". However, on review of title followed by abstract many were eliminated as they were not relevant. Details of this stage of the search are provided in table 1-2.

Database	Number of initial "hits"	Number rejected at title	Number rejected at abstract	Full articles reviewed
CINAHL	6119	6095	6	18
BNI	56	52	0	4
AMED	8	8	0	0
MEDLINE	143	135	1	7
PSYCHINFO	41	39	0	2
Totals	6367	6329	7	31

Table 1-2: Phase two literature search

A broad based search strategy was used; this could have been refined. However a low success rate in finding relevant studies is perhaps an additional indication that research involving people with dementia remains far from mainstream. Location of relevant studies was problematic in that many studies that appeared suitable at title, or even at abstract, were found to be guidance on how to undertake research with this group rather than completed studies. Those studies rejected at title or abstract clearly did not involve people with dementia.

Full studies considered included thirty-one from established databases supplemented by a more fruitful search of the Electronic Library for Social Care database, the grey literature, a hand search of Dementia: The International Journal of Social Research and Practice with a subsequent search of reference lists of articles that met the inclusion criteria. Articles were rejected at this stage for one of three reasons: if they included the experiences of people with dementia only as an adjunct to the views of others; if they had a major focus on quantitative methods and used qualitative approaches as a secondary method and, finally, if papers were summary reports that did not contain sufficient information to allow them to be assessed. It is acknowledged that application of these exclusion criteria is largely based on the subjective opinion of the researcher and that this will have influenced the selection of studies reviewed. A number of promising studies are unpublished and unavailable. It is acknowledged that this review is not exhaustive. However, it does offer an insight into the progress to date on research in this specialist field.

A total of forty-five studies were identified for full review. These studies do not lend themselves to a traditional systematic review methodology which, as Booth (2001) notes, suffers from the characteristics of "institutionalised quantitavism". The non-conventional approach taken for this phase of the review has been influenced by the concept that attempting to imitate quantitative review methods with qualitative studies may compromise much of the progress that has been made in developing the credibility of qualitative research over the last few years. This idea is echoed by Jones (2004a) who suggests that attempting to apply quantitative terminology to qualitative reviews leaves qualitative researchers at risk of losing much of the ground that they have gained over the last decade.

A number of tools are available that propose various models for evaluating research studies using qualitative approaches. Such guidelines provide useful information in terms of reviewing many studies. However, research with people with dementia has its own unique methodological and ethical considerations and, for this reason, a set of criteria was developed specifically for use with this type of study. Production of these criteria was influenced by the work of Popay et al (1998), Department of Health (2001a), McCormack (2001a), McCormack (2002), Bartlett and Martin (2002), Webb (2003) and Jones (2004a). A rating scale of level one to level three has been used to assess how closely identified papers met the criteria. Papers categorised as level one met the criteria most closely whilst level three studies were least consistent. It is recognised that some studies will have been published in more detail elsewhere and that omissions may be due to constraints of word limits.

Popay et al's (1998) assertion that flexibility rather than standardisation is the hallmark of good qualitative methodology influenced the approach taken to this review. The value in taking a pragmatic approach lies in its inclusionary nature which is vital particularly when considering a disadvantaged group whose voices are not often clearly heard. It is argued by Jones (2004a:97) that using qualitative methods for review embraces the "richness of human experience" and allows a full hearing of groups that are frequently marginalised. In addition to considering review methods, qualitative researchers are also becoming much more aware of the value of meta-synthesis. Considerable debate exists in the literature about the extent to which qualitative research is amenable to meta-synthesis. Sandelowski et al (1997) argue that summarising qualitative findings has the potential to destroy the integrity of individual studies. Equally, there is a strong counter argument from authors including Sherwood (1999), Silverman (1997) and Britten et al (2002) that if qualitative researchers do not begin to develop their capacity in meta-synthesis there is a risk that they will continue to accumulate an ever growing number of studies which will remain in isolation and fail to influence either strategy or practice. In this era of evidence based health care, Thorne et al (2004) suggests that there is a real need to develop understanding and application of meta-synthesis to qualitative work. Whilst fully accepting this proposition, the review of these studies reveals that they focus on diverse aspects of dementia with the result that there is an insufficient body of work on any subject to indicate that meta-synthesis would be of real value.

Phase two provides a review of work in the area of researching with people with dementia. The following section addresses ways in which these studies have managed some of the central tenets that have been identified in the criteria as contributing to conducting ethical and meaningful research involving people with dementia. As stated, findings are summarised rather than synthesised as the volume of work in each area remains low.

Aims and Participants

Studies were assessed against criteria which required that the aims of the study should be clearly stated and justified. Participants should have been selected in a way that allowed the best chance of answering the research question. Recruitment processes should be sensitive to the needs of this group and adopt an inclusive philosophy.

Aims

In every case the researcher had documented a clear aim for the study. All aims were framed in terms that implied that the researcher was investigating from the perspective of the person with dementia. This demonstrated that in each case the research could only reasonably be conducted with people with dementia.

Methods of Recruitment

Recruiting people with dementia to a research study demands a level of sensitivity beyond that required in many cases. Key issues exist that need to be considered early in the process. It is essential to ensure that an inadvertent disclosure of the diagnosis of dementia is not made during recruitment. Researchers also need to consider the way that participants are selected to ensure an element of inclusivity. It is crucial to achieve a balance between using a recruitment process that respects the individual whilst not causing them undue anxiety or concern.

Recruitment processes generally involved purposive or convenience sampling, which is reasonable for studies of this nature. Only the study by Aggarwal et al (2003) claimed to use random selection, although the procedure is not described. Discussion of the sampling and recruitment process is notably absent in several cases (for example Sabat 2002a, Proctor 2001, Snyder 2003). A number of studies selected participants who used services specifically for people with dementia, for example Pearce et al (2002) selected people attending memory clinics; Phinney et al (2002) recruited participants from a geriatric research centre and an early diagnosis support group; Katsuno (2003) worked with people attending a dementia specific adult day and residential care centre. Although it can be argued that attendance at a dementia care facility does not ensure that the person with dementia is necessarily aware of their diagnosis it is suggested that this is a higher probability than would be the case when selecting people from other areas.

Other authors are less explicit about how potential participants were selected. Werezak and Stewart (2002) recruited from unspecified agencies and Proctor (2001) reports only that participants were attending a day hospital. Two studies investigated care of people with dementia in acute hospitals used totally different approaches. Tolson et al (1999) used a strategy of asking all older people who were consecutively admitted to medical or care of older people wards to complete a cognitive assessment. People who produced two low scores were invited to be involved in the next stage of the study. This method of selection is not justified in the paper and does raise questions about labelling of people with acute physical health problems as having dementia. It is not entirely clear whether this label was shared with participants. Norman (2003a) recruited patients in an acute hospital on the basis that they had been labelled as having memory problems either by nursing staff or in the medical or nursing notes. Norman provides a sound justification for her choice in stating that patients labelled by staff as having dementia, whether this is accurate or not, were constructed in terms of this label and would therefore be treated in a similar way to those with a formal diagnosis. The latter approaches could be considered to increase the risk of inadvertent disclosure, whether confirmed or not, during the recruitment process.

When working with people with dementia there is a need to balance respect for the individual with using recruitment processes that are inclusive and do not cause undue anxiety and concern. Most studies used some type of "third party" during the first stage of recruitment, most commonly these were care staff or family members. A number of researchers asked care staff to identify people using their service who would be suitable to participate (for example Bamford and Bruce 2000, Mills 1997). This process could be viewed as assisting appropriate selection; equally it has the potential to introduce an element of bias through staff selection. Bamford and Bruce (2000) addressed this issue by allowing other interested users to join their discussions. A small number of researchers would only recruit participants who had a next of kin or spouse who was willing to take part (for example Phinney 2002a, Pearce et al 2002). Recruitment into the study of Graneheim and Jansson (2006) involved seeking consent from relatives. Participants were not informed of the study in advance, although they are reported as not objecting to being interviewed. Such approaches bring into question the respect for an individual's personhood and belief in the value that they bring to the study.

A study by Svanstrom and Dahlberg (2004) investigating the lived experience of dementia for spouses where one is diagnosed with dementia, recruited people with dementia from a range of local services. These authors state that it was the healthy spouse who made the decision to take part in the study and no mention is made of the feelings of the person with dementia. Again, this brings into question the extent to which the personhood of individuals was respected.

Use of a "third party", who already knew participants, was used frequently. Initial information was provided by care staff in studies by Pratt and Wilkinson (2001), Werezak and Stewart (2002) and Mason et al (2005). This process could be seen as reducing coercion and so may be considered good practice. One drawback is noted by Pratt and Wilkinson (2001) who report that it led to an exceptionally slow period of recruitment. It is notable that following first contact from a "third party" many researchers chose to communicate directly with people with dementia, for example Mason et al (2005) attended a support group to explain their study in more detail. Other studies, for example Burgener and Dickerson-Putman (1999) recruited via family care givers. It may be suggested that this approach borders on paternalistic and compromises the personhood of individuals. In addition, it makes the unfounded assumption that people with dementia and their carers have good relationships (Pratt 2002).

Inclusivity

Inclusion of people with dementia is becoming well established as a necessity. It is noted by Keady (1996) and Downs (1997) that researchers have tended to concentrate their work on those in the earlier stages and this approach remains evident. A number of studies reported the level of cognitive impairment of the participants with most using the Mini Mental State examination (MMSE) (Folstein et al 1975). Most participants had recorded MMSE scores of eighteen or above indicating mild to moderate dementia. Exceptions were Sabat (2002a) who engaged with a person with an MMSE of nine and Marzanski (2000) who included people with MMSEs ranging from seven– twenty nine. Some researchers made a conscious decision not to investigate the level of cognitive impairment of participants. This may have been on the grounds that MMSE score does not necessarily correlate with an ability to communicate one's views. The fact that most of this type of research concentrates on people with less severe dementia is highlighted by several authors including Hubbard et al (2003), Phinney et al (2002) and Bamford and Bruce (2000) who suggest that methods for inclusion of those with more advanced impairment need to be developed further.

It is evident that most researchers in these studies have given considerable thought to the selection and recruitment of participants. Some have used strategies such as the "third party" to minimise risk of anxiety or feelings of coercion. Equally, a small number of studies have employed processes that are questionable particularly in terms of selecting people who are likely to be able to answer the research question and in terms of ensuring participant choice. Virtually all participants had a relatively high level of cognitive function and several authors point to the need to include people with more advanced dementia. These studies indicate that there is a value in involving people with a pre-existing relationship with potential participants in the recruitment process. However it is argued that this approach must be carefully balanced in order to prevent inadvertent exclusion or paternalism. It is recognised that there is a need to expand the scope of research to include people with more advanced dementia.

Research Design

Criteria related to research design concerned the extent to which the method selected was appropriate to the research question. A high level of flexibility, particularly in terms of data collection, was required in order to accommodate the potentially varying needs of participants. The process of moving from data to interpretation should be explicit.

Research Method

Methods used in the studies varied considerably, forty used purely qualitative methods whilst five employed mixed qualitative and quantitative techniques. Use of predominantly qualitative methods may be a reflection of the professional backgrounds of the researchers many of whom worked in the arenas of nursing or social care and research. It is suggested that this group are likely to be conversant with qualitative methods and therefore be better equipped to engage in person focused enquiry. Only one researcher was noted to be from a medical background, Marzanski (2000) who worked as a Specialist Registrar in Old Age Psychiatry. He bravely stepped from the biomedical model into the qualitative paradigm. However, the study perhaps indicates some discomfort with this approach in its apparently fairly rigid application.

Explanation of the detail of research design is mixed. Bamford and Bruce (2000) explain each step of their research in detail, an approach followed by Pratt and Wilkinson (2001) and Gillies (2000). Other authors provide a much less comprehensive explanation, for example the work of Sabat (2002a) and Snyder (2003) give only a perfunctory overview of the research process.

Data Collection

Data were most commonly collected through interviews. Several studies used other methods of data collection to supplement interviews. For example periods of observation were completed by Phinney (1998, 2002a), Phinney et al (2002), Norman (2003a) and Nygard and Starkhammar (2007); Bamford and Bruce (2000) and Mason et al (2005) engaged in group discussions; video recording was used by Mason et al (2005), Vernooij-Dassen et al (2006) and Daniels et al (2007) whilst Tolson et al (1999) chose to review clinical documentation. Positive and negative attributes of these data collection techniques are not debated in detail in any of the papers. It is suggested by Clarke and Keady (2002) that there are key criteria that need to be met to ensure effective data collection with people with dementia. They consider that it is vital that the approach of the researcher is positive and creative and that the process enables enough engagement between researcher and participant to allow confirmation of issues.

Effective methods for conducting interviews with people with dementia have been the subject of much debate in the literature. There are a number of issues that need to be taken into consideration when conducting any qualitative interview. There are others that are particularly pertinent to interviews with people with dementia. These include whether the person should be interviewed alone or whether to have another person present to offer support, ways in which questions are asked and the number of interviews required.

It is suggested by Pratt (2002) that carers can be valuable collaborators in dementia research whilst equally cautioning against assuming that the person with dementia will want to be accompanied. Pratt suggests a compromise position of combining interviews with and without carers. This idea is supported by Preston et al (2007) who interviewed twelve people of who five chose to be accompanied by their spouse. In these interviews the spouses were encouraged to make their contributions after the interview, presumably to ensure that they did not detract from the primacy of the person with dementia. Most interviews were conducted with participants unaccompanied but it is not always clear if they were given the choice to include a supporter. Phinney (2002a), Pearce et al (2002) and Clare et al (2005) chose to interview people with dementia and their partners separately. These authors made it a prerequisite that partners had to be willing to be involved and imply that partners' interviews were used to corroborate the information supplied by the person with dementia. Whilst having a different perspective may have added depth to the data it may be considered that Phinney's (2002a) request that partners report what they thought the person with dementia was experiencing does appear rather speculative. In the case study of Hellstrom et al (2005) a couple were interviewed separately but asked about the same themes. Following this the couple joined in the process of co-construction which provided an agreed account that reflected their experiences. This approach could be viewed as epitomising respect for each individual in enabling each to give their own view and then collaboratively agreeing on the final version.

An alternative approach was taken by Daniels et al (2007) who conducted a single case study into the marital relationship of a couple, one of whom had Alzheimer's disease. Each of the three interviews were joint and the focus was very much on the marriage with the couple being left to begin to talk about the Alzheimer's disease when they felt it was appropriate. Again, this approach showed a high level of respect for both the individuals and their relationship. It is noted that there are potential pitfalls when including others, in this case the main visitor, in the interview process. These are identified by Tolson et al (1999) who report that the presence of the visitor, generally a family member, detracted from the ability of the person with dementia to communicate fully.

Interviewing people with dementia is clearly a venture that requires skill and sensitivity. It is noted that some still question the value in seeking the views of this group. This is highlighted by authors including Goldsmith (2002) and Clarke and Keady (2002). These authors are adamant that people with dementia, even in the more advanced stages, have a desire to communicate and that it is the responsibility of the researcher to find ways in which this can be enabled.

A range of interview styles have been suggested. Keady and Gilliard (2002) advise that largely unstructured interviews can be used to build a trusting relationship between participant and researcher which may enable the participant to reveal sensitive information. A semi-structured approach using a set of predetermined questions is discussed by Harris and Durkin (2002). They suggest that this can be valuable in ensuring some parity when interviews are being conducted by different researchers. An example they give is of interviews by two researchers, one of whom was a clinician and one of whom had Alzheimer's disease. A direct questioning stance is advocated by Young (2002) who states that when involving people with early dementia this approach can show a genuine desire to find out their views and thus enhance their self esteem.

Studies reviewed employed a variety of interview techniques. Style of interview varied from the very structured approach used by Burgener and Dickerson-Putman (1999) and Marzanski (2000) both of whom delivered a consistent set of questions, through the semi-structured approaches of Pearce et al (2002), Mason et al (2005) and Werezak and Stewart (2002), to the unstructured format of Sabat (2002a) and the counselling base adopted by Mills (1997). Extracts of data suggest that perhaps the skill of the interviewer is more critical to success than the interview approach used. For example Pratt and Wilkinson (2001) used interviews with a clear topic guide. They had planned to interview people twice but due to various constraints this was not always possible. However, the data they present demonstrates how, with the right approach, people with dementia can be assisted to provide rich insights into their experiences. Participants in a study of involvement in activity by Phinney (2006) enabled participants to express their views by supporting them to give narrative accounts of their own experiences. The counselling approach to interviews is advocated by Mills (1997) who used it to good effect in illuminating the narratives of eight people described as having moderate to severe dementia. Nelson-Jones (1993) discusses the concept of using counselling skills in qualitative research suggesting that transferable skills include altruism, humanism, intellectual curiosity and people orientation. Although these facets are not discussed, they are clearly represented in the work of Sabat (2002a) in his interaction with a person with relatively advanced dementia. To enhance engagement and stimulate discussion, Aggarwal et al (2003) and Norman (2003a) both used "prompts" such as photographs to trigger conversations with participants.

Most interviews are reported to have been tape-recorded with permission of the participants. This appears to have been relatively unproblematic with no researchers documenting particular concerns. This may be due to the fact that most participants had a relatively high level of cognitive functioning and so retained a sound memory of this type of equipment. In contrast, video recordings appeared to require a greater level of explanation and it is possible that older people involved in the studies were less familiar with this slightly more modern technology. Video recordings were used by Mason et al (2005) in a study of support groups and Daniels et al (2007) when interviewing a couple. Use of this technique is investigated in detail by Cook (2003) who used video recordings with older people with dementia in a residential care setting. Cook (2003) graphically describes her work in ensuring that the participants were familiarised with the equipment and her sensitivity in recording. Mason et al (2005) video recorded entire support groups but the way in which this was introduced and the impact that it had on group dynamics is not discussed in detail.

A number of studies involved a series of interviews, although this does not appear to be an absolute pre-requisite to achieving engagement with resulting rich data. This is evidenced by the work of Gillies (2000) who interviewed most participants only once but clearly enabled participants to express their views in considerable depth. Other researchers used multiple interviews, such as Phinney et al (2002) who conducted three interviews with each participant to the extreme of Mills (1997) who undertook between thirteen and twenty five interviews. It does not appear that more interviews necessarily leads to increased quality of data.

Data collection largely involved interviews with participants. Styles ranged from highly structured to conversational approaches and the number of interviews conducted varied from one to twenty five. Involvement of significant others in the interview process has been discussed and advantages and disadvantages noted. Literature offers some fairly prescriptive guidance on the way in which interviews with people with dementia should be conducted. However the guidance is, in places, contradictory. An idea that emerges from these studies is that, whilst guidance is available, the key element that enables effective data collection, regardless of espoused style, is the personal manner and approach of the individual interviewer.

Data Analysis

Whilst there is a wealth of guidance about how to include people with dementia in research, there is a marked absence of work that focuses on data analysis. None of the papers reviewed cite the analysis process as a particular challenge. Quality of explanation of the approach to analysis ranges from virtually absent (for example Marzanski 2000, Sabat 2002a) to comprehensive (for example Pratt and Wilkinson 2001, Phinney 2002a). It is noted that the lack of detailed description of the analysis process does not necessarily detract from the findings presented, although, it clearly leaves a question as to how the findings have been developed.

Both qualitative and quantitative methods of data analysis have been employed. Quantitative work generally uses fairly simple statistical approaches and, on the whole, straightforward techniques have been used to analyse data that supports qualitative findings (for example Katsuno 2003). Qualitative data has mainly followed well established methods. It is noteworthy that Mason et al (2005) are unique amongst these studies in paying detailed attention to the non-verbal communication of participants. This is perhaps surprising given the assumed difficulty that people with dementia have in expressing themselves verbally.

Interpretation of data does not appear to have caused major concern. Several authors returned to participants to check their understanding, for example Werezak and Stewart (2002) used second interviews to "validate" categories and Mills (1997) took emerging themes back to participants to deepen understanding. Steeman et al (2007) initially used grounded theory to analyse their data. They concluded that this was not wholly satisfactory and subsequently added elements of narrative analysis. This had the effect of strengthening their analysis considerably, providing a new level of understanding. It is perhaps surprising that, almost entirely, mainstream qualitative approaches to analysis have been used. It may be considered that other methods to aid the expression of the thoughts of participants would have been explored, such as the use of poetry, as demonstrated in the work of Killick (2001, 2002).

It has often been implied that people with dementia have little or no contribution to make to research (Rodeheaver and Daton 1988). Data generated in these studies strongly suggests that this is not the case. Quality of data and the apparent ease of data analysis may be explained in two ways. Firstly, it may be suggested that the researchers have been skilled in their approach to data collection and effectively enabled the articulation of views. Secondly, it may be that the tendency to recruit people with less severe cognitive impairment has allowed the generation of data that is more readily interpreted than that which may be produced with the inclusion of people with more advanced disease.

Research design of these studies has largely emanated from the qualitative paradigm which is established as appropriate for this type of work. Quantitative approaches have been used to provide some supplementary evidence. However their lack of utility in person focused work is acknowledged. Most studies have used interviews to collect data and it has been identified that the crucial factor in conducting interviews is the approach of the individual rather than the adherence to any particular style. Data analysis, when described, generally appears to be a straightforward process. It is likely that as people with more advanced dementia begin to be involved in research, alternative approaches to analysis, such as the use of poetry, to analyse interpret and disseminate research may become more common.

Personhood and Ethics

Several issues need to be considered in relation to personhood and ethics in dementia research. These include a justification for research with this vulnerable group, obtaining the required ethical approval and issues of consent and respect for personhood in terms of researcher-participant relationships. Ethical components of selection and recruitment have been discussed earlier in this chapter.

People with dementia have been described as one of the most excluded groups in society, experiencing the double jeopardy of being old and having a cognitive impairment (Rodeheaver and Datan 1988). In terms of research, although progress is being made, this group still tend to be a silent voice (Wilkinson 2002). For many years dementia has been considered as a neurological disease which leads to the gradual erosion of the person. This idea is challenged by Kitwood (1997a) who argues that the course of dementia is also influenced by societal attitudes and treatment. He describes malignant social psychology which together with neurological deficits gradually undermines the personhood of the individual. Although Kitwood is considering dementia care as a whole in his work on personhood the principles can equally be applied to dementia research. These principles are also closely allied to the ethical standards that should be applied to all research studies.

Justification

Each of the studies aimed to discover more about the experiences and views of people with dementia. It is clear that in each case there was a minimal knowledge base around the research question. This provides a clear justification for inviting people with dementia to participate. Only those with the condition can explain what it is like. For many years proxy reports have been used (Brooker 1995) but, even with the best intention, these are unlikely to reflect the thoughts of the person with dementia.

Ethical Approval

Ethical approval from the required bodies has been documented by some writers (for example Menne et al 2002, Werezak and Stewart 2002). It may be assumed that all studies that have been published would have gained ethical approval as this is a condition for publication in many journals.

Consent

Approaches to consent involved consideration of a number of issues including consent by people with dementia or proxies and use of verbal or written consent. All authors appear to have attempted to provide participants with sufficient and fairly standard information using written or verbal material, although little reference is made to confirmation of understanding. Gillies (2000) was unusual in providing tailored information to meet the needs of individuals. Length of time that people had to decide whether or not to take part is discussed infrequently. Participants in the study of Werezak and Stewart (2002) appeared to have little time to make a decision as an interview was conducted on the same visit that consent was taken.

The choice of whether or not to obtain written consent is debated in the literature. Bartlett and Martin (2002) suggest that for people with dementia the requirement to sign a consent form may induce feelings of anxiety and insecurity. Many researchers used written consent; this may have been influenced by the fact that for many Research Ethics Committees in the

United Kingdom written consent remains essential to the research process. Treatment of consent as a process (Milton 2000) rather than as a one off activity is noted in a few cases. Pratt and Wilkinson (2001) revisited consent on each occasion that they met with participants to ensure it remained valid. A similar approach was used by Phinney (2006) who gained informed consent from participants, which was repeated at subsequent interviews if participants had forgotten previous consent. An alternative approach was taken by Bamford and Bruce (2000) who rejected written consent in favour of verbal and behavioural consent. This method was chosen in order to minimise anxiety for participants.

A number of authors involved next of kin or proxies in the research study. Phinney (2002a) and Pearce (2002) excluded people who did not have a significant other who was prepared to be involved. Such an aproach must raise questions about the value that the researchers attached to the personhood of people with dementia. Other writers used next of kin in a more supportive role such as Aggarwal et al (2003) and Moore et al (2003) who involved them without apparently detracting from the primacy of the person with dementia. Gillies (2000) describes a four tier hierarchy that includes informal carers in the consent process but also ensured consent from participants themselves. This may be considered best practice in terms of involving carers, thereby potentially protecting participants whilst acknowledging that no-one can give consent on behalf of another adult (DoH 2001a, HMSO 2005). Two studies explicitly sought proxy consent, Werezak and Stewart (2002) and Burgener and Dickerson-Putman (1999) obtained written consent from proxies. It is noted that these studies were conducted in Canada and the United States which are governed by quite different approaches to research.

Awareness of diagnosis is an issue in research with people with dementia. Level of insight of participants is not widely considered, although some writers document that participants had previously been informed of their diagnosis (for example Phinney et al 2002). Risk of inadvertent disclosure of diagnosis is recognised by Pearce et al (2002) who deliberately did not mention the terms “dementia” or “Alzheimer’s disease” unless they were first used by the participants. Most researchers recruited only participants with an established diagnosis of dementia that had been confirmed by a specialist facility (for example Pearce et al 2002, Phinney et al 2002, Burgener-Putman 1999). As discussed earlier, the diagnosis of participants in studies by Norman (2003a) and Tolson et al (1999), involving acute hospital care, are based on slightly tenuous grounds with a presumed increase in risk of inadvertent disclosure.

Ethical issues around consent from people with dementia remain contentious. It is acknowledged that attitudes to the subject vary across continents. It is suggested that the approach to consent should be tailored to meet individual needs and beliefs. However, the constraints of research governance and ethics committee protocols, whilst necessary to protect participants, make any degree of flexibility hard to achieve.

Personhood

Personhood as a concept emanates from three major areas: transcendence, ethics and social psychology. In transcendence, the ideas that "being" alone is sacred and life is to be revered are powerfully presented. An ethical viewpoint considers that each individual has an absolute value and that we all have an obligation to treat each other with respect. Social psychology offers a broader explanation which is generally associated with issues of self esteem and with the stability, continuity and integrity of the sense of self. These concepts of personhood have been integrated and refined by Kitwood (1997a) to produce a definition that is central to the "new culture" of dementia care. Kitwood (1997a:8) states that personhood is "a standing or status that is bestowed upon one human being, by others, in the context of relationships and social being. It implies recognition, respect and trust. Both the according of personhood, and the failure to do so, has consequences that are empirically testable". Personhood in relation to nursing is considered by McCormack (2004) in an exploration of literature on person-centred care. McCormack (2004) acknowledges that systematic investigation into person-centred care is poorly developed. From available literature he draws out four concepts that underpin person-centred nursing: being in relation, being in social world, being in place and being with self. McCormack (2004) links each of these concepts with the work of Kitwood (1997a) to further develop the notions of knowing the person, the essential nature of values, biography and relationships and the absolute need for authenticity in preserving and respecting the personhood of the individual.

The concept that people with dementia should be central to the research process is becoming well established. It is stated by Clarke and Keady (1996) that the person with dementia cannot be regarded as an object to be examined. There is a need to move from a model of "research on" to "research with" this group (Riddell et al 1998). A requirement to develop and maintain effective relationships is noted by many authors.

Autonomy of participants is central to ensuring ethically sound research. It is recognised that the principles of autonomy need to be reviewed when researching with people with dementia. McCormack (2001a) proposes a model of autonomy based on interconnectedness. McCormack acknowledges that autonomy may be different for people with dementia but argues that they are still able to make decisions. Interconnectedness is grounded on open and honest communication with specific attention being paid to facilitation of decision making, recognition of the importance of individual values in the decision making process, explicit sharing of intentions and motivations and the creation of a culture that respects the views of the older person.

Researcher-Participant Relationships

Ethical considerations and respect for personhood in these studies are inevitably closely intertwined. To some extent the fact that researchers are seeking to hear the voices of this group is a testament to their belief in personhood. However, ways in which researchers demonstrate recognition, respect and trust in relation to participants are varied.

Mills (2003) suggests that for many people research can be seen in three stages: beginning of the study when levels of anxiety may be high, middle when they may begin to tire and the end when they may feel sadness as the relationship ceases. Initiating relationships has been considered by most researchers in terms of selection and recruitment of appropriate participants and in providing them with sufficient information to make a choice about whether or not to participate.

Despite careful preparatory phases, building of relationships with participants prior to data collection is rarely discussed. This may be due to constraints for researchers who are limited in terms of resources, particularly time. Equally it may be felt that it is wrong to expect to take more time than is necessary from participants. An exception to this finding on building relationships is provided by Sabat (2002a) who states that he developed a long term and trusting relationship with the participant prior to data collection. This was perhaps more readily achieved with the single participant involved. Sabat (2002a) acknowledged the participant as a thoughtful and insightful person and this assertion is supported by the way in which he leaves space in the conversation for the participant to express herself whilst facilitating her when necessary. To a lesser extent Harman and Clare (2006) built a relationship with participants by meeting them prior to interview to explain the research and seek consent.

Although most researchers did not explicitly establish relationships with participants prior to data collection, their respect for personhood is evidenced in their approach to this process. Bamford and Bruce (2000) commenced their study with a clear plan for data collection. However, during the initial stage they realised from the responses of participants that a more flexible approach would enable the articulation of different views according to how the participants were feeling. To this end the researchers reconfigured their plan. Pratt and Wilkinson (2001) demonstrate the value attached to personhood, partly through the depth of interaction that could not have been achieved unless a respectful relationship had been forged. The value that was attached to participants in a study about relationships in which one member had dementia was evidenced by Hellstrom et al (2007). Their study was conducted over a five year period and between interviews the researchers regularly telephoned participants to "keep in touch" with what was happening in their lives.

A small number of studies provide less clear evidence of attempting to maintain personhood. In an ethnographic study, which involved a researcher spending several hours observing people with dementia in their own homes using everyday technology, Nygard and Starkhammar (2007) provide no evidence of how the researcher-participant relationship was established and managed. Burgener and Dickerson-Putman (1999) used qualitative and quantitative data collection methods. In interviews they asked set questions that may have limited participants' opportunities to express their thoughts. Participants had all undergone quantitative tests prior to diagnosis and some reported that these had undermined their self esteem. Despite this, they were still subjected to a raft of quantitative measures. Marzanski's (2000) approach may also have lacked flexibility and limited the capacity of participants to express themselves fully as he chose to use standard questions. It is not possible to assess from the paper how these were delivered. Difficulties in obtaining data were acknowledged by Lindstrom et al (2006) who reported that people with dementia struggled to answer questions that focused on the future. It is notable that although this issue is raised the researchers do not explain if, or how, it was rectified.

Ending of research relationships is rarely discussed. It may be that this is not an issue for participants with a higher level of cognitive function and who had limited interaction with the researcher. However, in studies such as that by Mills (1997), which involved between thirteen and twenty five interviews with people described as having moderate to severe dementia, the feeling of loss at the end of the study may have been acute. Mills (1997) states that participants appeared to have enjoyed the interviews but does not document how the relationship was brought to an end. Closing the research relationship was an issue in the study of Ward-Griffin et al (2007). Inclusion criteria in this study stated that participants must have a standardised MMSE of over seventeen. In the time between the two interviews the scores of two participants fell below this figure but no indication is given about how this situation was managed. The only study that appeared to have contact with participants post data collection was that of Harman and Clare (2006) who offered the opportunity to discuss results. Four participants responded to the invitation and agreed that the model used accurately represented their personal experiences.

Respect for personhood is one component of these studies that is relatively difficult to judge. It is evident that respect for personhood exists in light of the depth of data collected. It is suggested that the quality of data in the best papers is unlikely to have been achieved if participants had not felt valued as individuals. There is an implication that researchers demonstrated a genuine interest and encouraged the sharing of thoughts. Respect for personhood has been found to be an implicit quality. Papers that document the concept are not necessarily those in which it is most powerfully discerned when reviewing the studies.

As suggested earlier, researchers who choose to involve people with dementia almost inevitably have some belief in the value that contributions by this group can make to the body of knowledge about dementia. The extent to which researchers consider the specific issue of dementia in studies can be placed on a continuum: from those who do not consider that people with dementia can give consent and need their narratives to be corroborated by others; through those who make few allowances for the impact that dementia may have on individuals to those that appear to have a genuine, inherent empathy and respect for this group and thus a capacity to gain valuable insights even from those in the more advanced stages.

Findings and Evaluation

Criteria in this section are concerned with the extent to which evidence for and against the interpretation have been considered, impact that the researcher has had on the study, evidence that supports the conclusion and ways that these are integrated with current knowledge and contribution to the body of knowledge. Studies reviewed can be grouped into broad subject areas including personal experience of dementia, religion and spirituality, receiving the diagnosis, outcomes of services or treatments and the use of technology. The extent to which the studies meet the criteria is explored under these headings.

Findings

Findings of these studies have been instrumental in beginning to illuminate the experiences of people with dementia from their own perspective. Most researchers state that their findings are not generalisable as the number of participants in each study is small. However, each study has produced further insights and it may be argued that the findings have transferability (Lincoln and Guba 1985). That is, the findings in one context can be transferred to similar situations or participants.

The Personal Experience of Dementia

A number of studies have investigated the personal experience of dementia. Sabat (2002a) explored the relationship between personal experience of Alzheimer's disease and Social Construction Theory. In his conversations with a person with quite advanced dementia he deduced that Self 1, the self of personal identity and Self 2, mental and physical attributes and related beliefs, may alter but remain intact. Sabat discovered that Self 3, the social personae, becomes vulnerable particularly in the way in which others respond to the new dysfunctional Self 2 which may lead to the person being restricted to the role of patient. Sabat links his findings with the work of Brody (1971) who suggests that dysfunctional treatment could lead to excess disability. He also makes links with the writing of Kitwood and Bredin (1992) who propose the idea that malignant social psychology, the way in which others can depersonalise and invalidate the person with dementia, can lead to the erosion of their personhood. In his study Sabat (2002a) skilfully demonstrates the way in which these concepts impact on the wellbeing of an individual. This makes salutary reading. The experience of dementia from a masculine perspective was investigated by Bartlett (2007) who suggests that social exclusion may be an issue for some men. As her work is based on one, albeit very insightful, case study this researcher acknowledges the need to explore this phenomenon further.

Experience of dementia is also explored from the perspective of maintenance of personal narrative. Capacity of people with dementia to maintain their personal narrative is studied by Mills (1997) who spent a considerable time span interviewing participants to elucidate the extent to which they preserved their personal narrative through the course of their illness. Mills indicates that personal narrative is something that she witnessed gradually decline in participants as the severity of their dementia increased. Proctor (2001) presents four case studies which imply that, given the right approach, people with dementia are able to retain and communicate at least some semblance of narrative. These studies indicate the value of working with people with dementia to maintain their narrative not only for their own sake but also because of the value it has in reinforcing attitudes of respect, understanding and acceptance in others who are influential in helping to maintain personhood (Mills 1997).

Narrative as a concept is also pertinent in a number of studies that consider how individuals cope with dementia, including their desire to maintain a sense of self. Experience of dementia and how people manage their situation is explored in several studies. Menne et al (2002) investigated the day-to-day experience of dementia and concluded that individuals wanted to continue with their established lifestyle as far as possible. Pearce et al (2002) considered appraisal and coping processes of men with early stage dementia. They highlight seven key themes relating to maintaining a sense of self and seven themes concerning reappraising and reconstructing self. Ways in which these themes have been developed is clearly charted. Gillies (2000), in a study of the experience of dementia, discovered that participants had a tendency to rationalise dementia as an inevitable part of normal aging. They were sensitive to their own "failings" but also recognised these in people around them. This author describes some coping strategies employed by participants, most common was resignation and acceptance of circumstances that they felt were beyond their control. Gillies also uncovered some disturbing evidence of the suffering experienced, including descriptions of how participants find the effects of dementia unpleasant, humiliating and undermining. Suffering associated with dementia is also recognised by Macquarrie (2005) who describes the dichotomy between agency and objectification experience of people with mild to moderate dementia. Participants in this study are reported to live with a feeling of both acknowledgment and resistance of their condition. This can result in a dialectical struggle which people used a range of strategies to overcome.

Phinney (1998) investigated the meaning of symptoms to people with Alzheimer's disease. She discerned two main themes, being unsure and trying to be normal. This author revisited the subject four years later finding that symptoms are not always salient to the experiences of dementia but that fluctuating awareness could lead to the breakdown of the illness narrative (Phinney 2002a). This author implies that a breakdown in illness narrative severely hinders an individual's ability to tell their own story. This could be contested as presumably the breakdown of the narrative is an integral part of the experience of dementia. In a further study, Phinney et al (2002) again considered ways in which people with dementia understood the meaning of their symptoms. In their phenomenological work, which included some quantitative measures, they found that simply measuring symptom awareness was not helpful. As with previous studies they found that this phenomenon tended to fluctuate and lead to a breakdown of the illness narrative. They imply that a discrepancy between the interpretation of the person with dementia and clinicians can prove challenging due to a lack of shared understanding.

Learning to live with early stage dementia was explored during interviews conducted by Werezak and Stewart (2002:80). Theory that has been constructed from this study revolves around the concept of a "continuous process of adjusting to early stage dementia". This process comprises five stages: antecedents, anticipation, appearance, assimilation and acceptance. It is suggested that this process evolves as the awareness of self and the outer world changes. Experience of coping strategies of people with dementia was explored further by Gilmour and Huntington (2005). These authors elicited views of participants and concluded, in common with other studies, that there is a need for ongoing, skilled, well paced and sensitive information together with a requirement to provide support for active coping strategies.

A comparable study was undertaken by Van Dijkhuizen et al (2006) who focused on how a group of women made sense of, and attempted to cope with, early stage Alzheimer's disease. These researchers developed three higher order themes from the data that they tentatively link with a "Level of Connectedness" model. They suggest that there is a need for further development of psychosocial interventions which consider well-being from the interpersonal perspective. Experience of early stage Alzheimer's disease has also been investigated by Clare (2002) who identified and conceptualised coping strategies used by participants; a continuum from self protection to integrative responding is proposed. Self protection embraced the themes holding on and compensating whilst integrative responding, which was less frequently discerned, included the themes fighting and coming to terms. Clare (2002) suggests that these accounts imply that there is a need to reconsider approaches to helping people with dementia by incorporating a range of elements that can be selected and adapted according to individual need. Relationships between participants' responses and Clare's (2002) suggestion for improving practice are clearly explicated. In a further paper Clare (2003), using the same group of participants as before, investigates the understanding that people with dementia have of their own situation. Clare (2003) proposes that their awareness can be placed on a continuum from self maintaining to self adjusting. Self maintaining is concerned with attempts to normalise their situation and minimise difficulties. Self adjusting comprised attempts to confront difficulties and adjust the sense of self accordingly.

Langdon et al (2007) investigated the lived, subjective experience of people with early stage dementia. This study considered the individuals' own experience and embraced their perceptions of how others responded to their diagnosis of dementia. Participants reported that when people became aware of their diagnosis they started treating them differently, resulting in a feeling of loss of social status and role. This experience led some participants to be cautious about the extent to which they disclosed their diagnosis, particularly to a wider audience.

Aggarwal et al (2003) sought to elicit the views of people from residential and day care settings about their experiences of having dementia and about the care they received. Participants reported that care offered limited levels of social stimulation, choice and independence. It is postulated that a wide range of factors may influence this perception. The experience of having dementia, in common with studies by Menne et al (2002) and Pearce et al (2002), painted a picture of the feelings of loss endured. Participants in Aggarwal's study are reported to have valued the opportunity to explore their experiences with people who were interested. This was wide ranging and ambitious study but the findings generated have a real value in informing care and further research.

A different perspective on the concept of living with dementia is explored by Moore et al (2003) who investigated the experience of people with dementia living in a locked unit. Their study involved interviewing seven veterans who described feelings of being bewildered by their apparently unjustified captivity and the acute, visceral distress this caused. As described in other studies these participants used coping mechanisms, in this case seeking respite either through searching for activity or by trying to understand the reasons for the restriction imposed on them. Living with dementia and disturbing behaviour was explored by Graneheim and Jansson (2006). These researchers worked with three participants in a residential home and discovered that they experienced profound feelings of being surrounded by disorder, being trapped by restriction and being set aside as well as being included.

Relationships with others following a diagnosis of dementia are explored by Ward-Griffin et al (2006). These authors investigated the relationships between mothers with dementia and their adult daughter care givers. Relationships from the perspective of the mothers are reported. Each mother expressed gratefulness for the care provided by their daughter, but equally they experienced a sense of guilt about being a burden. Four themes emerged from this study. "Doing care" was concerned with the mother's perceived capacity to self care; "undemanding care" related to the mothers desire to limit requests for assistance; "determining care" indicated the tension between wanting to be independent and needing assistance and "accepting care" occurred when mothers submitted to care from their daughters whether they felt they needed it or not. A further study on mother-daughter relationships was conducted by Ward-Griffin et al (2007). This research, which used a similar approach, identified four types of relationship: custodial, cooperative, combative and cohesive. It is interesting that such a different set of themes was generated from an ostensibly similar research question. These authors highlight the need for further research into this area as, given the increasing prevalence of dementia, this type of relationship is likely to become more common.

Support processes in professionally-led dementia groups were considered by Mason et al (2005). Eight themes emerged from their study: a useful group, I do find it difficult, all talking together, keep the pot boiling, attending to see if you can get it, there isn't one that's like another, outside on your own and the business of dementia. Whilst this study investigated support groups it is notable that a number of the themes are congruent with those found elsewhere. Feelings of social isolation are also reported by Aggarwal et al (2003) and Bartlett (2007). Participants' perceptions of their failings, and their recognition of this in others, has many parallels with the work of Gillies (2000). When describing the business of dementia, participants elucidate many of the issues that are highlighted in other studies of the experience of dementia such as the work of Menne et al (2002) and Pearce et al (2002).

Personal experience of dementia has been shown to be distressing for many individuals. There is a recognition that the way in which others relate to the person with dementia is linked to their ability to maintain their personhood and self narrative. Ways in which people cope with dementia has commonalities in that they may strive to maintain a semblance of normality and some people attempt to rationalise their situation. It has been shown that coping strategies are developed but these vary according to stage of dementia and personal beliefs and circumstances. It is clear that the knowledge base around the personal experience of dementia remains poorly developed, particularly in relation to more advanced dementia. However, the personal experience of dementia is perhaps one the most fully explored area of research involving people with dementia. The body of knowledge is rapidly growing and there are a number of themes that emerge recurrently. It is possible that synthesis of these studies is now timely.

Religion and Spirituality

Religion and spirituality in the lives of people with dementia is considered in two studies. Katsuno (2003) investigated spiritual experiences of people with dementia and explored the relationship between personal spirituality and perceived quality of life. Findings indicated that many participants had a strong faith in God and tended to use religion as a coping mechanism. Although it is reported that a strong faith was present in many, negative cases are also presented. Snyder (2003) also examined the role of religion and spirituality in the lives of people with dementia. This author is more circumspect about drawing conclusions. She claims only to have provided an introduction into some spiritual themes addressed by people with dementia and goes on to highlight the need for further investigation.

It may be argued that it is not surprising that the people who would be willing to participate in this type of study would be those who possessed a spiritual belief or faith. However, these studies are both successful in providing a balanced insight into spiritual and religious considerations of people with dementia. These and other similar studies provide some broad insights into the ways in which individuals experience dementia. One of their prime strengths is the way in which they demonstrate the depth of thought and ability to articulate that is retained by people, certainly in the earlier stages of the disease process.

Receiving the Diagnosis

Experience of being diagnosed with dementia is a subject of investigations which allude to the care and sensitivity that is required to ensure that this process causes the minimum distress to individuals. Marzanski (2000) questioned thirty participants with cognitive impairments ranging from mild to severe. He found that, despite having been told of their diagnosis, two thirds of patients reported that no-one had ever talked to them about their illness, although many were able to give an accurate description of their condition without using the term dementia. Effects of being told of a diagnosis of dementia are also considered by Pratt and Wilkinson (2001). Their study provides a rich insight into what it is like to be a person receiving a diagnosis of dementia. Through extracts of conversation, these researchers illuminate some of the feelings of participants and demonstrate some of the stages they may go through post diagnosis. Findings have been developed into a model which gives practitioners guidance on the possible reactions to, and implications of, receiving this diagnosis. A wealth of literature exists on sharing the diagnosis, most of this is written from the perspective of health care staff with some additional reflections from lay carers. Marzanski (2000) and Pratt and Wilkinson (2001) have both generated new insights from the perspectives of people with dementia which may be used to inform the debate.

Extensive research has been conducted into disclosure of diagnosis from the perspective of health care staff and lay carers. Pratt and Wilkinson (2001) discuss the advantages and disadvantages of disclosure whilst acknowledging that the debate around this issue is far from being concluded. Studies of current practice show that two thirds of general practitioners in Scotland do not tell patients of their diagnosis (Downs and Rae 1997). This practice was also discovered by Vassilas (1999). A study of Old Age Psychiatrists showed that they almost invariably told carers of the diagnosis, people with severe dementia were rarely told of their diagnosis and disclosure to people with mild or moderate dementia was variable (Rice and Warner 1994). Reasons for non-disclosure are examined in detail by Wilkinson and Milne (2003) who cite as influencing factors concern about accuracy of diagnosis, the limit of therapeutic options, a perception of inevitable decline and causing distress to individuals. Whilst it is accepted that medical treatment for dementia remains limited, it is argued that failure to disclose diagnosis, possibly for theoretically justifiable reasons, denies individuals the ability to access services that are available and opportunity to put their affairs in order while they are still able. Non-disclosure is viewed by Monaghan and Begley (2003) as compromising the autonomy of the individual. Current knowledge base around disclosure of diagnosis from the perspective of the person with dementia remains extremely small. However there are tentative indications that a diagnosis, if delivered in a sensitive and individualised way, may be better than not knowing.

Outcomes of Services or Treatments

Outcomes of services or treatments have been the subject of several studies. The idea that people with dementia and their carers should be involved in determining outcome measures rather than being dictated to by professional staff is becoming more widespread. It is supported by Traynor et al (2004) and Gibson et al (2004) in terms of needing to develop person-focused outcomes for the evaluation of drug therapies. Outcomes in terms of community and acute hospital care have also been investigated.

Bamford and Bruce (2000) consulted fifteen community living service users from a resource centre for older people with dementia to identify their desired outcomes of community care. Current outcome measures include cognition, behaviour, mood and psychiatric symptoms, physical health status, functional and self care abilities, family and staff caregiver outcomes, service use and costs and quality of life. In their discussions, Bamford and Bruce (2000) uncovered two types of outcomes that were considered important by people with dementia and their carers, quality of life outcomes and service process outcomes. Quality of life outcomes centred on having access to normal activities and having a pattern of life that maximised feelings of choice and control. Service process outcomes related to how services were delivered and the extent to which participants could influence the service. This study graphically demonstrated that outcomes that participants wanted bear little relation to the outcome measures that are commonly used to evaluate community services.

Tolson et al (1999) examined what people with dementia considered to be the components of best nursing care in the acute setting. Unfortunately this study was not wholly successful in discovering the views of people with dementia. This may be because interviews were conducted with patients and their main visitors who were possibly quicker and provided more articulate answers. Input of patients could also have been limited by the influence of the physical illness that led to their admission. Despite a lack of success in answering the research question, this study provides a laudable attempt to examine what is important to this group and has provided useful insights into how future studies may be conducted. Norman (2003a) investigated dementia care in the acute setting from multiple perspectives including gaining an insight into the knowledge base and educational needs of nursing staff and eliciting the views of patients and carers of their experience of acute hospital care. As a result of this study Norman (2003b:3) developed the core category "the nurse, individual interaction map (with external impacting factors)". Elements that have been used to construct this category are explicated in detail and from this work Norman has developed a set of guidelines for practice.

Needs and desires of people with dementia relating to services that are provided are clearly under investigated. Preliminary studies indicate that there is a dichotomy between the outcomes currently used and those that are important to service users. Experience of people with dementia of acute hospital care is barely investigated at all. The increasing number of people accessing this service points to an urgent need to consider how people with dementia view their care and consideration of ways in which care could be enhanced in the future.

The Use of Technology

Use of technology is a relatively recent addition to the dementia research agenda. Nygard and Starkhammar (2007) investigated the use of everyday technology by people with dementia in their own homes. They constructed a four point taxonomy of the difficulties that were encountered. These authors suggest that this tentative taxonomy needs to be validated. A more specialised study by Hanson et al (2007) explored the capacity of older people with early stage dementia to be involved in the planning, design and evaluation of information technology programmes for their use. The study indicates that such a level of involvement is possible and that the majority of participants were fully engaged. Participants reported that the project enhanced their self confidence, stimulated thought and was very enjoyable. It is perhaps surprising that there are not more published research studies concerning the use of the various types of technology that are now used by people with dementia.

Evaluation of Phase Two Studies

Studies have been reviewed which provide an overview of research actively engaging people with dementia. Qualitative methods have generally been appropriate to address the research question. Quantitative methods have successfully been integrated in some studies. In each case they have provided some insight into the views and experiences of this group. A number of authors have asked extremely broad questions about what it is like to live with dementia. These studies have provided a wealth of insights on a wide range of topics. Other studies have been more focused such as those investigating aspects of diagnosis. The focused nature of these studies has been valuable in that the specific information generated is more readily available to be used to influence practice. It is noted that a narrower focus does not necessarily capture more pertinent information, as is apparent in the two studies about acute care.

Researchers have predominantly identified the limitations of their studies, often in a fairly harsh manner. Ways in which studies were conducted is variable. As noted earlier, a large amount has been written giving advice on how people with dementia should be included in research. It is evident that in each of the studies some thought has been given to how people with dementia can be ethically and meaningfully included in the research process. Reviewing studies from the last decade has indicated that researchers are gradually developing increased expertise in effectively engaging people with dementia in the research process.

Key Learning

Forty five studies reviewed in phase two reveal some important issues relating to ethical and meaningful research involving people with dementia.

- Qualitative research methods are more congruent with person-focused dementia research.
- Whatever research method is chosen, it is imperative that it is applied flexibly to meet the needs of individuals.
- Selection and recruitment processes need to protect participants from undue anxiety or coercion. However this needs to be balanced against paternalism that may erode the personhood of individuals.
- There is clear evidence that, given the right approach, people with dementia are able to communicate their thoughts and feelings.
- Skill, expertise and manner of the researcher are central to the credibility of the study.
- Indications are that, rather than feeling anxious, many participants enjoy the opportunity to tell their story to an interested listener.
- The body of research that involves people with dementia remains relatively small, particularly with people in the more advanced stages.
- It appears that over the last decade there has been a rapid rise in the number of studies that actively engage people with dementia. Review of these studies indicates that researchers are now more likely to document the ways in which they have ensured that such involvement is ethical and meaningful.
- There is a significant lack of studies that seeks the views of older people with dementia about acute hospital care.

Conclusion

In phase two a set of criteria have been used to judge the quality of studies. Of the forty-five studies reviewed three studies were found to have met the criteria most closely and so were allocated to level one, thirty seven were judged to be at level two and five at level three. It is evident that the body of knowledge on the subject remains small at present and for this reason findings have been summarised rather than attempting meta-synthesis. This phase has revealed a number of key learning points about how ethical and meaningful research can be conducted involving people with dementia. As noted earlier in this review it is suggested that there is an element of subjectivity in judging how closely the research meets the criteria. On reflection, it is considered that ways in which decisions have been made may not be entirely transparent. It is considered that using a detailed set of criteria to measure qualitative research studies produces a rather fragmented result which detracts from acknowledging the value of studies in a holistic sense. This thought led to phase three of the review.

Phase Three

Phase three of this review revisits the three studies that were judged to be at level one in phase two. They are the papers that most closely met the criteria for research involving people with dementia. Phase two of the review employed an ostensibly qualitative approach based on the work of authors who are all situated in the qualitative paradigm. However, it is suggested that the criteria used in phase two, whilst aiming to be a measure of qualitative work, is unintentionally based on the essence of quantitative work. Use of conventional systematic review processes for qualitative reviews is questioned by Jones (2004a) who argues powerfully that attempts by qualitative researchers to imitate quantitative colleagues has led to a degree of "mission drift". It is suggested that this phase of the review has succumbed to an element of "mission drift" and, whilst theoretically qualitative approaches have been applied this has failed to explicate the contribution that the level one studies have made to research involving people with dementia.

As stated earlier the approach to this review is somewhat unorthodox. On completing phase two there was a feeling that there were factors that had led to papers being allocated to level one that were not entirely transparent. This idea is one that has been identified to some extent in the work of Edwards et al (2000). These authors propose a model of review described as "signal" and "noise" in which "signal" represents the relevance, applicability and value of the study whilst "noise" represents the strength of evidence and design weaknesses. Edwards et al (1998) suggest that the "signal" and "noise" approach is more inclusive in systematic reviews as it involves assessing the "weight of evidence" thus reducing the risk of losing potentially important literature. The technique is broadly designed to legitimise utilisation of qualitative work in traditionally conducted systematic reviews. It may be suggested that, given the intended use of the "signal and noise approach" it presents an uncomfortable mismatch with this review. Further evidence from the work of the authors (for example Edwards et al 1998, Edwards et al 2000, Higginson et al 2002) indicates that the application of this model to date draws on a positivist approach. However, the idea that there is a value in reviewing research using differing and flexible approaches is particularly resonant at this stage of the review. It is recognised that the papers judged to be at level one in phase two all produced an exceptionally high signal; that is they were considered to be of particular value in the field of research involving people with dementia. The reason for these papers being selected is subtle and perhaps not amenable to the use of a set of criteria to evaluate their quality.

Three papers demonstrated a high signal and so were deemed worthy of further review. It was evident that using Edwards et al (2000) model would be inappropriate as it is embedded in quantitative beliefs. It was considered that a review method that was true to qualitative philosophy needed to be identified. Jones (2004a) advocates a return to the roots of the qualitative paradigm arguing convincingly that the fundamental concepts of qualitative research methods should be extended into the realms of review and synthesis. He states that narrative is the cornerstone of qualitative work and can be used valuably in reviews. Jones identifies four relational qualities that should be considered in reviewing studies: dialogue, experience, reflection and narrative. Detractors of qualitative work may argue that such an approach to reviews is intangible and largely based in the experiential and intuitive domains. Whilst positivists may view this negatively, it is argued that intuition is likely to be based in expert knowledge. Scheff (1997) argues that the great advantage of intuition is that it exposes interpretive accounts of the real rather than seeking truths in the positivist sense.

Qualities identified by Jones (2004a) were applied in reviewing the level one studies. The purpose of this stage of the review is not to summarise or synthesise findings but rather to attempt to synthesise what has been learnt about the ways in which people with dementia have been included in the first fragile and tentative steps into a vast and relatively unexplored area. Each of the studies is reviewed individually.

Study One

An exploration of the effect of being told the diagnosis of dementia from the perspective of the person with dementia was conducted by Pratt and Wilkinson (2001) in a study funded by the Mental Health Foundation. An overview of dementia research, particularly that relating to disclosure of diagnosis, is provided. It gives a clear justification for the study and also contextualises it for the reader.

Presentation of this report is logical and comprehensive. Equally it is presented in language that is easily accessible. Details of participants are summarised in a table which is elaborated on by a full case study of each person. This gives a detailed description of each individual and their context and is written in a mixture of the words of researchers and participants which give a powerful feeling of authenticity.

In their interviews the researchers aimed to discover how participants felt about the way they were told of their diagnosis. Readers are alerted to the idea that diagnosing dementia can be a lengthy process which may involve high levels of emotion. It is explained that the researchers asked participants about disclosure of diagnosis in different ways, suggesting that questions framed in terms of disclosure in a wider sense were more easily answered than more targeted questions. Themes are developed around the disclosure of diagnosis and are justified and supported by extracts of text that are of sufficient length to allow readers to comprehend how they have been categorised and begin to appreciate the experiences that participants have been through. Research processes and difficulties, for example barriers to recruitment, are presented in detail allowing readers to follow the story.

Respect for personhood is evident at every stage of the study. Researchers chose to make initial contact via professionals that had a pre-existing relationship with the individual. Unusually they did not seek information regarding memory assessment and chose to rely on professional judgment about what constituted the early stages of dementia. This choice ensured that people were not excluded from the study on the grounds of memory capacity, recognising that this would not necessarily correlate with the ability to discuss their feelings. Researchers were aware that not all referrals met the inclusion criteria as it became clear that, contrary to the belief of referring agencies, not all participants were aware of their diagnosis. In these cases the interviews continued with the focus being either on memory problems or a general topic that the participant chose to talk about. Some of these interviews still provided useful information and only two were excluded.

Readers are drawn through the study gradually, building up a picture of how participants felt about their experiences which are then used to develop a model of the process of receiving a diagnosis of dementia. Two case studies are presented which demonstrate how the model is relevant and useful in understanding what may happen to individuals. The report concludes with a description of feedback and consultation which involved people with dementia, carers and service providers. Preliminary findings were presented by participants and researchers. Workshops were used to generate recommendations for practice. Quotes are used powerfully to bring to life the very "ordinariness" of people with dementia and illustrate that whilst some issues may be specific many will produce a sense of empathy in readers:

> "If I'm given a lot of information at one time I can't take it all in, where if I'm just given a bit of information at a time I don't have to maybe remember what's been said ......" (Pratt and Wilkinson 2001:30).

Remarkably little information is offered about the researchers. There is little hint of reflexivity and their input in the interviews is rarely reported verbatim. It is currently suggested that reflexivity is a crucial component in qualitative studies (Finlay and Gough 2003). However its absence in this paper has produced an impression of direct communication from participant to reader which has been enhanced by the researchers providing signposts and interpretations which encourage readers to think more deeply.

A compelling style of writing is used in this study. It is absolutely clear that the key players are participants and that the role of the researchers has been to enable them to tell their stories. It could be suggested that some of the information that is regularly reported in qualitative studies, for example the setting for interviews, has not been discussed. However, it can be argued that such detail would be extraneous in this paper where respect and care for individuals is implicit throughout. The researchers have been skilled in providing readers with a narrative that embraces stories of a group of individuals.

Study Two

A report of a small consultation with people with dementia and their carers to identify the desired outcomes of community care has been written by Bamford and Bruce (2000). The scene for this research is set effectively, drawing on a range of literature. It is noted that key limitations of many current outcome measures for people with dementia is the marginalisation of the perspectives of this group. This study begins to address this gap. Some of the issues they encountered during the study are addressed and show the flexible approaches the researchers adopted to overcome these. This has a particular resonance for other dementia researchers as it indicates how principles of good practice can be applied. For example, data gathering processes evolved from the planned six formal group discussions to a more inclusive approach using informal and formal groups and individual interviews. Topic guides, vignettes and prompts such as photographs were used to aid discussion. As in the study by Pratt and Wilkinson (2001) participants were identified, by staff with previous knowledge of them, for their ability and desire to communicate rather than on the basis of a memory assessment score. Half the participants were described as having mild dementia and half moderate.

Ways in which participants were recruited and encouraged to share their story in whichever way was most readily achieved, together with the researchers espoused concern to understand rather than report the "truth" of what was said, all indicate their desire to maintain the personhood of participants. This must provoke a sense of shared endeavour with other researchers who are engaged with people with dementia.

Again, in this paper the voice of the participants has primacy; quotes used are much shorter than those of Pratt and Wilkinson (2001) but still convey a message that the researchers have genuinely sought to elicit their views. One example is when a researcher asked a person who used services if they thought that the home care service was good:

> "I do in some cases, but if you can do it, I don't think it is. Because it takes your jobs away from you that you'd occupy your time with……but if you're not feeling well or anything like that, well then it's a godsend." (Bamford and Bruce 2000:555).

Little information is provided about the researchers and their pre-existing stance on the subject other than that they acknowledge that there is a need to discover more about service users views. Vulnerability of individuals is recognised and a strong sense of justice and caring enough to find ways in which they can express themselves permeates this study. Bamford and Bruce also focus mainly on views of participants although this is slightly more tempered with their interpretations. The paper has a stronger flavour of the researchers conveying the story of participants to the reader than there being a direct line of communication. Nevertheless the story remains effectively told using this different style. Narratives make sense and are described in sufficient detail to allow readers to believe the findings which are linked to current knowledge. Conclusions of this study, that the desired outcomes identified by service users bear little relation to outcome measures currently used to evaluate community care services, are transparently derived from the views of participants. This study provides a real and credible story which is easy to follow; the only interruption felt is when text detective, an annotation tool, is used with relatively little explanation.

Study Three

Sabat (2002a) explores relationships between the experience of an individual with Alzheimer's disease and Social Construction Theory. He explains the value of the study in terms of assisting people to understand the concept of loss of self (Cohen and Eisdorfer 1986), or what Tobin (1999) describes as the deselfing of Alzheimer's disease, need to be challenged. Sabat describes the single participant in his study in a level of detail that allows readers to form a clear picture of the person. He then describes the relationship that had been built between the participant and himself over a two year period and explains how the relationship has developed from researcher-and-patient to person-to-person. The participant is noted to have moderate to severe Alzheimer's disease and to experience severe word finding problems.

Skill is shown in achieving a dialogue with the participant and in recognising her as an individual with her own personal narrative:

> Researcher: "You're not just any ordinary person who has some problems finding words. You're a person for whom words, words to you are kind of like a musical instrument."
>
> Participant: "Um hum, um hum. That's exactly right."
>
> Researcher: "And so the kind of frustration you feel would be greater than for a person whose focus in life was not so literary ….."
>
> (Sabat 2002a:29)

Whilst it could be construed that Sabat was putting words into the mouth of the participant, this is patently not so as is shown in subsequent extracts of conversation. Sabat is skilfully using conversation to enable the participant to express her views rather than engaging in a more challenging style of interview. This researcher takes an approach to story telling that is quite different to that of Pratt and Wilkinson (2001) or Bamford and Bruce (2000) in that he appears to invite the reader to join the conversation and certainly generates a feeling of wanting to know more of the thoughts of the participant. Ways in which he describes the participant again evokes a feeling of "ordinariness", he presents her as a person rather than as a "case", and in doing this he exposes the idea that this could be any one of us and thus produces a story with which many readers could engage.

This is the only one of the three papers that provides relatively lengthy extracts of conversation from both researcher and participant. Little is explicitly exposed about the researcher and his views but they are powerfully demonstrated in these extracts in that they show his genuine desire to help this participant to make readers aware of just how much of her self is left intact. Analysis of conversations in this study is used to draw conclusions that should begin to reshape the way in which readers view selfhood in dementia.

A second review of the three studies has generated insights that were not revealed in phase two. This lends weight to Jones (2004a) assertion that qualitative reviews should be based on the fundamental concepts of qualitative research. This approach allows studies to be viewed holistically, thus reducing both the risk of fragmentation and loss of the essential message that are an inherent risk when using methods that have been adapted from quantitative approaches. Revisiting these studies using Jones (2004a) approach has reinforced the belief that they may be considered as being at the forefront of research involving people with dementia.

A significant contribution to research involving people with dementia has been made by these studies. It is suggested that what sets these papers apart from others is the way in which research was conducted rather than purely the value of the findings. The mindset of the researchers appears to be grounded in a powerful belief in, and application of, the concepts of genuine respect for older people and those with dementia that are articulated in the work of McCormack (2004) on person-centredness, McCormack (2001a) on autonomy and Kitwood (1997a) relating to personhood. The difference in these studies is that the thoughtfulness and flexibility of the researchers in their approach to people with dementia and their openness to the idea that even people in the advanced stages can communicate, given the right support, appears to be woven through the fabric of their research. Other studies, whilst acknowledging these concepts, give the impression of a far more formulaic application. A remarkable lack of detail is provided about the researchers themselves despite a growing trend towards inclusion of reflexivity in qualitative research. However, the effect that lack of acknowledgement of self has in these papers is to reinforce the primacy of participants. This approach leads to real engagement between reader and participants which is supported rather than led by the researchers. In some cases the thought that has gone into the design and execution of the three studies is implicit rather than explicit but can readily be identified by likeminded researchers who have been sensitised to relevant issues. Although not necessarily transferable, findings of these studies are believable and transparent enough to generate further research into these important areas.

Conclusion

This review has used a rather unorthodox approach to systematically reviewing person-focused dementia research. Approaches whilst non-conventional have succeeded in setting person centred dementia research within the context of dementia research as a whole. In phase one the trajectory of dementia research over the last three decades is plotted. This identifies the predominance of biomedical studies with a small growth in person-focused studies in more recent years. In phase two forty-five person-focused studies have been reviewed using a set of criteria based on the work of other qualitative researchers. These studies covered a range of subjects; some asked very broad questions about what it is like to live with dementia whilst others have been more focused on specific issues such as disclosure of diagnosis and the experiences of people with dementia in acute hospitals. Findings from these studies are disparate due to the wide range of perspectives that have been studied and are therefore not wholly amenable to meta-synthesis. It has been discovered that the use of fixed criteria to evaluate studies can lead to fragmentation and loss of the central message. It has been revealed that most studies have applied many of the central tenets of producing ethical and meaningful research involving people with dementia. Reflection on studies that were allocated as level one indicated that using a set of criteria for evaluation detracted from the value of the study as a whole as there was a tendency for the study to be fragmented as individual criteria were applied. A method for reviewing studies that was faithful to the qualitative paradigm was identified and applied in phase three. The three studies that were reviewed again in phase three can be regarded as being at the cutting edge of dementia research in view of the skilful ways the researchers have conducted ethically sound and meaningful research and has allowed the voice of people with dementia, some in the more advanced stages, to be heard.

One element that all the studies in phase two and phase three have in common is that they provide evidence that people with dementia do have something worth saying. It is clear that this remains an under researched area and virtually all papers point to the need for further studies. This conclusion, together with the virtual absence of research about the experiences of older people with dementia in acute hospitals, powerfully supports the need to conduct this study. A critical element in ensuring that the study is both meaningful and ethical is in selecting and using appropriate research methodology. This concept is discussed in more detail in chapter two.

CHAPTER TWO

METHODOLOGY

Introduction

Chapter two provides a rationale for the choice of critical, interpretive ethnography as the predominant research methodology for this study. Reasons for incorporating elements of the narrative approaches are examined. The research process is explained and methodological decisions justified. Issues around ethics and reflexivity are explored.

Methodology

The fundamental aim of this research is to explore the experiences of individuals in relation to the care of older people with dementia in the acute hospital setting. It is acknowledged that research with people with dementia can be challenging. It involves a group who can be considered vulnerable and who may be seen to hold low status in society. For these reasons it was considered early in development of the study that this research subject was not one that could be taken in isolation. It was essential to begin by setting it within the broader social and political context.

Political and Social Context

Older people with dementia in acute hospitals are the primary focus of this study. It is suggested that being an older person in Western society is not always a comfortable position to be in. Despite the demographic shift towards an older population (Department of Health 2001b) it is stated by Bytheway (1995) that many societies are suffused with ageism which views older people as incompetent, ugly and burdensome and discriminates against them on a personal and structural basis. Nolan (2003) reiterates the concepts of ageism suggesting that there are three major "isms" in society: sexism, racism and ageism. Nolan states that the difference with ageism is that anyone who lives long enough is likely to experience these complex and subtle phenomena. A moving illustration of this experience is provided by Bennett (2005) in his description of the way in which his mother's personhood was gradually eroded during her stay in a residential home.

Bernard and Phillips (2000) consider the current and future status of older people in Britain. These authors trace social policy developments concerning older people over the last five decades. They argue convincingly that there is a need to move from the concept of "old age" to one of "ageing", a phenomenon that will be experienced by all and is potentially less divisive. Bernard and Phillips (2000) identify four key concepts that they consider should influence development of social policy that avoids ageism. These include a positive, inter-generational life course perspective, combating discrimination, enhancement of empowerment, citizenship and voice and, finally, critical commentary and action. It is evident that, to some extent, society is attempting to reduce ageism. In some cases older people have challenged professionals to review their practice and find new ways of working "with" rather than "for" older people (Ogg et al 1998).

It could be argued that, to a degree, the United Kingdom Government has attempted to improve the situation of older people. A range of initiatives has been implemented to enable voices of older people to be heard, for example through Patient and Public Involvement in the New NHS (Department of Health 1999b) and a range of Better Government for Older People (Department of Health 1999a) bulletins. An example of this approach includes the work of Thornton (2000) who provides clear advice on how older people may be involved in influencing service development but the extent to which this has happened in practice is not entirely clear. Autonomy of older people may have been enhanced by the Mental Capacity Act (HMSO 2005) and, theoretically, health care has been improved through the implementation of the National Service Framework for Older People (Department of Health 2001b), although the absence of financial support for this may have hampered progress.

Despite attempts to reduce ageism it is suggested that Garner and Ardern's (1998) assertion that we continue to live in a youth centred, youth dominated culture in which the prospect of being old, dependent and ill could be terrifying, retains some validity. It is suggested that older people remain marginalised and undervalued in society although moves are being made to alter this situation. It is argued that older people who also have dementia find themselves in an even more invidious position. Kitwood (1997a) suggests that people with dementia are subjected to a particular kind of inhumanity. His description takes this treatment beyond the realms of “isms”. Kitwood (1997a) conjectures that people with dementia are treated poorly in response to the anxiety of others. He speculates that we are all afraid of becoming frail, mentally unstable and dependent. Being exposed to people with dementia activates these fears and, as a defence mechanism, this group are treated as a different species; their personhood is denied. The stereotype of people with dementia as senile old people who have “lost their mind” (Lyman 1998, Mills 1997, Sabat 1998) is still articulated and serves to reinforce a negative image and marginalisation.

Despite the fact that older people with dementia tend to be undervalued by society there is a growing body of evidence that this group are advocating their own needs and are committed to improving care and promoting change. Examples of this include the Scottish Dementia Working Group (2008). The aims of this group of people with dementia include: influencing public policies that affect the lives of people with dementia and their families, promoting improvement in provision of services and reducing prejudice and stigma attached to dementia. People with dementia are also campaigning to ensure their needs are met through the Dementia Advocacy and Support Network International. This worldwide organisation brings together people with dementia to improve quality of life. Specific aims of the organisation include: promoting respect and dignity, providing a forum for exchange of information and advocating for services (DANSI 2008). These are just two examples of the move towards recognition that this group are not helpless people with no future. Such groups clearly demonstrate that people with dementia are able to play an active role in shaping their future and those of others.

Whilst movement is being made to reduce negativity around both ageing and dementia it is argued that, at present, this group continues to experience the double jeopardy described by Rodeheaver and Datan (1988). This idea was reinforced recently in reports by the Alzheimer’s Society (2007) and the National Audit Office (2007) both of which noted a lack of consistent provision of health and social care services that are available to this group. The concept that older people with dementia are viewed as poor relations in the acute hospital setting is currently supported mainly by anecdotal evidence. It can be argued that caring for older people remains a “Cinderella” service that tends to attract less attention than higher profile, more technologically advanced specialities. A small number of studies have considered views of acute sector staff of people with dementia. Dewing (2003) suggests that staff have a tendency to speak about patients using language that can be detrimental to their personhood and therefore dehumanising. Gerdner and Buckwater (1994) attempt some justification for this approach by stating that some staff depersonalise patients as a way of dealing with feelings of fear and inadequacy. An alternative interpretation is offered by Schofield (1986) and Meyer et al (1999) who state that older confused patients are perceived by health care providers as relatively unimportant and unworthy. This idea is supported by Norman (2003a) who observed that patients who had been labelled as having memory problems were treated differently to others by nursing staff. The value attributed to older people with dementia in acute hospital settings may be summarised by Marshall (1999:9) who quotes from harassed nurses who state "they should not really be here".

This brief review of the social and political context surrounding older people with dementia demonstrates clearly the powerless position they may occupy in society. Given this disadvantaged position, it was considered essential to use a research method that set the study within the broader picture and provided the best possible opportunity for participants to convey their experiences to a wider audience.

Ethnography

A review of texts reveals that ethnography has been through many incarnations since its beginnings in the early 1900s (O'Reilly 2005). It is a research method that remains resistant to absolute definition although its historical context and categorisation have been traced by many authors (for example Denzin and Lincoln 1994, Atkinson et al 1999). Whilst it is accepted that there is not one universal definition of ethnography, it is equally evident that a number of authors agree on the principle that ethnography includes certain key characteristics. It is generally acknowledged that ethnography embraces the following tenets.

- It is intended to provide a direct description of a group or culture (Creswell 1998, Spradley 1980, Holloway and Todres 2003).
- "Thick" description is used (Geertz 1973, Maggs-Rapport 2001).
- Data is collected through extensive fieldwork and interviews (Creswell 1998, Fetterman 1998, Savage 2000, Holloway and Todres 2003).
- The researcher is the major instrument of data collection (Clifford 1997, Coffey 1999, Fetterman 1998, Maggs-Rapport 2001).
- Key informants are sought (Rock 2001, Maggs-Rapport 2001).
- Emic and etic perspectives are considered (Creswell 1998, Fetterman 1998, Keating 2001, Hughes 1992).

- Ethnography is both process and product (Holloway and Wheeler 2002, Savage 2000).

It is the key concepts identified above that make ethnography a valuable research method for this study. A selection of these concepts is explored in more detail below.

Direct, "Thick" Description of the Group or Culture

The purpose of this study is to provide a description and interpretation of the complex and dynamic culture of older people with dementia receiving acute hospital care, a culture about which little is currently known. It is suggested that the provision of "thick" description (Geertz 1973), with accurate descriptions that include accounts of matters with which readers are already familiar, adds authenticity and enables them to judge its completeness and recognise any bias (Stake 1995).

Data Collection through Observation and Interviews

Use of differing methods of data collection has particular value in this study. The use of both observation and interviews offered the best opportunity of capturing a holistic picture of dementia care; using interviews alone caused some concern for a number of reasons. I believed that this method had the potential to produce a series of relatively uni-dimensional views that would not fully capture the critical complexity of the inter-relationships between the various groups involved. A further consideration was that interviews may generate data that reflects a situation that is quite different from the reality of life and that may not explicate the nuances of everyday practice. A final thought was that some participants, particularly those with dementia, may find interviews anxiety provoking or simply impossible. Although it is well documented that people with dementia can be involved in meaningful research interviews the majority of these have been conducted with people in the earlier stages (Keady 1996, Downs 1997). Participants in this study included people with more advanced dementia who could have found formal interviews distressing and uncomfortable or beyond their capability. Desire to ensure that a range of people, regardless of their status, were able to participate in this study led to the selection of a research method that included observation as well as interviews as methods of data collection.

The Researcher as the Major Instrument of Data Collection

A researcher being the major instrument of data collection is an idea that can be viewed as having both advantages and disadvantages. Until starting this study I was a senior nurse and professional lead for the study wards, together with many other wards, within the hospital. Advantages of this situation were that access was facilitated more easily and that I was able to "fit in" more readily. Equally, such familiarity with the research setting may have increased the risk of less rigorous questioning and potential "taking for granted" of what was being observed. It was also possible that my previous senior role may have made some junior staff wary. It was clear that role management was vital to the success of this study and ways in which this was achieved are discussed in subsequent sections of this chapter.

It is apparent that the central tenets of ethnography fit well with the aims of this study. The need to set the research within the broader context led to the selection of the subtype of critical interpretive ethnography.

Critical Interpretive Ethnography

Ethnography remains open to a number of interpretations and within such interpretations a number of sub types have evolved. Number and definitions of subtypes vary considerably from one author to another but are perhaps expressed most succinctly by Holloway and Wheeler (2002) who distinguish between descriptive or conventional ethnography and critical ethnography. Descriptive ethnography focuses on descriptions of a culture and, using analysis, explicates patterns and categories. Critical ethnography is more political in nature. Thomas (1993:4) defines critical ethnography as "conventional ethnography with a political purpose".

Within critical ethnography there are variations on the critical theme (Thomas 1993), again a range of subtypes are offered by different authors (see Hammersley 1991, Van Maanen 1988). Thomas (1993:23) proposes a continuum from "armchair reflection" to direct political action. This author states that postmodernists tend to be "armchair radicals" in that they aim to change ways of thinking rather than attempting to action change. At the other end of the spectrum are the radical Marxist orientated approaches which advocate replacement of existing forms of social organisation. In this study an "armchair reflection" approach is taken for three major reasons. Firstly, little is currently known about the experiences of people with dementia in acute hospitals. For this reason a major aim is to open the minds of readers to new ideas and interpretations and generate interest and further investigation into this poorly researched area. Secondly this relatively uncontroversial style has been chosen because it is felt the intended practitioner audience is more likely to be influenced by rational, thoughtful work which is set in a broader context rather than by a highly political polemic. Thirdly there is a need to be realistic about the power and influence of a single researcher. Whilst it is reasonable to believe that recommendations may be made to improve practice, the goal of restructuring the organisation is perhaps too ambitious within the confines of this study.

It is evident that the subtypes of ethnography each have their own value and are appropriate to different situations. The approach to ethnography is one that must be chosen by each individual ethnographer based on the subject being studied together with their underlying personal philosophical assumptions. There is agreement amongst authors of several research texts that it is vital the ethnographer defines and makes explicit their position in relation to the subtype of ethnography that is selected (Streubert Speziale and Carpenter 2003, Creswell 1998).

This study draws on the philosophies of both critical and interpretive ethnography. As is often the case in ethnography, this choice has been made based on a "purposeful and deliberate kind of eclecticism that can offer complementary explanations" (Lett 1987:124). Choice of a critical interpretive approach is based on three fundamental beliefs that I hold.

- To be of value this ethnography needs to be set within the broader political and social context.
- The intention of the study is to enable the voices of this vulnerable group to be heard.
- The purpose of the study is to produce knowledge that may be used to influence future practice.

Each of these beliefs and the context that they create for the study are discussed in more detail below.

Political and Social Context

As discussed earlier in this chapter it is thought that conducting this research without considering the wider picture would risk reducing its impact on readers. The group being studied tend already to be in an invidious position which may then be compounded by admission to an acute hospital. It was therefore vital to consider the study in a broad context.

Enabling Voices to be Heard

In a broad context it has been seen that older people with dementia occupy a relatively difficult place in society in which their views may be poorly represented because of their relative powerlessness. The aim of this study was to provide participants with an opportunity to tell their stories to readers; this aim is congruent with gradual social and political changes that support enabling consumers' views to be heard (Thornton 2000).

Knowledge to Influence Practice

Reflection on the purpose of this study led to a review of three epistemologies outlined by Meleis (1999): correspondence, coherence and pragmatism. Specific ethnographic epistemologies of the emic and etic perspectives are also considered.

Historically, the aim of much research has been to present readers with the "truth" about the subject being studied. Definition of what constitutes truth has long been problematic. In positivist terms, at the most simple level, truth is described as correspondence to a fact. A broader interpretation suggests that truth consists in a relation to reality (Stanford 2005a). This concept of truth relies on the assumption that an objective reality exists (Im and Chee 2003) in which researcher and participants are rigidly separated and which is independent of the social and psychological aspects of reality (Lomborg and Kirkevold 2003). Whilst this realist position may have a value in some quantitative studies, it is clearly incongruent with the multiple world view beliefs of most qualitative researchers. The qualitative paradigm demands a more flexible and broader perception of "truth".

Coherence theory perhaps moves towards a wider perspective suggesting that the truth of any proposition relies on its coherence with a specified set of propositions (Stanford 2005b). Truth is viewed as transient, if the proposition is sufficient now then it is considered that there is truth in it (Meleis 1999). The idea that it is the coherence of a belief with a totality of beliefs that provides a reason to assume that the belief is true is advocated by Rorty (1979). This theory seems plausible and more congruent with the qualitative paradigm but alone it lacks the embracing, practice-based philosophy that was sought for this study.

A third epistemology suggested by Meleis (1999) is pragmatism. Pragmatism is a term derived from the Greek word meaning action. The words "practice" and "practical" are also derived from this source (Doane 2005). In contrast to other epistemologies the aim in pragmatism is not to search for truth but rather to consciously set aside concerns about how evidence represents the world (Davidson 2001) and concentrate instead on the usefulness of evidence derived from different sources. Berman (2000:198) captures the idea that truth is not an absolute; he proposes that the aim in research is ongoing inquiry rather than the establishment of a final truth:

> "in the nomadic mind …. the road to truth is always under construction; the going is the goal …. for nomads 'truth' is a verb, something you live. No sooner are you at one point than an elaboration or revision suggests itself".

Pragmatic inquiry acknowledges the inherent inseparability of theory and practice.

Fundamental concepts of pragmatism as described by its originator Charles Pierce in the 1870s include respect for the views of others and the notion that conversations rather than universal truth are the basis for developing beliefs (Warms and Schroeder 1999). These original ideas have been revived and refined by Rorty (1987) who states that the values of pragmatism include tolerance, respect for the opinions of others, willingness to listen, reliance on persuasion rather than force and emphasis on communication over truth. Rorty (1987) also stresses the need to leave room for alternative narratives.

Pragmatists' view of truth and reality embrace the concepts that inquiry is a continual reweaving of different views of the truth which incorporate new ideas and better explanations in the context of human encounters (Warms and Schroeder 1999). This idea is supported by Freshwater and Avis (2004) who suggest that inquiry should generate evidence that can be integrated with current knowledge to enable discovery of better ways of living our lives. The practical nature of inquiry is emphasised by Rorty (1987) who states that arguments about truth versus falsity and objectivity versus subjectivity are unhelpful. Rorty suggests that our aim should be to listen to as many suggestions as possible and then find the best solution for that time, place and situation. Key thoughts in pragmatism are clearly summarised in a series of questions posed by Doane (2005).

- What practical difference would it make to anyone if one notion rather than another was true?
- What concrete difference would any theory make to anyone's life?
- What experiences would be different?
- What is the value of theory in experiential terms?

It is noted that pragmatism is not without its critics. Pragmatism rejects the traditional philosophical concept of the pursuit of truth (Mounce 2000). Absence of seeking an absolute truth has led to the accusation that pragmatism is "a position of diminished responsibility" (Barnett 1997:84) in which there is "an allegiance to 'anything goes'" (Barnett 2000:122). Badley (2004a) argues cogently that many of Barnett's criticisms of pragmatism are simply ill conceived and that his espoused beliefs and pragmatist ideology are in fact closely allied. A more proactive stance is taken by Freshwater and Avis (2004) who acknowledge potential pitfalls of pragmatism but state that these may be minimised by the researcher taking responsibility for their own authority. This requires an awareness of one's own discriminatory processes, personal beliefs and how these originate and are embedded in the broader context. Freshwater and Avis (2004) suggest that taking a critically reflexive approach throughout a study ensures that the researcher fulfils their responsibility to examine the internal and external consistency of the beliefs thus negating the criticisms of Barnett (1997, 2000) and other like-minded writers. Use of reflexivity is discussed more fully later in this chapter.

Whilst the epistemology of pragmatism remains controversial it fits well with this study in which the aim is to capture multiple truths with a view to discovering ways in which to improve practice. Warms and Schroeder's (1999) description of the pragmatist as a person who is open to listening to multiple ideas or versions of the "truth" to better solve problems is wholly congruent with my personal philosophy.

Ethnography offers two alternative but complementary epistemological bases, the emic and etic perspectives. In this study I have chosen to present a predominantly emic viewpoint, that is the insiders view. It is acknowledged that this choice is not without difficulty. Capacity of any researcher to present the views of participants is challenged by Clifford (1986:2) who argues that ethnography is "always caught in the invention, not the representation of cultures". This author implies that any element of interpretation by the researcher detracts from accurate representation of the participants.

Holloway and Wheeler (2002) define the interpretive paradigm as a research approach in which the focus is on humans and ways in which they interpret and make sense of their own reality. The aim is to reflect and reconstruct what the researcher sees and hears and thus provide an interpretation of the actions of participants. Use of the interpretive approach is questioned at a fundamental level by Josselson (1996b) who suggests that the researcher's interpretations may be seen as an uninvited intrusion into participants' lives which deprive them of the opportunity to make sense of their own lives. In line with Josselson's assertion, Stanley and Wise (1983) argue that participants should always retain the right to self definition. More specific criticisms of interpretivism are levelled by other authors. Savage (2000) claims that such interpretations could potentially be unverifiable whilst Clarke (1992) is dismissive of this approach, stating that interpretation and the relative importance attributed to different issues is at the whim of the researcher.

Whilst these criticisms may have some validity, it is argued that interpretation is an inevitable part of ethnography. What is important is that it is made clear the product presented is the researcher's own interpretation (Lerum 2001) in which the aim is not to present an entirely subjective or entirely objective account but rather to mediate the "two worlds through a third" (Germain 1993:19). It is suggested that what is vital in ethnography is that in order to make interpretation transparent and open to scrutiny by others a clear audit trail must be incorporated (Koch 1998). This style of interpretation, in which the researcher makes themselves visible in the text (Chase 1996) and therefore exposes their interpretation, should help to diminish the power of the authorial voice (Josselson 1996a) and ensure that interpretations are able to be challenged (Dingwall 1992).

It is vital that views of participants represent the major voice in this ethnography. However it may be suggested that this view in isolation may not be sufficient to produce any change in practice. It is felt that there is therefore a need to combine the predominant emic perspective with aspects of the etic view, the outsider's perceptions. It is suggested that the researcher may discern patterns and ideas of which participants themselves are not aware (Katz 1997) and that these perspectives may prove to be a valuable addition to the study if clearly represented as an alternative view.

Criticisms of Critical Interpretivist Ethnography

Although ethnography is well established in the qualitative research community, as with all research methods, it remains open to criticism. Fundamental conflicts and tensions between qualitative and quantitative paradigms are well rehearsed in the research literature (for example Holloway and Wheeler 2002) and will not be repeated here. It is argued that ethnography is a wholly appropriate research method for this study. Ethnography as a whole is open to a number of criticisms, perhaps the most significant of these is that ethnography is just story telling, that it is a particularly costly research method and that it is not generalisable.

Addition of the critical element adds further to the criticism by raising the issue of researchers taking to their political soapboxes.

Story Telling

The idea that ethnography is viewed by some as mere "story telling" with no scientific grounding is raised by Koch (1998). This author notes that, despite the reservations of some, story telling has its own unique value and has long been used as an effective means of communication. Benefits of story telling include the ability to make core health care practice visible (Hendricks et al 1996, Nelms 1996). Additionally listening to patients may reveal ways in which practice could be improved (Koch 1994, Koch et al 1995). Story telling can be therapeutic (McDaniel et al 1995) and has been shown anecdotally to be beneficial in research involving people with dementia (Mills 1997, Sabat 2001). It is suggested by Van der Staay (1994) that stories can influence social policy and by Gabriel (1995) and Yanow (1995) that they can facilitate change in organisations. These claims almost certainly remain contentious in relation to contemporary health care settings. The major advantage of story telling in this research is that it allows marginalised groups to have a voice (Biddle 1996, Turton 1997); this is an opportunity that is particularly valuable when researching with a group that is often excluded by society.

Katz takes up the idea of story telling in terms of presenting people's lifeworld; he poses the questions that if all ethnographers have to offer is a description of everyday experiences of participants, a description of day-to-day reality, then "so what?", "who cares?" (Katz 1997:392). In answer to this idea it is argued that at present very little is known about the care of people with dementia in acute hospitals. It is suggested that those providing care are so involved with delivering the required service that they rarely have time to step back and reflect. It is acknowledged that there is a remarkable paucity of research that investigates acute care from the perspective of people with dementia or their carers. Katz (1997) continues his discussion of ethnography by suggesting that people from outside the culture being studied can only view it through a "veil of mystery" (Katz 1997:394), a strangely similar metaphor to Sabat's (2001) tangled veil of dementia. These metaphors perhaps point to a need for research that may begin to illuminate what is going on behind these veils.

Cost

Ethnography is deemed to be costly and time consuming (Savage 2000). This is a fair criticism as ethnography demands a high price in terms of the researcher's time to gather data through extensive periods of observation and interviews, followed by the translation of this data into a text that is of interest and value to others. However, it is argued that this investment is worthwhile in terms of answering this research question and indeed it would be difficult to construct a research method that yields the richness and depth of data required to discover more about this complex subject about which little is currently known.

Generalisability

It is contested that ethnography is not generalisable, an argument that can be levelled at any qualitative study. Generalisability is frequently judged to be the hallmark of good science (Murphy and Dingwall 2001b) and this is therefore often used as a way of disparaging qualitative research (Morgan 1983).

It can be suggested that ethnographers fall into three broad camps concerning their views on generalisability. One group are those that reject the whole concept of generalisability as an appropriate goal (for example Denzin 1983) even to the extent of describing it as being "unimportant, unachievable or both" (Schofield 1993:201). An alternative view is taken by Stake (1995) who argues that the purpose of ethnography is particularisation rather than generalisation. This author suggests that the researcher's aim should be to understand the uniqueness of each participant and offer readers a vicarious experience of each. Examples of how such vicarious experiences have been enabled are presented in chapter four. Stake (1995) describes readers as being invited to engage in a process of "naturalistic generalisation" as they relate written stories of individual participants to their existing knowledge of other settings. Whilst there is clearly a value in readers making their own generalisations about research, Stake (1995) also suggests that researchers must choose the extent to which they organise their analyses and interpretations to provide propositional generalisations or assertions which allow readers to work with existing propositional knowledge and modify existing generalisations.

A third view is taken by researchers such as Koch (1998) who approaches generalisability from an alternative perspective stating that transferability (Lincoln and Guba 1985), that is the capacity to transfer findings to other similar settings, is more pertinent in ethnography. This type of approach is comparable with the views of Morgan (1983) who suggests that ethnographers should concern themselves with identifying generic processes and phenomena through which participants construct and understand their realities. Morgan (1983) argues that this identification of the generic factors is illustrated through the evidence of individual examples or archetypes so evidence is likely to be evocative rather than comprehensive.

In this study the aim has been to accurately and thoroughly present stories from the participants that include enough raw data to allow readers to consider their own interpretations. Whilst it is acknowledged that data from individuals cannot simply be generalised to other people (Holloway and Jefferson 2000), effort has been made to identify generic processes and patterns that may be used to inform and influence practice and, as Savage (2000) states, identify ground breaking questions for further research.

The Political Soapbox

Although the need to present this research within its political and social context is justified, equally there is a need to avoid being so overtly "political" that the passion of the researcher supersedes the primacy of the voices of participants. The issue of the "jargon trap" is raised by Van Maanen (1988:28) who states that this can lead to overblown claims and distorted conclusions. Thomas (1993) proposes that the researcher should aim to lead the reader through data that is presented in sufficient detail to allow them to be convinced by the power of the illustration rather than the persuasiveness of the researcher. Thomas (1993) states that axe grinding should also be avoided by remaining faithful to the data rather than producing polemics that may alienate readers.

Research Questions

To guide the initial stages of the study a number of ethnographic questions were developed as outlined below.

- What is it like to be a person with dementia in an acute ward?
- What are lay carers' beliefs about the care received by people with dementia on an acute ward?
- What informs the care that is delivered by health care staff?
- Are the beliefs of health care workers congruent with the care they deliver in practice?

- What areas need to be explored further in interviews?

Selection of critical interpretivist ethnography is based on the premise that the research is intended to acknowledge relevant social and political context, give voice to participants and be of value in influencing future practice. It is suggested that these aims can most readily be achieved using this approach.

The Research Process

Research design was ethnographic with data being collected through participant observation, conversations and interviews. The study was conducted in a specialist older peoples unit in an acute hospital. Three wards were involved; two specialised in acute medicine and one in orthopaedic rehabilitation. Each ward was led by a senior nurse supported by a team of registered and non-registered staff. Therapy staff were unit based however physiotherapists tended to work predominantly on specified wards. Each ward had two allocated medical consultants with their associated teams. Social work staff were allocated on a case by case basis. Wards all ran at maximum bed occupancy with a constant pressure to expedite discharge.

This section provides an overview of the research process. Issues that needed to be considered in preparation for data collection are discussed, namely access to the field and my role in terms of participant observation and insider versus outsider roles. Processes of data collection are considered including levels of participation, recording of information in the field, duration of observation and interviews, selection of participants and review of documents. Approaches to data analysis are explored. This section closes with review of ethical considerations and reflexivity.

Preparation for Data Collection

In ethnography it is clearly recognised that the researcher is an integral part of the research process. Until the study began I was in the unusual position of having been a senior member of nursing staff in the clinical settings being studied. This position required careful consideration in terms of the influence that it had on the research process.

Access to the Field

The study was undertaken on three care of older people wards in a large acute hospital. Initial stages of gaining access to the field involved selecting appropriate wards for the study. This choice was influenced by two factors. Firstly, whilst working for the Trust, I had undertaken a series of audits to establish the number of people with dementia in the hospital at specified time points. Two wards consistently had a relatively high proportion of people with dementia and including them would increase the chance of recruitment to the study. Secondly whilst working for the Trust I had developed respectful working relationships with staff from all disciplines on these wards which would be valuable to the study. Addition of a third ward is explained later in this section.

Once the study wards had been selected the process of obtaining approval from a National Health Service (NHS) Research Ethics Committee, an NHS Research Governance Committee and an information governance manager was undertaken. These approvals were all granted between March and May 2005. The next stage involved seeking approval from the General Manager, Director of Nursing, Medical Consultants and Senior Nurses. These clinicians and managers were gatekeepers (Hammersley and Atkinson 1983) and had the ability to open up or block routes to information. Fortunately, they gave their approval wholeheartedly. The most influential players had been contacted whilst I was working in the Trust and therefore were already familiar with plans for the study.

Whilst approval was given readily by senior members of the organisation the reaction of ward level staff was slightly more circumspect. Theoretically they were interested in the study and could see its value but senior ward staff expressed concerns about potential impact on their own workload. One study ward had experienced a prolonged period of instability in leadership with senior staff being "shuffled" around the older peoples' wards to maintain some leadership during a time of poor recruitment. This led to the ward experiencing over a year of temporary leadership and a relatively low sense of ownership of the ward. Gaining access was therefore initially quite challenging and frustrating. Whereas I could totally appreciate the enormous strain that senior staff were under, particularly having until recently been part of the equation, their inability to commit to the study was disappointing. At this stage I considered the work of Rock (2001:33) which states that "no one will ever be as interested in one's work as one is oneself". This idea, whilst seemingly obvious, led me to a period of reflection about the approach to accessing the field and also to my own experiences of being researched in practice. Rock (2001) suggests that for participants the researcher is not an important person and that generally there is little reason why people should choose to take part. This idea had great resonance. I had not always given priority to the work of other researchers in practice as in my mind this activity had always been secondary to the provision of clinical care. One aspect of access that proved difficult was that only a matter of months before I would have had an automatic right of access due to my previous role, having to work so hard at it now seemed alien. A period of reflection was useful in resetting my mindset. At this stage a new Senior Nurse was appointed to a substantive post on one ward. This leader could see clear benefits to the research and felt that ward staff should have pride in the fact that they had been selected. I had spent some time talking to staff about the study and one established nursing assistant with considerable personal power and influence was particularly enthusiastic about the study. Support from these two individuals eased access to the field. Lessons learnt from gaining access to the first ward were useful when approaching the second ward. Again key staff assisted the process through their interest in the work and their influence with other staff.

Fetterman (1998) suggests that the use of intermediaries is particularly valuable when accessing the field as the trust that participants have in these people will approximate to the trust that they initially place in the researcher. Having intermediaries with different spheres of influence led to me gaining free access to the field and a relatively high level of acceptance by participants. An honorary contract with the host organisation was secured.

As the study progressed on the first two wards questions began to emerge about the extent to which people with dementia were offered rehabilitation opportunities. This thought led me to include an older peoples rehabilitation ward in the study. Access to this third ward proved much more fraught, to the extent that data collection was abandoned relatively quickly.

The Role of the Researcher

The Role in Participant Observation

Participant observation is an essential feature of ethnographic research (Fetterman 1998, Savage 2000, Holloway and Todres 2003, Coffey 1999) with a researcher being the major instrument of data collection (Clifford 1997, Maggs-Rapport 2001). Participant observation is open to a number of interpretations. It is described by Emerson et al (2001) as a core process of ethnography in which a place is established in the field for a relatively long period of time in order to allow the ethnographer to investigate, experience and represent the social life and processes of that culture. It is suggested by Savage (2000) that participant observation should be considered as more than merely a method of data collection and should be given explicit theoretical attention.

In traditional ethnography there is an assumption of a duality between researcher and participants in which the researcher adopts the role of ignorant outsider (Coffey 1999) whose aim is to provide a comprehensive description of a little known culture (Denzin and Lincoln 1994). This approach is clearly not appropriate for this study, both in terms of my prior knowledge of the field and because of the belief that the emic perspective should be predominant. Denzin (1997:xviii) supports the notion of a post modernist ethnography that discovers methods of "feeling our way into the experiences of self and other …. an evocative epistemology that performs, rather than represents the world". This post modernist ideology which supports a joint, multi-vocal production (Savage 2000) between ethnographer and participants is far more congruent with the aims of this study.

Savage (2000) raises the possibility of parallels between the process of knowledge production in participant observation and nursing. She cautions that knowledge generation must be tempered by acceptance that there is no guarantee of a reciprocal perspective between ethnographer and participants, that the subject is inevitably transient and that it may require the translation of non-verbal knowledge into language. These concerns have been, to some extent, addressed by Lawler (1991) who describes nurses' understanding of the patient's experiences as "somology". This concept of understanding is based on the epistemological assumptions that there is a possibility of reciprocal perspectives or the availability of one person's lived experience to another and that experiences that are communicated non-verbally can be translated into meaningful language.

I believe that my nursing experience has enabled me to develop a level of intuition about behaviours in health care that were used during participant observation to gain an understanding of the world view of others using data derived from all the senses. Equally, I maintained a high level of awareness that my preconceived ideas and intuition should not cloud the opportunity to view the field from a new perspective.

Processes of participant observation and how these may be successfully accomplished are considered in the literature. It is likely that any person who is to be the subject of observation is likely to experience some level of apprehension. As Fetterman (1998) suggests, concerns of participants may be reduced by the use of intermediaries who are already known and trusted by participants. Equally, it would be unrealistic and potentially limiting for the researcher to rely substantially on a small number of people to establish them in the field. It is therefore vital that researchers begin fieldwork by building relationships with participants (Germain 1993). Berg (1998) stresses the importance of developing interpersonal relationships with participants in order to gain trust and co-operation. Hammersley and Atkinson (1995) support this idea stating that these relationships are at the core of knowledge creation in ethnography.

The idea that the researcher should develop a rapport with participants appears superficially to be a common sense issue; unless some understanding, trust and reciprocity exist, it is unlikely that the researcher will be able to observe anything that is close to everyday practice. Rapport as a concept is moved to another level by Springwood and King (2001) who suggest that rapport when applied to ethnography involves the researcher "getting there" and "being there" and makes powerful claims to understanding, authenticity and authority. This is a vast claim and in this study rapport was primarily concerned with establishing a new relationship with participants in which they had an understanding of the process and purpose of the research and in which I was recast in an academic-practice role rather than in my previous role of professional leader. Whilst the centrality of researcher-participant relationships in ethnography is acknowledged, it is argued by Harrington (2003) that accounts of establishing such links are infrequent and fragmented in the literature. Establishment of relationships in this study focused on ensuring that participants were aware of why and how the research was being conducted, identifying my role, causing minimum disruption and discomfort in the field and sharing the concept of creation of knowledge. Interpersonal skills I had gained during many years in clinical practice generally supported the development of effective research relationships. These relationships had to be continually nurtured through the data collection phase. On the first two wards this was relatively unproblematic. I remained alert to signs that participants may need to temporarily withdraw from the study and negotiated this on a regular basis. On the third ward staff appeared to find it exceptionally hard to grasp the idea that my aim was simply to observe what really happened in practice. A number remained convinced that my role was to judge or criticise their work. This made relationships extraordinarily difficult to establish. On each ward I attempted to begin to build a rapport with participants from the stage at which I introduced the research that was sustained throughout the study until eventual disengagement from the field.

It is advised by both Germain (1993) and Fetterman (1998) that ethnographers should enter the field using a low key approach that minimises their unsettling effect on the culture. The aim is to preserve rather than control the culture and to become effectively integrated. Rock (2001) suggests that ethnographers should remain on the margins at first and not place too many demands on participants. This was particularly key as in my previous role I tended to be viewed as someone who deserved virtually automatic attention in light of seniority and there was a need to dispel this idea. My aim was to adopt the stance of listener and learner (Fetterman 1998) and follow the advice of Gehring (1973) who stresses the importance of watching and listening initially before attempting to interpret what is observed.

Fieldwork initially felt somewhat uncontrolled but this experience is recognised as relatively common in ethnography (Fetterman 1998). At the outset I concentrated on getting a feel of the culture in a holistic sense. This stage was particularly important in this study as I needed to enter the field in a new and substantially different role; there was a need to acclimatise to this perspective before considering more specific issues. It is suggested by Fetterman (1998) that once the researcher has some familiarity with the field work of participant observation can become gradually more refined. This idea is supported by Germain (1993) who states that whilst fieldwork is often exciting and intriguing the researcher needs to maintain some goal orientation. This author suggests that every two hours of fieldwork is likely to generate around eight hours of notes thus justifying the need to use time in the field to best effect. Whilst some degree of goal orientation in field work is advised by both Germain (1993) and Fetterman (1998) they also advocate a level of flexibility that allows capture of significant events that arise.

Roles taken by researchers in ethnographic participant observation are widely acknowledged to be critical to the success of the study (Pellatt 2003, Preston 1997, Koch and Harrington 1998). Participant observation is a complex undertaking that has been comprehensively discussed in the literature in terms of the insider-outsider dichotomy and the participant-observation continuum. These issues are considered below.

Insider versus Outsider

The insider-outsider dichotomy was particularly pertinent in this study in view of the alteration in my role. As stated previously, I was the professional lead for nursing for the Directorate of which the study wards were a part. It may be assumed that this role would automatically have conferred insider status but certainly my perception was that, even in this role, engagement with potential participants was peripheral as the role, if not myself, was regarded as part of "the management" and therefore somewhat distanced from reality. It could be argued that working in the field for a protracted period actually increased the perception of me as an insider. Literature suggests an array of advantages and disadvantages for insider and outsider roles. Allen (2004) argues that only insiders who are truly immersed in a setting can produce an authentic account. Equally, this author raises the issue that researchers in a familiar setting may make assumptions about what is being observed without seeking clarification. Kanuha (2000), in a discussion about native and non-native roles, identifies a potential drawback of insider status as being a tendency to be accepting of vague statements and points to the need for insiders to consciously pursue such statements to ensure shared understanding. Benefits of being an outsider are perceived as including potential production of a less biased report (Allen 2004) and the opportunity to make the strange familiar (Pugh et al 2000).

It is suggested by Spradley (1980) that a researcher with a dual role as insider and outsider is vulnerable to role confusion. In this study I was situated towards the midpoint of the continuum in the initial stages and tended to move along the continuum at different times during the study. Previous work in the area gave a degree of insider status and offered the advantages of having some understanding of the culture and an ability to "fit in". Equally, there was a need to maintain a conscious awareness that the field needed to be viewed with an open mind and that seemingly obvious questions needed to be asked to prevent me relying on my own assumptions. Conversely, I may also have been viewed as an outsider being relatively or totally unknown to some participants and no longer working for the organisation. Whilst this status offered opportunities to see the culture in a new light it also reinforced the need to build research relationships at each stage.

Burgess (1984) disputes the notion that there is an absolute polarisation of insider and outsider roles. This author states that it is rare for a researcher to be either totally familiar or completely unfamiliar with a setting. It may be argued that entering into a lengthy debate about one's position as insider or outsider is unlikely to be fruitful. The concept of an insider-outsider continuum, along which the researcher travels, seems reasonable. Hammersley and Atkinson (1983) add weight to this idea proposing that it is an existential fact that we are part of the world we study, thus being a complete outsider is impossible. It is suggested that a more contemporary approach to the insider-outsider debate is through authentic presentation of self in the research setting; this idea will be explored more fully in the reflexivity section of this chapter.

The Process of Data Collection

There are three major methods of data collection in ethnography: participant observation with recording of field notes, interviews and review of documents (Wolcott 1994). The first two of these were used as explained below. A review of documents was not completed. Reasons for this choice are examined.

Level of Participation

Fetterman (1998) describes the process of participant observation as a delicate balance between participating in the lives of the people being studied and maintaining sufficient professional distance to ensure adequate observation and data recording. In terms of the role in observation, researchers have a number of choices to make. Gold (1958) identifies a range of roles which include complete participant, participant-as-observer, observer-as-participant and complete observer. Junker (1960) identifies the same range of potential roles and suggests that the complete participant deliberately conceals their research activity from participants. It is unlikely that this approach would be considered ethically sound in the current climate. Participant-as-observer role supports the research being openly conducted but research activity is considered subordinate to the primary role of the individual. Observer-as-participant approach allows the role to be publicly known and supports a level of interaction between researcher and participants. A complete observer engages in no interaction with participants. Junker (1960) describes these roles as a continuum through which the researcher is likely to oscillate in the course of the study.

In this study it was essential to achieve a balance between acknowledging that I am a practitioner with many years of experience, with the reality that my role had changed to researcher in practice. The concept of being a complete observer was likely to lack validity given that I was known to a number of participants and that avoiding interaction would not only be extremely difficult but would also compromise effective data collection. A role of complete participant was untenable for practical and ethical reasons. A realistic approach was to adopt a role of social-participant-as-observer in which I was open about the research activity. I was clear that the research was my primary pursuit but also actively participated in actions that might reasonably be expected to be part of social rather than clinical interaction. Examples of these activities included assisting with bed making, helping patients to eat and drink and assisting with recreational activities.

Two thoughts influenced selection of this approach. Firstly it provided a level of authenticity in that it acknowledged my previous clinical role whilst respecting the fact that this role had changed. Secondly it is noted by Germain (1993) that good fieldwork relationships are built on a degree of reciprocity between researcher and participants. This idea is supported by Harrington (2003) who states that there should be some exchange, some level of the researcher giving back to the participants, although it is noted that ways in which this can be achieved is not often stated. In this study, the fact that I demonstrated a readiness to assist participants, albeit in a very small way, encouraged their willingness to participate. It was acknowledged that the role of social-observer-as-participant was appropriate in terms of the research process, professional accountability and indemnity issues. However, it also proved frustrating when I had to resist being more actively involved in care delivery. This was a role to which I had to consciously adapt.

In practice this role proved challenging. My desire to be involved in care was difficult to overcome, particularly as clinical staff tended to include me in their communication despite efforts to remain on the periphery. Inclusion by staff occurred on a number of occasions. Examples of this included me being asked during a ward round, in which I was not involved, to provide an update on the progress of a participating patient towards nursing home placement. Another incident concerned the medical staff needing rapid, expert clinical advice on the management of intravenous fluids for a patient who was critically ill. Both these events, and many others, tested the boundaries of the research and professional roles and forced me to be flexible within reasonable limits.

One issue in participant observation that had not been anticipated was the feeling of physical awkwardness experienced when first entering the field. Having spent many years as part of a ward team, the feeling of utter conspicuousness was difficult to manage. Coffey (1999:73) describes this sense accurately suggesting that it is "often difficult to know what to physically *do* in the field in order to look natural, comfortable, engaged and welcoming while not appearing bored, threatening or judgmental". The extent to which I felt at ease varied considerably between the wards. On the first I spent long periods of time sitting at the ends of bays in chairs designated for visitors. This allowed good views of what was going on whilst not causing disruption to the activities of participants. Gradually participants became accustomed to my presence, as they grew more confident that I was not going to ask them "difficult" questions they slowly began to include me in their work and conversations. This was the ward that allowed me to achieve the highest level of participation, being content for me to be involved in day to day activities such as bed making, providing drinks and completing menus. This relaxed approach allowed me to gather great volumes of rich data. The second two wards were smaller and I found it much more difficult to be unobtrusive. I felt that the staff were more wary of my presence and would sometimes actively avoid coming into a bay if I was present. I remained alert to this possibility to ensure that I did not compromise patient care.

Although the role of the researcher can be carefully planned prior to undertaking ethnographic research it was recognised that the nature of such a study is grounded in inter-relationships between researcher and participants and so needs to be adaptable within ethical and professional confines. In this study there was an ongoing need to clarify and negotiate my role so that it was understood and agreed by all parties. Practical issues of what I could actually do were considered and adapted on a regular basis.

Recording of Information in the Field

Field notes are generally acknowledged as being one of the central methods of collecting data in ethnography (Wolcott 1994, Emerson et al 2001, O'Reilly 2005). It is suggested by Emerson et al (2001) that the ways in which information gathered in the field is recorded and valued as part of the research process vary from one researcher to another largely based on the researcher's underlying assumptions about ethnography and also influenced by personal preference.

I left the decision about what should be recorded in field notes open until the field work began as it was extremely difficult to anticipate what might be observed. It is suggested by Emerson et al (2001) that field notes are inevitably selective, the researcher writes down things that seem significant whilst omitting other matters. From this perspective field notes never provide a complete account (Atkinson 1992). In reality I found myself generating vast quantities of field notes. I recorded every interaction between participants with dementia and participating lay carers and staff members. I felt that it was vital to document these interactions verbatim as I did not want to lose the nuances of the communication. The only reason that this level of recording was possible was the marked infrequency of such interactions. Other field notes focused on communications between staff about participants with dementia, some of these involved lay carers. I also recorded field notes concerning the long periods of time in which the participants with dementia were alone and not engaged in activity or communication. I make no claim to have produced a complete account as I made a conscious decision to absent myself from certain situations and clearly was only observing for fixed time periods.

In this study field notes were central. They constitute what Fetterman (1998:114) describes as the "brick and mortar of an ethnographic edifice". Field notes were the major tool of data collection reflecting the interactions and relationships between participants and between myself and participants.

Methods by which I recorded and managed field notes were carefully considered. A need to record accurate field notes is not disputed. However, Emerson et al (2001) warns researchers against "participating-in-order-to-write" suggesting that too much concentration on writing may impede their capacity to become immersed in the field and so appreciate the full picture. The way which field notes were recorded evolved during the course of the study. I initially envisaged that I would record jotted notes in the field as an aide-memoire for preparation of fuller notes. I had informed participants that I would be making notes. My plan was to record them in relative privacy on the assumption that the sight of me constantly writing would be inimical to the development of trusting relationships. Using jotted notes I quickly found that I was losing the subtleties of what I was seeing and hearing; the notes did not quite capture the detail that was so important. I began to openly write notes as I was observing and in reality participants rapidly grew used to me writing and did not appear disturbed by this. I found that writing fairly full notes contemporaneously ensured far more accuracy and depth of recording than was achieved with jotted notes. I engaged in many "opportunistic" conversations (Costello 2002) with participants during the observation phase. These meetings were recorded in writing either in real time or as soon as possible after the event. Field notes were transcribed verbatim onto a template that allowed me to add further pertinent information in a separate column. Field notes recording observation in practice were also supported by a reflective diary that recorded my own thoughts and interpretations. This is discussed in more detail in the reflexivity section of this chapter.

Management of field notes is described in some detail by several authors (for example Fetterman 1998, Schwandt and Halpern 1988, Bogdan and Biklen 1982) who provide relatively prescriptive advice on how this may be achieved. Emerson et al (2001) offer an alternative perspective accepting the field notes may be "messy" and unintelligible to others. These authors imply that the way in which field notes are recorded and managed is something that is highly personal to the ethnographer and an activity that evokes a deep level of ambivalence. I certainly found this quite a daunting prospect as a novice ethnographer. I used some key aspects of advice, such as ensuring that notes were written up as soon as practicable after the event to prevent the loss of vital detail. However, other aspects of field note management were developed on a personal basis as field work progressed.

Duration of Observation

Amounts of time spent in participant observation vary considerably according to the size and scope of the study. It is suggested by Fetterman (1998) that a period of observation in which the ethnographer is in residence for around six to twelve months would allow for immersion in a culture. It would seem that this advice is directed towards studies where ability to reside within a culture and time limits are not issues. A more pragmatic view is taken by Germain (1993) who advises that length of time in the field should be based on the amount of time it will take to build up a relationship with participants, how readily significant data can be accessed and of any seasonal and cyclical variations that may be relevant.

A brief review of comparable studies reveals some unity in the amount of time needed for data collection. In a study of terminal care, Costello (2000) completed 160 hours of participant observation over nine months. Tutton and Seers (2004) undertook 130 hours of observation whilst investigating the comfort of older people on one ward. A study by Coombs and Ersser (2004) considering staff relationships in an intensive care unit included 200 hours of observation in two phases. In view of my familiarity with the setting, I anticipated completing between 100 and 150 hours in practice. After completing 125 hours of observation I reviewed the situation and concluded that I could continue to gather new and fascinating data ad infinitum. However in practical terms I had a huge amount of data to be analysed within a finite timescale and therefore chose to end the data collection phase. I initially expected to undertake observation as five-hour blocks three or four times per week over a period of several months. In the event I had to be far more flexible in light of difficulties in recruiting people with dementia, levels of activity on the ward and my own capacity to maintain high levels of concentration. Periods of observation lasted for between two and six hours and were completed over the course of a year.

Interviews

Observation and interview processes were iterative. In order to supplement and clarify periods of observation, participants were invited to be interviewed. Interviews were used as they offered the opportunity to facilitate participants to say what they wanted to, in their own language and using their own concepts (Sapsford and Abbott 1992).

A total of eighteen formal interviews were undertaken with patients, lay carers and staff representing all disciplines and a range of grades. Approaches to interviews developed as the research progressed, all were conducted on an individual basis using styles that were acceptable to participants and met ethical guidelines. Interviews took place within the Trust in an area in which the participant felt comfortable and that afforded a level of peace and privacy. They were arranged at times that were convenient to participants and did not disrupt care delivery. I aimed to create a safe and comfortable forum in which the participant and I became "conversational partners" (Rubin and Rubin 1995). A small number of participants were interviewed on more than one occasion in order to enhance the quality and depth of the data (Pratt 2002). Interviews were audio taped with permission of participants. Notes were written as soon as possible following interviews to capture any pertinent observations and thoughts (Mulhall 2003).

Initially the purpose of the interviews was to explore issues that had been observed in practice. The aim was to conduct relatively open interviews in which participants had the opportunity to air their views. I used participant observation to generate an interview schedule using predominantly open-ended questions. Even as I was conducting these interviews I was aware that they did not feel right. On reflection I realised that use of fairly fixed questions was limiting the ability of participants to express themselves fully. Reviewing the interview transcripts proved disappointing as they appeared to lack depth.

When considering other approaches to interviewing I was attracted by the narrative methods. It had become clear that my own assumptions were clouding participants' opportunity to express themselves freely. I decided to change technique and ask a single narrative inducing question (Wengraf 2001), this tended to start with "tell me your story about your involvement with ...." I felt significantly more comfortable with this approach as it generated much richer and more person-focused data. At times I sensed that some participants were not wholly comfortable and I sometimes needed to offer supportive prompts in order to avoid participants stopping prematurely or being left feeling inadequate. Despite my occasional interruptions data proved fascinating. It is possible that the participants in this study found the narrative approach difficult as I was, to some extent, asking them to talk about another as much as themselves. In virtually all the interviews I found that I had to work hard to convince participants that they each had a genuinely valuable contribution to make to the study.

Selection of Participants for Observation

Participants belonged to one of three discrete groups: patients, lay carers and health and social care staff. The patient group comprised older people with dementia as a pre-existing condition, who were in-patients on the study wards. Initially I felt that it was important that patients met certain criteria, including specific memory test scores. Parameters selected were that they should have a documented diagnosis of dementia, be over sixty five years of age and have a mini mental state examination (MMSE) (Folstein et al 1975) score of below twenty three which would indicate a range of impairment from mild to severe (George et al 1991, Dick et al 1984). At a very early stage in the study it became clear through observation and conversation that there was remarkably little correlation between MMSE score and the ability to communicate. This finding is supported in the work of Pratt and Wilkinson (2001) who recruited people on the grounds of their ability to communicate rather than a test score. It was also noted that the MMSE score quoted by staff sometimes bore little relation to the mental state that I observed. It is likely that patients' scores may fluctuate, particularly in view of their superimposed physical illness. In light of these thoughts the inclusion criteria for patients were amended to include anyone over the age of sixty-five with a documented diagnosis of dementia; MMSE scores were recorded for information only. Lay carers of any patients who met the inclusion criteria were also able to participate. Health and social care staff of any grade or discipline who provided direct care to patients on the study wards were included.

Selection of Interviewees

A purposive selection strategy was used, that is participants were selected for a specific purpose (Coyne 1997). Participants were chosen because they were recognised during participant observation as able to provide the rich data (Patton 1990) required to produce meaningful findings.

Interviews involved the three groups outlined above. Particular care was taken when involving patients and their carers to avoid unethical practice. The fact that they may, or may not, be aware of having a diagnosis of dementia had to be managed with tact and sensitivity. Interviews were conducted with the patient and carer together or separately as they chose. Health and social care staff of any discipline or grade that provided direct care to patients were interviewed. Key informants were identified during participant observation and purposeful sampling was used.

Key informants are described by Holloway and Wheeler (2002) as those within the field who can provide specific, detailed information about the culture. In this study key informants included those in roles such as Ward Sister and Lead Medical Consultant who exerted considerable influence in the setting. Whilst it is important to recognise and utilise the contribution of key informants, Rock (2001) warns against attaching too great a value to this and advocates that researchers should remain aware that such informants, in common with all others, only present their own embedded view of a complex world.

Review of Documents

It is suggested by Wolcott (1994) that a review of documents may be valuable in data collection. Documents that may have proved useful in this study included the case notes of patient participants and local guidelines, policies and procedures relating to dementia care. The idea of reviewing case notes was considered but I made the decision that, whilst interesting such a review represented an unnecessary intrusion into patients' privacy. Therefore on ethical grounds the idea was rejected. A review of guidelines was not undertaken as such documents simply did not exist.

Data Analysis

Data collection yielded many thousands of words from observation, informal conversations and interviews. Data collection and analysis were iterative processes; analysis has occurred throughout the study. The majority of early analysis identified key themes and questions for further investigation. It also pointed to the need to refine data collection techniques. Two attempts at more formal analysis were tested. In the first, data were coded and categories generated. This approach had the effect of fracturing the data and largely losing the essence of the people involved. In the study individuals were all surrounded by powerful stories and trying to break these down into codes and categories and then rebuild them into a meaningful whole was not successful. A further approach was to present the complete story of one individual, this was slightly more successful although the telling of the story may be seen as a rather crude attempt.

Data collected have proved complex to analyse. Kvale (1996) suggests that it is relatively common for qualitative researchers to find themselves with a mass of data wondering how best it should be analysed. Kvale poses a range of questions that are valuable in focusing the mind of the researcher on the task of generating writing that provides a unity between the original data, analysis and the final report. Data in this study have been gathered from a range of patients, lay carers and health and social care staff. As data have been collected in an acute hospital setting it has been patchy as patients are often transferred to other environments with little warning. At times it would have been useful to explore episodes of care in more detail and to follow up having had time to reflect on interviews. However, the nature of work in acute care and time pressures on staff has meant that this has not always been possible. Data are therefore fragmented in places. Whilst this may be frustrating from a research point of view it does accurately represent much of the care that I have witnessed.

The nature of the data has generated a huge amount of thought about how it could be analysed and presented to meet the aims of the study. Initial attempts at coding and categorising and ethnographic description did not do justice to the individuals involved. Having experimented with these approaches I decided to clarify in my own mind what I was trying to achieve in data analysis and presentation. The following were my major aims:

- Ensure that participants with dementia remain central.
- Enable the voices of the participants with dementia to be heard in whatever way possible.
- Give equal value and credence to data collected through observation, informal conversation and interviews.
- Present fair and authentic accounts of the care given to people with dementia in the acute hospital setting.
- Ensure that the findings remain firmly grounded in the richness of the data.
- Reflect upon the findings of this study in the context of existing literature.
- Relate the findings of this study to the wider social and political picture.

Having elucidated my aims I began to look for alternative methods of analysis and presentation. I was attracted by the idea of narrative analysis and a review of key texts indicated that it could have some merit in this study. Principles of the narrative approach include the concepts that:

- Individuals make sense of their world most effectively by telling stories (Bailey and Tilley 2002).

- It can democratise the experience of teller and listener (Jones 2003).
- It avoids the pre-determined assumptions in the researchers questions (Priest et al 2002).
- What people have to say about their lives is far more enlightening than any research question will reveal (Chamberlayne et al 2000, Wengraf 2001).
- The gestalt of the story is maintained if the story teller is not interrupted. Gestalt is defined as "a whole which is more than the sum of its parts, an order or hidden agenda informing each person's life," (Holloway and Jefferson 2000:34).

Integration of narrative approaches to data collection led me to reflect on whether they would work for data analysis. There is fairly extensive literature on narrative analysis. There are a number of key themes in many of these writings but many of them appear to be at least moderately contentious.

Definitions of narratives are not uniformly agreed upon. It is proposed by Riessman (1993), Polkinghorne (1988) and Elliott (2005) that a narrative is a story with a beginning, a middle and an end with a logical temporal sequence. The idea that a narrative is greater than and more structured than a story is suggested by Priest et al (2002). It could be argued that this debate is a matter of semantics and that the story or narrative is what the teller says it is. What actually constitutes a narrative is also open to debate. Whilst some authors focus on oral narrative (Holloway and Jefferson 2000), others state that narrative can include any form of textual data (Priest et al 2002). Polkinghorne (1988:13) suggests that narrative can be defined as "any spoken or written presentation".

The concept that learning through narratives is inherent in humans is supported by White (1981) who suggests that communication through story telling is a natural human instinct. It is suggested by Priest et al (2002) that narrative knowledge is essential to enable people to make sense of the world. This idea is supported by Bruner (1986) who states that narrative knowledge is as valuable as paradigmatic knowledge, that is knowledge gained from science, in enabling better understanding of the world.

It emerged from the review of literature on narrative approaches that narrative analysis has no single methodology or heritage (Priest et al 2002) and that it's epistemological foundations are unclear (Redwood 1999). It is evident that development of narrative analysis has been influenced by philosophy, anthropology, sociology, psychology, sociolinguistics (McLeod and Balamoutsou 2000) as well as ethnomethodology and literary criticism (Torode 1998).

In common with other forms of qualitative data analysis, narrative analysis does not have a standard set of procedures for researchers to complete (Riessman 1993, Ekman and Skott 2005). There are frameworks available for analysis, for example Priest et al (2002) reviews the approaches of Emden (1998), McLeod and Balamoutsou (2000) and Gee (1986, 1991) in analysing narrative. Each of these methods has a clear value but it could be argued that they all appear to focus on interview data and take a "micro" approach focusing very much on the fine detail of words. This process is not entirely consistent with this study where a broader more inclusive style is needed. The bibliographic narrative interpretive method described by Chamberlayne et al (2000), Wengraf (2001) and Jones (2003) also appeared to have some merit. The idea that stories are unique and individually constructed wholes and that what people tell us about themselves is far more enlightening than anything we may glean from more overt questioning was resonant with my thoughts.

Whilst it is accepted that it is probable that no story is ever truly complete, it was evident in the work of Jones (2003) that narratives he analysed were extensive stories told by participants and that Jones used opportunities to complete second and even third interviews to generate rich and detailed data from individuals. The very exhaustive analysis of narratives that Jones and his colleagues used to analyse his data would not fit with the data I had collected. It was felt that any method of narrative analysis that focused more on language than plot may not work in this study as much of the data from participant observation is constructed in my own language as well as that of the participants themselves. Another concern with Jones's approach when applied to this study is that members of the analysis team who had not collected the data would be seeing the words in isolation. This may be very effective when working with participants who are able to articulate their ideas clearly. One of the strengths in using ethnographic methods of data collection is that it allowed me to "be there" and contextualise the utterances of people, some of whom had profound communication difficulties. My aim was to assist with the articulation of experiences which some participants may struggle to put into words but which they communicated in other, often very subtle, ways. It is noted that Riessman (1993) describes narratives as interpretations in themselves. These stories then require interpretation by the researcher as they are not artefacts that "speak for themselves". It is suggested by Ayres and Poirier (1996) that this view on narratives may lead to doubts about the credibility of analysis. This argument is countered by Woods et al (2002) who states that as long as analysis has been undertaken responsibly and remains faithful to the data then conclusions produced may be considered a valid interpretation. Despite misgivings I was convinced that some form of narrative analysis would work in this study.

There were two particular issues that suggested a flexible approach to analysis would have to be developed. One concern was that the narratives that were available were not always coherent and in places far from complete. I was doubtful about their internal strength. If it is accepted that a narrative should have a beginning, a middle and an end it could be said that this data is somewhat lacking. The stories are, because of circumstance, patchy with different characters being involved at various times. Data could be described as having something of "veil of mystery" (Katz 1997:394). Words alone will not illuminate the story sufficiently and my task is to attempt to raise the "veil of mystery" for readers. The data as a whole has parallels with Sabat's (2001) tangled veil of dementia, it often looks like a tangled veil of individuals doing their own work, frequently overlapping but rarely coming together as a coherent whole. Starting and ending points of the narratives are not clear cut but most are linked to admission and discharge from hospital. A second and perhaps more important issue to be considered was the extent to which people with dementia can be said to have a personal narrative. Whilst some researchers have demonstrated that people with dementia do retain at least an element of personal narrative (Mills 1997), it is argued that dementia often with superimposed acute physical illness can lead to breakdown of the personal narrative.

Chatterji (1998) raises the concept of personal narrative; she questions whether problems of communication that may be experienced by people with dementia may lead to the loss of the only means we have of gaining access to their stories. It is suggested by Desjarlais (1994) that people who live at the margins of society under conditions of deprivation may experience an existence of successive events that cannot be reproduced as a temporally coherent narrative. In acknowledgement of the idea that narrative may not be possible for some people, Chatterji (1998) suggests using the term "voice" rather than "narrative" suggesting that voice is "premised on the act of listening" (Chatterji 1998:357). Whilst accepting Chatterji's thoughts on narrative it is notable that by using an ethnographic approach to data collection and narrative approach to analysis she has successfully woven a convincing and well crafted story about one man with dementia and the various people involved in his care. Chatterji (2006) describes her approach to analysis as being influenced by phenomenology, the illness narrative literature and systems theory. Her published work is not explicit about how these influences have been used in practical terms; however the outcome of her approach is that she effectively presents a commentary supported by extracts of data that link her findings with existing literature. The story she presents is clear and powerful.

At this stage I felt that, whilst the actual techniques that had been reviewed would not work with the data, the principles of narrative analysis had considerable credence. The idea of McLeod and Balamoustou (2000) that "how to do it" manuals are not helpful and that researchers must create their own method encouraged me to pursue narrative analysis as the principles were congruent with my own aims. A review of narrative analysis has demonstrated some of the advantages and disadvantages of its use in practice. Major advantages are its recognition that, given an opportunity, most people will tell a story that is far more interesting, revealing and insightful than would be produced with data that is infused with the researcher's assumptions and questions. Difficulties of using narrative analysis in this study are noted. However it is felt that by drawing on current methods to create one that is specific for this work (McLeod and Balamoustou 2000) and that is faithful to the data (Woods et al 2002), the aims of this work may be fulfilled.

Following review of ethnographic and narrative approaches to data analysis I finally chose to use elements of both techniques. Data were analysed in two distinct ways, these are presented as discrete entities in chapter three. Part one of the chapter begins with a brief description of the study setting which is intended to set the scene for readers. This is followed by a series of narratives which concern the five patients with whom I was able to spend most time. The purpose of these narratives is to enable the reader to gain an insight into the lives of these individuals whilst they were in hospital. Narratives are inevitably only snapshots developed from many hours of observation. However, hopefully they allow a small entry into the worlds of the individuals. It is important for me both personally and ethically, to try to describe the experiences of people and therefore, as Ashworth and Ashworth (2003) suggest, reinforce the idea that these individuals are people and understandable as such.

Development of the narratives was guided by the work of Polkinghorne (1995) who advises that the following components contribute to development of "a story line or plot that serves to configure or compose the disparate data elements into a meaningful explanation of the protagonist's responses and actions," (Polkinghorne 1995:17):

- Description of cultural context
- Nature of the main person in the plot of the study
- Identification of important, significant others in affecting actions and goals of protagonist
- Explanation of relationship between main characters
- Concentration on the choices and actions of the main character
- Attention to previous experiences
- Production of a study with a beginning, middle and end.

Although Polkinghorne's (1995) criteria for developing a narrative appear reasonable they do present some issues in this study. In particular the identification of important, significant others in affecting actions and goals of protagonist is problematic in that in each case the protagonist has, to a greater or lesser extent, lost their capacity to define their own goals and actions. Ability to pay attention to previous experience is also compromised as knowledge about the main characters before their admission to hospital is limited. The reasons outlined above led me to adapt Polkinghorne's components to include:

- The person
- The cultural context
- The plan
- Enactment of the plan.

This approach sets the person with dementia firmly at the centre of the narrative.

It is acknowledged that production of these narratives is in itself interpretive in nature and readers of them will interpret them again within their own frameworks of understanding. However it is anticipated that they will begin to illuminate what it is like to be a person with dementia in an acute hospital.

Ethnographic analysis was influenced by the work of Chatterji (1998) and Thomas (1993). Thomas (1993) in writing about critical ethnography encourages researchers to guide readers through the data providing enough detail to ensure that they are convinced by the power of the data rather than the opinions of the researcher. Whilst wanting the data to remain central there was also a need to link it with current knowledge and set it within the broader political and social milieu. To achieve this narratives are followed by shorter extracts of data from other patients and carers. Part two of the chapter explores the current state of practice as it was observed. This data is linked with existing literature, an approach that is used effectively by Chatterji (1998). Data is also considered within the broader social and political context; this is described by Thomas (1993) as an intellectual responsibility and an ethical obligation.

Approaches to data analysis and presentation are firmly grounded in the traditions of critical ethnography and narrative analysis. Joining these two approaches could be considered to move this work into what Rapport et al (2005) describe as the edgelands of research. This type of flexible method is supported by Holloway and Todres (2003) who advocate a "third position" that allows flexibility as well as consistency and coherence. It may be suggested that as research that actively engages with people with dementia becomes more prevalent, there will be an increasing need to consider innovative and flexible methods that meet the needs of individual studies.

Following reflection on the analysis to this point I began to have reservations about my work. I achieved my aim in that I had presented data that were evocative and that health and social care staff could relate to in terms of their everyday work. Equally I started to feel that I had fallen into the trap that frequently catches ethnographic researchers. I felt that my data analysis was very much open to two criticisms. Firstly, although the analysis had met many of the criteria suggested by Katz (2001) for a "good'" ethnography, for example the data presented is rich and varied, it describes poignant moments and it reveals social forces in action. I had not at this stage addressed the theoretical relevance or the potential of the research (Snow et al 2003). Secondly I had used intuitive rather than strictly systematic procedures for analysing the data. These two points left the study open to dismissal as "nice read, but no theoretical implications" (Snow et al 2003:183). It could be claimed that I had addressed the "what" and "how" but had neglected the "why" that is essential in every ethnographic analysis (Katz 2001). In many ways it could be argued that the "why" element is the key to good ethnographic research, it is the component that enables the development of theory and thus the potential to change practice. The "why" in this research is presented in chapter four which supports the proposition that in this work the analysis is in the interpretation.

Ethical Considerations

At the very early stages of planning this study I addressed one critical question, should older people with dementia be included in the study? Until a decision was made on this question the study could not progress. A review of literature presented two broadly opposing points of view. On one side there is a vast amount of literature from the biomedical field (for example Volicer and Ganzini 2003, Wong et al 2000, Shah and Dickenson 1999 and Marson et al 1997). These authors and many others focus on the impairments in abilities and functioning that may be experienced by people with dementia. They present these people as a homogenous group (Norman 2003a) and tend to imply that the onset of dementia inevitably leads to a loss of capacity to make decisions (Shah and Dickenson 1999). It is notable, that while these papers broadly suggest that people with dementia are unlikely to be able to make rational decisions, they offer remarkably little coherence in their definitions or measurement of decision making capacity (Kim et al 2002b). It is suggested that this view of the ability of people with dementia to participate in research does much to reinforce negative stereotypes of incapacity (Wilkinson 2002) and allows the idea to flourish that this group are senile old people who have "lost their mind" (Lyman 1998, Mills 1997, Sabat 1998, Sabat and Harre 1992).

There is an increasing alternative view that supports people with dementia being involved in research (for example Cotrell and Schulz 1993, Downs 1997, Wilkinson 2002). It is argued by Wilkinson (2002) that a social model of research should be adopted that focuses on social and cultural processes and policy frameworks that systematically disable people rather than on medical problems and deficits. In deciding whether to involve people with dementia in this study I considered two questions that Wilkinson (2002) frequently encountered in her research endeavours: why bother and is it possible? Once these issues were addressed the final question was how people with dementia can be included in a way that is both ethical and meaningful.

The question of "why bother?" has a number of fairly straightforward answers:

- There is a need to redress the power imbalances between researchers and people with dementia (Reed and Payton 1998). Traditional research has produced studies "on" people with dementia and there is a need to undertake research "with" this group.
- It is only by researching with people with dementia that we will begin to understand their lived experience. No amount of proxy reports will provide a real insight (Wilkinson 2002).
- Excluding people with dementia on the grounds that they may not have the capacity to consent using traditional approaches would be morally wrong as they would then remain as a silent and excluded

voice (Wilkinson 2002) and be denied the opportunity to shape future services.
- There is increasing acknowledgement that service users should be able to influence services as stated in documents such as Patient and Public Involvement in the New NHS (DoH 1999b) and the National Service Framework for Older People (DoH 2001b).
- At national level the need to include people with mental incapacity in research is being considered, particularly in the Mental Capacity Act (HMSO 2005).
- The inclusion of people with dementia demonstrates respect for the personhood of individuals (Kitwood 1997a) which is one of my fundamental desires.

The question of whether it is possible to include people with dementia in research has been conclusively answered; a review of such studies has been provided in chapter one. A number of researchers have demonstrated remarkable success, the only proviso being that most have tended to work with people with early dementia and there is relatively less evidence of success in working with people in the more advanced stages. Answers to the questions "why bother?" and "is it possible?" led me to the conclusion that people with dementia must be involved in this study. The challenge was to find ways that this could be achieved that were both meaningful and ethical.

In any study the researcher has a duty to uphold the ethical principles of beneficence, respect for human dignity and justice (Farsides 2003). The principles of beneficence encompass the concepts of doing no harm, preventing harm and doing some good (Beauchamp and Childress 1989). A major ethical concern in this study was the wellbeing of the participants. There are three groups of participants in this study: people with dementia, their lay carers and hospital staff. Whilst these may be considered as three discrete groups it is argued that many of the principles of conducting ethically sound research will be applicable to all. For this reason the approach to all participants is broadly parallel. This choice was also influenced by a powerful desire not to treat people with dementia as a separate and alien group. The process of inclusion is outlined in figure 2-1.

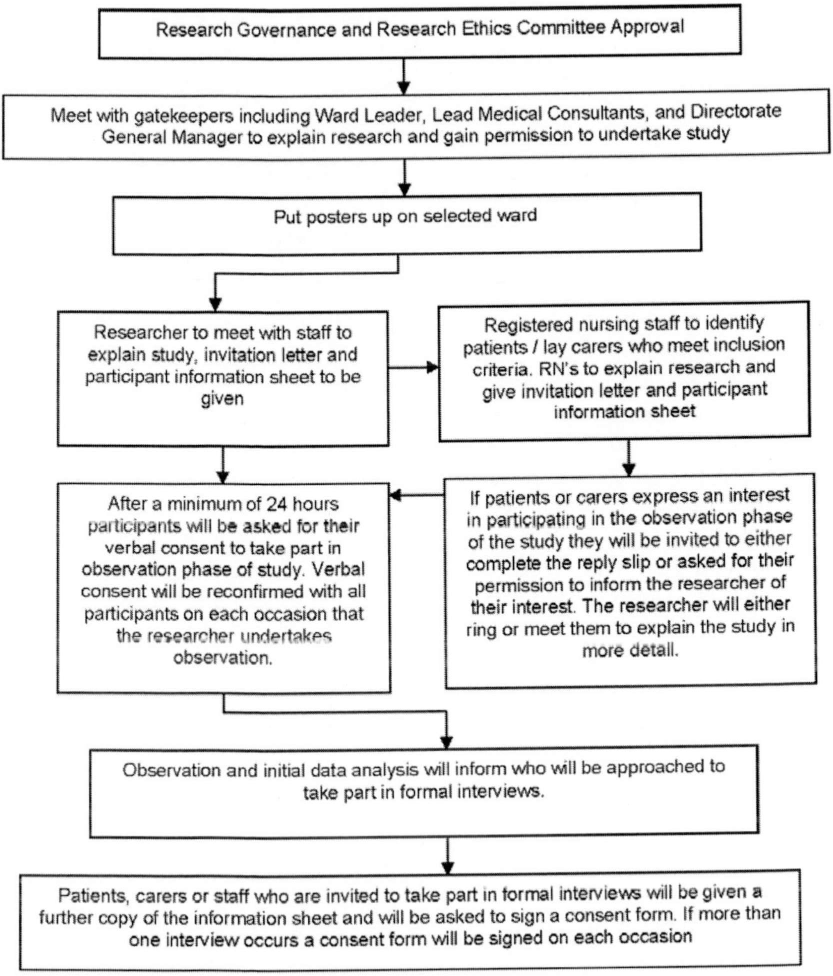

Figure 2-1: The Process of Inclusion

The aim of this process was to gain voluntary consent from each participant. Staff were given verbal and written information and sufficient time to consider their participation. Most staff agreed to participate and those who declined cited two reasons. Some stated that they could not bear to be watched, others said that they had not been trained to work with people with dementia and were therefore worried that they would be found to be "doing it wrong". In some respects I was relieved that staff of different grades and disciplines declined with relative ease as this provided reassurance that my approach and previous role were not proving coercive. Patients and lay carers were initially approached by registered nurses on the study wards. Costello (2002) suggests that this tactic enables a decision to be made without undue pressure. Patients and lay carers who expressed an interest in the study met with me to discuss it in more detail. In the case of patients, their next of kin were approached and asked for their agreement to invite the individual to participate. This caused me some concern both in terms of potential detriment to personhood and because the action may be interpreted as asking for proxy consent which is not valid (Department of Health 2001a). On balance it was considered to be good practice to involve the next of kin and is also now a requirement of the Mental Capacity Act (HMSO 2005). This style of consent is congruent with the negotiated model espoused by Grout (2004) which acknowledges that consent from older people with mental health problems may not fit with the dominant bioethical model.

During the observation phase a process model of consent (Milton 2000) was used. This choice was based on the premise that a single act of gaining consent was inappropriate for a study that continued over many months. Verbal consent was gained from each participant at the beginning of every period of observation to ensure that they were willing to continue (Reed and Payton 1996). Consent from patients was based on the inclusionary approach of Dewing (2002), Grout's (2004) negotiated model and on the principles of interconnectedness espoused by McCormack (2001a). I spent some time with patients and staff developing relationships before attempting to include patients in the study.

Participants who agreed to take part in interviews were asked to sign a consent form. This choice was justified as interviews were more formal, discrete episodes for which "one off" consent was valid. It is recognised that asking people with dementia to sign a consent form may be counter-productive as it may induce feelings of anxiety (Hubbard et al 2002). During the observation phase I achieved a level of interconnectedness (McCormack 2001a) with patients that enabled only those who appeared to understand and be at ease with the research process to be selected for interview. Appropriate staff and lay carers helped to inform this decision. It was made clear at every stage that participants were able to withdraw from the study without detriment.

Whilst ethical aspects of this study were well planned and had the approval of all the required bodies my experience in the field was not so straightforward. The process of trying to explain the study to people with dementia proved even more difficult than anticipated, trying to find the right words without being patronising was challenging. Conversations with patients led me to believe that they were willing to share their experiences. A number of this group said clearly that they were willing to tell me what they knew. However, despite every effort to explain that this was a research project I remained far from convinced that these participants comprehended this. My unease was compounded by concerns that were expressed by some staff about the inclusion of people with dementia. This led to several interesting debates about whether it was more ethically sound to attempt to gain the views of this group, albeit with a limited level of informed consent, or simply to assume that they had no valuable contribution to make. A small number of staff remained uncertain about engaging with these patients. I spent many hours agonising about whether it was really ethical to include these participants but eventually concluded that it could be justified on the following grounds:

- The research was highly unlikely to do participants any harm.
- Participants appeared to positively enjoy having periods of undivided attention.
- Findings may improve the care for people with dementia in the future.

Despite rational justification I continued to feel a slight unease about the ability to gain informed consent and remained vigilant for verbal or non-verbal signs that participants wished to withdraw.

Reflexivity

In much of the literature concerning ethnographic studies the importance of reflexivity is recognised. Indeed Flood (1999:35) goes as far as stating that "without some degree of reflexivity any research is blind and without purpose". However, reflexivity is a contentious issue as it is subject to an array of interpretations. These interpretations vary amongst authors but may broadly be divided into two camps. Firstly there is the type of reflexivity that focuses primarily on the researcher; this fits with the category that Finlay (2002b) describes as reflexivity as introspection. This approach may be valuable in terms of self dialogue and discovery. Equally it may foster self-indulgence (Koch 1998, Marcus 1998) or even what Scott (1997:134) describes as "narcissistic preoccupation with self". The pitfall of over concentration on self is that the researcher's voice may become dominant to the detriment of participants.

An alternative view of reflexivity is provided by Northway (2000) who defines it as a means of promoting honesty and transparency in the research process, it can provide an audit trail and therefore indicate the rigour of the study. This approach is supported by Koch and Harrington (1998:882) who promote the use of reflexivity as an effective way of signposting “what is going on” in the study.

It is recognised that examination of self and personal motivations and beliefs are essential for rigorous qualitative research. However the purpose of reflexivity in this study is based on providing a clear account of how knowledge has been acquired, organised and interpreted (Althehide and Johnson 1998) and the influence that both myself and the participants have had on this. It is about situating the research and doing justice to the personal stances of both researcher and participants.

Reflexivity has been achieved in this study by critically examining each stage of the research process to ensure that the final product is both believable and plausible (Koch and Harrington 1998). A reflective journal has been maintained and “critical friends” (Northway 2000), including the supervisory team, have been enlisted to continually challenge my own assumptions. Reflexivity has been woven though the whole study rather than being treated as a separate entity and it is examined in more detail in chapter five.

Conclusion

This chapter has explained and justified the choice of critical interpretive ethnography as the predominant research methodology for this study. Reasons for incorporating elements of the narrative approaches have been examined. A need to employ flexible but coherent approaches to this relatively new branch of research involving people with dementia is justified. The research process has been explained in detail and issues around ethics and reflexivity have been explored.

CHAPTER THREE

THE COMMENTARY

Introduction

Chapter three combines both findings from the data and a discussion relating to these findings. The chapter comprises two main sections. Section one begins with a brief description of the study settings, this is intended to set the scene for readers. To provide a picture of what it is like to be an older person with dementia in an acute hospital, a series of narratives have been developed. These narratives are intended to provide authentic accounts of the experiences of the five people with dementia with whom I spent most time. Narratives include insights into the experiences of the carers and are followed by shorter extracts of data from other patients and carers. Section two explores the current state of practice as it was observed. Each section incorporates a discussion of how findings relate to published literature. Construction of the chapter has been influenced by my desire to meet the following aims:

- Ensure that participants with dementia remain central.
- Enable the voices of the participants with dementia to be heard in whatever way is possible.
- Give equal value and credence to data collected through observation, informal conversation and interviews.
- Present fair and authentic accounts of the care given to people with dementia in the acute hospital setting.
- Ensure that the findings remain firmly grounded in the richness of the data.
- Reflect upon the findings of this study in the context of existing literature.
- Relate the findings of this study to the wider social and political picture.

The approach to the production of this chapter is somewhat unorthodox in being influenced by the traditions of both critical interpretive ethnography and narrative analysis. This choice has been driven by my desire to meet the aims outlined above, particularly given that some of the participants in this study were in the more advanced stages of dementia. This approach is firmly grounded in accepted methods in that the ethnographic component identifies patterns and themes that constitute the culture and provide an account of people in their social and cultural context (Holloway and Todres 2003). Identification of patterns and themes involved a process of "defamiliarization" (Thomas 1993:43) in which I attempted to remove myself from "taken for granted" assumptions about the data and review it in a new light searching for similarities and contrary experiences. This long process identified a range of themes that are discussed later in this chapter. The narrative component adheres to tradition in enabling the stories of individuals to be told in such a way that meaning is given to the thoughts and actions of participants (Polkinghorne 1988). The choice to use narratives was driven by the acceptance that traditional analysis is about transferring information whereas my goal was to communicate with readers (Ellis and Bochner 2006). In order to do justice to the participants in this research I wanted to capture their stories and, as far as possible, give readers an insight into their worlds. My aim was to enable readers to feel the experiences of the participants rather than merely be presented with "disembodied words on a page" (Ellis and Bochner 2006:431).

Critics may argue that these approaches lack analytic rigour. There are those that argue that narrative research is merely storytelling with no scientific grounding (Koch 1998). Criticisms of lack of rigour are equally applied to ethnographic analysis (Snow et al 2003). As discussed earlier, other methods of analysis had previously been attempted such as coding and categorising data. These were not successful in that they had the effect of breaking data into small sections in which the essence of the experiences of participants was lost. I felt that this style of data analysis and presentation had the potential to "reveal meaning without committing the error of defining it" (Arendt 1973:107). I wanted to produce work that had a clear relationship to the everyday life of likely readers, words that would be evocative and that they could relate to. It is suggested by Ellis and Bochner (2006:435) that this "style of communicating has more potential to transform and change the world for the better [and] offers the possibility of opening hearts and increasing understanding of difference".

Within the written narratives are a range of photographs taken in clinical settings. Use of visual narratives is well documented in the fields of anthropology and sociology (Prosser 1998, Pink 2003). It is acknowledged that there is little evidence of this technique in health care literature (Riley and Manias 2003).

One of the major concerns in using images was the ethical implications. As Harper (1998) suggests photography is more intrusive than observational fieldwork. For this reason the majority of images are of inanimate objects. Only one picture includes a clearly visible person with dementia. The consent process with this lady was negotiated with care (Banks 2001). We discussed the use of photographs and, when they were taken, we reviewed them and together selected the one for inclusion in this thesis.

The photographs have been used at a simple level. Denzin (1995:25) argues that visual images can show "the real in all it's truth". My intention was not to try to demonstrate any sort of truth but rather to reinforce and elaborate on the words provided (Harper 2005). It is recognised that images are inevitably polysemic, that is they have a range of possible meanings and each viewer will make their own interpretation. It is anticipated that the pictures will prove evocative and capture the imagination of the reader. They are intended to add to the richness of the narratives and enable readers to connect with the study (Harper 2005).

It is the fusion of these approaches that move this work into what Rapport et al (2005) describe as the edgelands of research in which rigid frameworks are relaxed. This type of flexible approach, utilising a range of methods, is convincingly supported by Holloway and Todres (2003) who advocate a "third position" that allows flexibility as well as consistency and coherence. The value of this technique is that it allows the provision of the fullest and most authentic possible accounts of the experiences of the participants.

Ways way in which findings and discussion are depicted is based on the work of Polkinghorne (1995), Thomas (1993) and Chatterji (1998). Descriptions of the study settings have been included in order to set the scene in which the data were collected. Narratives were developed using an adapted version of a framework devised by Polkinghorne (1995). This author provides a clear outline of the information that is needed to compose a comprehensive narrative. However this approach was not wholly suitable for this study as it required a level of detail that was not available from all the participants. The framework was therefore simplified to include a description of the person, cultural context, plan and enactment of the plan. Reasons for this adaptation are explained more fully in chapter two. The purpose of including narratives is to provide an authentic account of the experiences of older people with dementia and their carers.

Presentation of this chapter has also been influenced by the work of Chatterji (1998) and Thomas (1993). Thomas (1993:63), in writing about the production of critical ethnography, urges writers to "lead the reader, step by step, through the data with as little prompting as possible by painting a picture in sufficiently sharp detail that readers will be convinced by the power of the demonstration, rather than the passion of the researcher". Whilst the desire for data to remain central is paramount there is also clearly a need to link findings with current knowledge. To achieve this extracts of data are followed by a discussion that links data with existing literature, a technique that is used so effectively by Chatterji (1998). Data is also considered within the broader social and political milieu. Thomas (1993) describes this critical approach as both an intellectual responsibility and an ethical obligation.

The final part of the chapter brings together findings and discussion and considers ways in which these may be used as a basis for practice development. It is felt that this approach to the presentation of findings and discussion, whilst unorthodox, meets the aims of presenting fair and authentic accounts of care received by older people with dementia in an acute hospital and setting it within the context of current literature and the social and political context. As discussed in chapter two the commentary essentially provides the "what?" and "how?" of this ethnography (Katz 2001).

Throughout the chapter direct quotes from participants and field notes are presented in italics, underlined words are those stressed by participants, underlined bold words are those said very forcefully.

The Study Setting

The study is set in a large acute hospital trust in the United Kingdom and involved three wards: "Freshwater", "Ventnor" and "Shanklin" which are part of a unit dedicated to caring for older people; this is in a separate building that is attached to the main hospital by a long and exposed corridor. Most patients enter the unit on beds, trolleys or in wheelchairs from the emergency department or from the admissions ward via this corridor. It gives the impression of taking people well away from the hub of activity in the main hospital buildings. The immediate impression of the unit is not one of welcome with a bare and institutional entrance area occupied by only a few people who move quickly between wards and departments.

Wards are similar in that they offer specialist care for older people, generally those over the age of seventy five, although people are admitted on the basis of need rather than age. Each ward is led by a senior nurse supported by a team of nursing staff both registered and non-registered. Wards also use temporary bank staff on a regular basis. Staff are mixed in terms of gender, race and age and the wards provide placements for nursing students. Much of the clerical and administrative work is undertaken by the ward clerks, the senior nurses also have access to some secretarial support. Wards tend to work predominantly with their two allocated medical consultants and their attached teams of junior doctors. Therapy staff are unit based, however physiotherapists tend to work primarily on specified wards. Social work staff are allocated on a case by case basis dependent on their workload and the geographical area in which the patient normally resides.

There is a ward round with each of the consultants at least once a week. Each ward also has a multi-disciplinary team (MDT) meeting each week largely to plan discharges. Ways in which these meetings are conducted is very much dependent on the mixture and grades of disciplines that attend and they may be led by any member of the team. Patients with complex problems or complicated discharge plans may have a case conference. These meetings may be attended by the patient, their lay carer and a range of staff from the MDT.

"Freshwater" and "Ventnor" wards provide acute care whilst "Shanklin" focuses more on rehabilitation although, in reality, these are not absolute distinctions as pressure on bed capacity leads to patients being allocated the next available empty bed. Wards all run at maximum bed occupancy and ward staff experience constant pressure to expedite discharge. Wards all have some patients for whom discharge is delayed, these patients are medically fit for discharge but remain in hospital awaiting either a package of home care or placement in a residential home.

The wards participating in the study, whilst superficially similar, actually have markedly different cultures. This is a phenomenon that I was aware of whilst working in the hospital but which was even more obvious when viewing the areas through the eyes of a relative "outsider". It was evident that care was influenced by the prevailing culture but that individual personal philosophies were equally powerful.

Data revealed that care was variable. Some was excellent whilst some clearly needed improvement. It is acknowledged that it may be more straightforward to capture examples of poor care. These tend to be more discrete and rapid episodes. The good care that was delivered was generally more consistent and appeared to be linked to the mindset and beliefs of individual practitioners. It was notable that those who appeared to deliver "good" care, that is care that preserved the personhood of individuals, were often unable to identify that their skills were greater than those of any of their peers. This explanation may, or may not, offer some mitigation to the apparent harshness of my observations.

The Narratives

A total of eleven patients were involved in this study. Length of involvement varied from a brief meeting to several weeks of participant observation and conversations. Duration of involvement varied for a number of reasons. One patient initially agreed to participate in the study but as I was talking to her I knew intuitively that this was an uncomfortable experience for her. She was clearly searching for the "right" thing to say and her anxiety at the thought of getting anything wrong was obvious from her expression. I therefore chose not to involve this patient any further. Other patients were involved for much longer periods but their participation often stopped abruptly as they were transferred to other areas or discharged with little warning. I was able to spend prolonged periods of time with five of the patients. This section presents their narratives, experiences of their carers are incorporated. Narratives are presented in newspaper format to signify that they are reports of the stories of individuals. Following the narratives a series of shorter extracts of data are provided which illuminate the experiences of other patients and carers.

The amount of information I was able to glean about the patients was limited. Details of age, mini mental state examination (MMSE) score and abode was generally available, information about next of kin (NOK) was sketchy and any insight into these patients as individuals was virtually absent. Brief details of the patients involved including approximate length and type of participation are provided in table 3-1.

Table 3-1: Information on Patient Participants

Name	Age	MMSE	Abode	NOK	Length of involvement (approx)	Type of involvement
Tom	84	7	Residential home	Daughter	3 weeks	Observation and conversation
Hilda	85	4	Own home	Brother	8 weeks	Observation and conversation
Phyllis	93	3	Own home	Son	2 weeks	Observation and conversation
Walter	92	4	Own home	Paid carers	3 weeks	Observation and conversation
Doris	80	1	Own home	Daughter	1 week	Observation and conversation
Anthony	94	0	Own home	Wife	1.5 weeks	Observation and conversation
Win	85	1	Own home	Son	1 hour	Observation and conversation
Dora	92	0	Residential home	?	4 weeks	Observation, conversation and interview
Ben	93	1	Own home	Daughter	3.5 weeks	Observation and conversation
Amy	88	0	Own home	Husband	2.5 weeks	Observation and conversation
Eileen	84	0	Own home	Husband	3 weeks	Observation and conversation

Hilda's Narrative

Introduction

Hilda was admitted to hospital having been found by the police in the street wearing her nightclothes. She stayed in hospital as a place of safety for nearly ten weeks until she was found a placement in a residential home.

The Person

Little was known about Hilda prior to her admission. It seemed that she had lived independently alone in her small bungalow. She was eighty five years old. Hilda had a mini mental state examination score of 4. She had no obvious medical problems. When she arrived on the ward Hilda had none of her own possessions, a situation that did not change for the duration of her stay. Hilda was a tiny lady with short, straight grey hair. She had lively, often alert blue eyes. Hilda could walk without help but always appeared to struggle with slippers that did not quite fit.

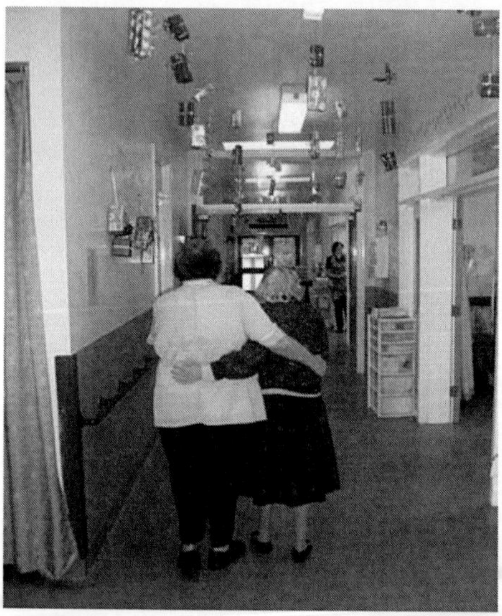

She was a quiet lady but clearly enjoyed company and would join in conversation initiated by others. When asked about herself, Hilda gave a very brief description. She explained that she usually lived in London with her parents and her twin brother, she missed them very badly and wanted to get home to them soon. She worried about how they were coping without her as she usually did all the housework and cooking. She said that she worked in a grocery until she was in her sixties. She never had children as she was widowed young and *"didn't really bother with that again"*. Hilda said that she was in hospital on the South Coast as she was here on holiday.

The Cultural Context

Hilda was on Freshwater Ward in a bay with five other patients, the bay was relatively bright and spacious. Hilda had a bed by the window out of which she enjoyed watching builders constructing a new section of the hospital. Hilda's bed space was very sparse, on her locker top were a wipe and a bar of soap. There were a few hospital clothes in her locker and a suitcase beneath her bed.

There was remarkably little interaction between Hilda and the other patients in the bay. Initially Hilda befriended another lady with more severe dementia, they would sometimes sit together in the afternoon and have a cup of tea and watch the work of the ward. The other patient died suddenly, Hilda told me how upset and shocked she was by this event as she thought the lady was going home soon. Other patients appeared to view Hilda with some concern. They indicated that Hilda could be restless at times and sometimes woke them up. The lady in the next bed talked about Hilda as though she didn't exist saying *"sometimes when she speaks she seems quite intelligent you know ... there seems to be more and more of them, I suppose we're living longer"*.

The Plan

From the time of admission it was recognised that Hilda did not have any acute medical problems. The focus of her care was therefore to help her to meet her personal care needs and to expedite her discharge. A decision was made rapidly that Hilda would be unable to return to her own home. Her brother agreed that she should go into a residential placement but did not feel able to be involved in the process due to his own poor health.

The Enactment of the Plan

Hilda's days quickly fell into a routine. She was woken early and had a cup of tea and some breakfast. At some point in the morning Hilda was invited to go out to the bathroom to have a wash. On the whole she was given a set of wash things and sometimes clean clothes and guided to the bathroom. It was not clear how able she was to wash herself, however it was clear from her words and actions that being clean and neat was very important to her. Once Hilda had finished in the bathroom she returned to the chair by her bed and dozed. Her day was then punctuated mainly by mealtimes, drinks rounds and visits to the lavatory.

The staff said they liked Hilda and found her easy to look after. Apart from one episode soon after admission when she tried to get into bed with another patient she exhibited little challenging behaviour. She took minimal time to look after and was unerringly polite. She was described by staff as "*happy in her own little world*" and as a *"cheerful little thing"*.

Hilda seemed to be quite aware that there was a definite routine to her days, she also communicated her thoughts about the various components of this routine. Hilda was able to make clear and decisive decisions about what she would like to eat and drink. She tended to forget that she had completed a menu and told me *"you just have to eat what is put in front of you"*. She said that most of the food was okay *"they feed you well as long as you like it"* she said pulling a face. I told Hilda that I thought she was losing weight, she said she needed to lose a bit, I told her not to get too thin and she smiled. Hilda had quite a high level of manual dexterity and enjoyed eating and drinking spontaneously. One nursing assistant routinely presented her with cereal and a jam sandwich for her breakfast "*I've made it into soldiers for you*". At this Hilda smiled benignly, her face painting a picture of someone who knew she was being patronised. As the tea trolley was wheeled round Hilda requested *"cup of tea please, no sugar"* without prompting. She carefully moved the cup to the windowsill by her bed.

Hilda was often left to wash herself, however her capacity to do this appeared slightly compromised. Hilda was clearly concerned about her personal hygiene. One nursing assistant had doubts about whether Hilda was managing to wash herself, this nurse offered Hilda a bath one morning. Hilda had a bath and hair wash which she said she really enjoyed. She spent a lot of time following this adjusting her clothes to her satisfaction. Hilda was discontent with the input of nurses on some occasions. One morning a nursing assistant accompanied her to the bathroom and stayed to help her wash. When Hilda returned from the bathroom I asked if she had enjoyed her wash. She walked past me muttering; when I asked her to repeat what she had said she replied clearly *"talk about a lick and a promise, not enough soap"*. Her clothes were badly marked. Hilda spent many minutes adjusting her clothes but seemed to remain dissatisfied with her appearance. The fact that Hilda had none of her own clothes also concerned the staff; they managed to find her a selection of ill fitting clothes. The staff regularly attempted to ensure that she was decently attired. Hilda had a skirt that was too big for her and the staff spent some time trying to ensure that it was secure. *A SN strides up to Hilda. She asks how she is today and Hilda says she is fine, the SN, who has a strong accent, starts to speak very quickly. It is clear from Hilda's face that she does not understand. The last bit is "your skirt, your skirt". The SN goes up to Hilda and lifts her cardigan, the nurse gives an affirmative grunt and walks away. Hilda says to me "I don't know why she wants to look at my fat". I tell her I think that the nurse was checking that the safety pin was still in her skirt so that it didn't fall down. Hilda nods but looks uncertain and mildly disturbed by this interaction.*

On another occasion Hilda seemed much more content with the approach of a nursing assistant. *An NA comes over to see Hilda, she's noticed that her skirt is slipping down so she comes with a bandage to use as a belt. She notices someone has already put a safety pin in Hilda's skirt, Hilda says this is fine. The NA approaches Hilda in quite a purposeful way and explains why she is doing what she's doing, Hilda's nod is much more positive this time, she appears to make sense of what the nurse is doing.*

Hilda spent some of her time tidying up her bed area. She acknowledged that she liked everything to be clean and in its correct place. She did not like to have her used cutlery and crockery on her bed table for too long. When a nursing assistant was collecting rubbish from each patient's bed space Hilda asked her to take her cup and glass away. She was told *"no, we don't take them now"* but was offered no further explanation. Hilda looked really dejected. When gathering Hilda's wash things one nursing assistant pulled her locker right to the far end of her bed and opened it facing the lady in the next bed.

She took out the contents; mostly hospital mugs and cup holders, there were very few of Hilda's possessions. The nurse said to the other patient *"I think we like hoarding"*, they both laughed.

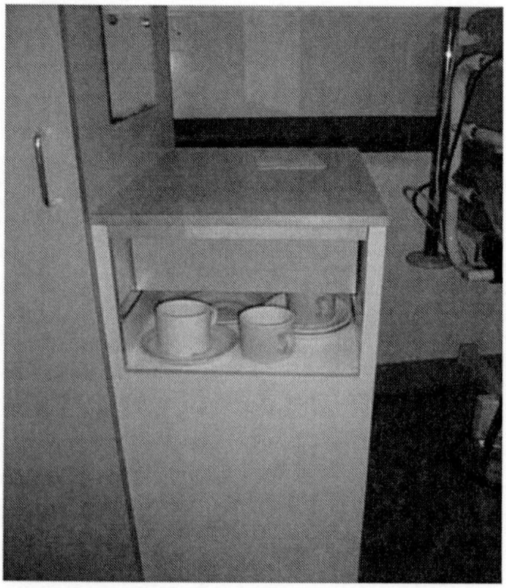

Hilda spent many, many hours sitting in her chair, sometimes dozing. When we talked about being bored she said that it was not really a problem as "*I watch what goes on*". The majority of her interactions with staff were short and purposeful in nature, for example Hilda being reminded to have a wash or someone helping her to complete her menus. She had her vital signs checked daily. *A nursing assistant comes over to Hilda and says "hello cheeky, we'll have to take your temperature under your arm now you've started your tea, we'll try and squeeze it in there". She puts the thermometer under Hilda's arm and goes back to another patient. She returns to Hilda and asks if she can take the thermometer out. Hilda says she can if it's still there, the nurse says "we'll forgive you", Hilda looks deeply puzzled.*

Hilda's care was primarily based on her physical needs although there were occasional episodes when there seems to be more of a person to person connection between Hilda and individual staff. One nursing assistant told me *"one day I think she'd spoken to her brother and then she was crying, she was having a very lucid moment as much as she did, she said there's nothing of mine here sometimes I want to write little notes and .... I can't, I don't have anything and the next day I bought in a little notepad and a pen and she was happy as happy could be but I don't think she* ever *wrote in it ..... but it was there".*

Hilda showed me her notebook. She seemed to derive some comfort from having it although she did say that she hadn't got around to writing in it. The act of kindness of giving Hilda a notebook was ridiculed by another member of staff

The nurse comes back from her break and goes through the things on the top of Hilda's locker again; she finds a notebook "this must be your little notebook .... (to others) not that there's anything in it", she puts it in Hilda's suitcase. Hilda did not appear to hear this comment.

Hilda rarely displayed overt emotion although she did become upset following contact with her brother. Hilda received a telephone call from her brother. She was clearly pleased to hear from him, she spoke to him for several minutes. One of the nursing assistants was sitting by Hilda while she talked to her brother, she seemed visibly shocked that Hilda was so upset and became tearful herself. The nursing assistant talked about the awfulness of thinking about Hilda being in a home. She described Hilda as a loveable person who she would like to take home with her. When Hilda finished the conversation she returned to her chair. She said that her brother was miserable because he was alone. She said she didn't want to go into a home. I said to her that it may be better than being here. Hilda said she liked it here, I asked why and she said she didn't really know, she's just used to the people. I said she may get to know some people in the home better as they stayed there for longer, Hilda nodded but was clearly not convinced. She said her brother would come to see her less now, I knew he hadn't visited since she'd been in hospital. Hilda said "*he's got his own car so he doesn't need other people's vehicles*". She said "*all I want is for him to come in and say that I don't have to go*". She sat back in her chair and gazed out of the window.

As the weeks went by Hilda began to look gradually more weary. One morning she looked particularly tired. When I asked her how she was she smiled broadly and told me that she had not been here long. I said that she looked a bit tired, she replied *"I don't sleep well in hospital"*. I asked her if she knew why, she said she didn't know. I asked if the bed was comfortable and Hilda replied that it was fine. I noticed that as time passed Hilda's attempts to communicate became less frequent and she gave the impression of slowly shrinking and becoming more tired both physically and spiritually. I noted *Hilda is fast asleep in her chair, she looks just a little thinner and a little more frail since last week. Again she looks as though she has faded just slightly over the last couple of days.*

Whilst Hilda lived through her daily routine of personal hygiene, eating, drinking and dozing the MDT worked on her discharge plans. Hilda remained clear throughout the process that she wanted to return home. The MDT decided that this was too much of a risk and a decision was made swiftly. Hilda's brother agreed that she should be found a residential placement but declined to be involved in the process due to his own frailty.

A social work care manager was allocated to Hilda. The care manager visited her on the ward on many occasions trying to build up a picture of Hilda and the type of placement that she might like. The care manager spoke of the burden of responsibility of having to choose a placement for someone else. Initially there was a plan that Hilda should visit a possible placement however it was decided that it would be too upsetting for her to leave the hospital and then return. Due to a number of issues the first placement was lost so the care manager viewed a number of other homes. She finally chose one on the basis that it was small and family run. It had a very friendly environment with lots of interaction between staff and residents. The care manager felt strongly that Hilda would be happy in this homely environment where she could be involved in some domestic activities and there was a large garden.

When Hilda talked about her future she said that someone wanted her to go into a home but that this was not what she wanted. She seemed unclear about why she was in hospital, she suggested that she had come in for an operation that had now been performed, she said "*I don't know how long I'm going to be here, I've been here for a while, I thought once I was back on my feet they'd send me home*". She regularly expressed great concern about her future and said that she never saw a doctor. On this occasion the consultant ward round had very visibly bypassed her. Hilda talked a lot about going home to her parents and her brother. She said she didn't get much time to herself because there was always a lot of housework to do. She used to enjoy reading the newspaper and playing darts when she had some spare time. She worried a lot about her brother being alone in London and felt she should be with him. We talked about what makes a good hospital, she said that this one is fine but that she prefers the one in London as it is nearer home. She said it's important that people get on and that no-one argues. She really didn't like arguing. Hilda looked frightened when she heard raised voices particularly when she couldn't see who was speaking, just the volume of a large group of people talking normally seemed to disturb her. When I asked her if she was happy in hospital she thought for a moment and said "*not really happy, but contented*". We agreed that perhaps contented is the best you can hope for in hospital. Each time the subject of going home arose Hilda became tearful and distressed. She pleaded with me to get the doctors to change their minds. She said "*the trouble is once you get into these places you rarely get out of them*". She said that some of her friends had gone in and never got out.

The medical staff communicated with Hilda in differing ways. Hilda said that she hadn't seen a doctor since she came into hospital but that someone would tell her what was going to happen to her. On the ward rounds Hilda tended to be passed by or discussed over the notes trolley. On one round the doctors said that Hilda was awaiting a placement in a home for people with mental health problems and bemoaned the fact that she was privately funded so they had no control over speeding up her discharge. A senior doctor commented that Hilda was never ill in the first place and so never needed to be in hospital. On occasion the doctors stopped and saw Hilda briefly. A doctor approached Hilda and said in a clipped tone "*you look worried, what's the matte*r", she rapidly turned away from Hilda and moved on to the next patient. Another conversation began "*you don't look so smiley toda*y" without waiting for a response the doctor started to tell Hilda that they were waiting for a place in a home for her. Hilda replied adamantly that she wanted to return to her own home. The more the doctor repeated the message the more distressed Hilda became. This led the doctor to back track using long and complex sentences including concepts such as preparing for the idea and trial placement. The conversation was curtailed abruptly as the doctor returned to the huddle of her colleagues around the notes trolley where they giggled slightly. The day prior to discharge a more junior doctor visited Hilda and asked her if she knew what was happening to her on the following day. The doctor explained that Hilda would be moving to her new home tomorrow. Hilda remained adamant that she wanted to return home, she cried pitifully. The doctor and Hilda continued to talk until they reached a natural lull, the doctor then turned to me and said that she didn't know what to say next. She wanted to tell the truth but was aware that this was distressing Hilda terribly. Her expression conveyed just how much this dilemma worried her. Following the conversation Hilda turned to me and pleaded "*can't you get them to change their minds*". The nursing staff described Hilda as a quiet, gentle person who was undemanding on their resources. Soon after one of the ward rounds a registered nurse came to see Hilda, she was plainly shocked to see Hilda crying. The nurse sat on Hilda's bed and rubbed her forearm, she spoke to her in a very soft voice peppered with sweethearts and darlings. She tried to rationalise with Hilda why she needed to go into a home but with each point the nurse made Hilda offered a reasoned counterargument. Eventually the nurse said simply "*I don't know what to say next*". The nurse opted to distract Hilda by getting her to tidy her locker; Hilda stopped crying. On the day of her discharge a nursing assistant sat on Hilda's bed and said "*do you know what day it is, you're going home today*" Hilda's face totally lit up but soon crumpled as the nurse added "*to a special home*". Hilda started to cry quietly. She seemed unable to settle and spent her day tapping the arms of her chair rather than having her usual naps. Eventually in the late afternoon an ambulance crew arrived to collect Hilda. She cried and said she didn't want to go but moved to the wheelchair without argument. She looked totally defeated.

I heard several weeks later from the care manager that she had visited Hilda in the home. She had settled in quickly and was enjoying being able to join in with some of the housework. Hilda contracted a chest infection and died in the home two months after her transfer.

Amy's Narrative

Introduction

Amy had been in respite care when she fell and sustained a complex fracture of her neck of femur. She was initially admitted to a trauma ward where she underwent internal fixation of the fracture. She was transferred to Shanklin ward where she stayed for five weeks until her transfer to a residential home.

The Person

Amy had been diagnosed with Alzheimer's disease two or three years prior to this admission. She had been offered anti-dementia medication but had absolutely refused this treatment despite the efforts of her husband and medical staff to get her to accept it. Amy's husband talked about how her condition had declined steadily since diagnosis. Her behaviour had deteriorated with increasingly frequent angry outbursts which, although quickly forgotten, were clearly distressing for him. Amy and her husband lived together in a ground floor flat. Over the last few months Amy had become less and less able to leave the flat. Her sleep pattern had become severely disrupted leaving her husband exhausted. She had become very noisy at night choosing to clean the flat in the early hours, this had led to several complaints from their neighbours. As her condition had worsened Amy needed an increasing level of home care. Her husband also employed a private cleaner. His physical health was failing and he was unable to do much around the flat.

Amy had begun to go into respite care periodically to allow her husband some rest. It was whilst in respite care that Amy fell and broke her hip. She was admitted to a trauma ward where she had the fracture internally fixated. The fracture was complex and the fixation only partially successful, this meant that Amy was left with an unstable and painful hip. Following surgery Amy was transferred to Shanklin ward.

Amy was tall and 'stick thin'. Her husband explained that her appetite was poor and that she tended to eat mostly crisps now. Her hair was beautifully cut and Amy took a pride in ensuring that it looked right. She had a range of cosmetics in her locker which she allowed staff to apply occasionally. She had her own clothes. Amy could walk a few steps with a Zimmer frame and the support of one or two nurses, the pain of this process was etched on her face. Amy appeared to be constantly agitated although her level of agitation fluctuated. She talked incessantly but it was extremely difficult to follow the thread of what she was saying. Amy spent much of her time looking through magazines or at some photographs that were on the ward. She seemed more at ease when she had some company.

The Cultural Context

Amy was being nursed on Shanklin Ward in a bay of four patients all of whom needed rehabilitation following trauma. The bay was clean, bright and airy. Amy had a lot of her own possessions around her. In particular she had a huge range of chocolates and biscuits which her husband brought in for her. She spent a lot of time rearranging these and offering them to other people, she rarely ate them herself. The beds in the bay were relatively far apart and there was little interaction between any of the patients. The other patients looked exceptionally frail and one also clearly had some cognitive impairment. Amy talked virtually all the time she was in the bay. One morning almost from the moment she woke Amy started talking to the lady opposite. First she asked the lady if she was still alive and then enquired why she had a mouse running across the top of her bed. Amy kept up a constant stream of questions and comments but received little response in return. The lady opposite nodded acknowledging what Amy was saying for a while but eventually muttered "*do shut up*" under her breath.

The nursing staff were aware that the other patients were finding Amy's relentless talking through both day and night very tiring. They were also aware that Amy appeared to enjoy company so she spent much of each day sitting in a wheelchair at the nurses' station talking to anyone who would listen. It transpired that Amy spent some of her nights out in the ward corridor as she got noisy and distressed and disturbed other patients.

The Plan

As Amy had sustained a complex fracture of her hip, the initial plan was to try and rehabilitate her as far as possible in terms of mobility. It rapidly became evident that the rehabilitation offered to Amy was minimal and the plan soon altered to focus on the provision of personal care and rapid discharge arrangements.

The Enactment of the Plan

Although the initial purpose of transferring Amy to a rehabilitation ward was to try to maximise her mobility, this aim was not followed through. On initial assessment by a registered nurse Amy was quickly labelled as someone who may not benefit from rehabilitation. The nurse said "*she had what I call a significant degree of Alzheimer's disease really in that she* can't, *we first noticed it in terms of her mobility and trying to rehabilitate her,* she can't, she can't and she couldn't *um, process any kind of detailed instruction for mobility so her only mobility, h'her sort of mobility abilities really is about that kind of automatic mobility"*. The doubts about Amy's capacity to rehabilitate were echoed by the physiotherapist who stated simply "*she's got no carry over*". The physiotherapist rapidly withdrew from Amy's care. This caused some concern for the nursing staff although one could see some justification stating that "*well the physio found that she couldn't really* actively *rehabilitate her so there was* no point *us giving her detailed rehab goals or working with her to detailed rehab goals 'cos she couldn't, she couldn't negotiate those goals, she couldn't* agree *those goals"*. This nurse went on to say that *"it's a shame to some extent that the physios have withdrawn from her"*. They withdrew from her because they said they couldn't actively rehabilitate her "*which seemed a bit* unfortunate *really because you believe that everybody's kind of capable of it"*. Another registered nurse commented "*she had no physio, she had no OT input, um, unless she would cooperate with it, they're so busy they're going to go to someone who cooperates aren't they?"* Both nurses attempted to rationalise why Amy received virtually no therapy input.

Amy's active rehabilitation quickly ceased. Her care then focused mainly on daily activities such as personal hygiene and eating and drinking. The nurses had differing ideas about how Amy's personal hygiene needs should be met. One registered nurse took a flexible approach suggesting that "*we don't have to have a routine with this little lady do we, why do we have to get her up and wash her at a certain time, let's do it when we can"*. Other nurses had differing beliefs, one nursing assistant stated that all patients must be washed in the morning "*they have to be finished by twelve so we can go to lunch*". This nursing assistant entered Amy's bay, Amy asked if she could go to the loo. The nurse said "*you want to go to the toilet"*. Amy didn't answer immediately, the nurse stood in the doorway of the bay with hands on hips and said "*do you want to go to the toilet or* not". Amy looked a bit surprised and still did not offer a quick reply. The nurse said *"***come along then** *the breakfasts arrived ten minutes ago*". The nurse walked with Amy to the loo, the nurse sighed and raised her eyebrows. Amy said "*if only it didn't hurt so much*", the nurse did not respond and Amy limped a little further towards the bathroom. She said again how much her leg hurt. The nurse told her it would hurt less if she just kept walking "*so you won't be standing on it for so long"*. The mornings were particularly difficult for Amy, as she sat in her bed one morning trying to reach her breakfast she said clearly "*I can't get out of bed at all now*" her face was a picture of pain and frustration. Her breakfast was removed largely uneaten with no comment. Another day Amy was more successful with her communication "*I need you to help me,*" the nurse replied gently "*I will"*.

One morning a registered nurse hurriedly washed Amy while she was still in bed, when she had completed the wash she said "*are you going to get up now, everyone is up now in their chair, come along, good girl"*. Amy responded "*I ache all over so don't make it too difficult*". The nurse realised that Amy had not taken her morning medication including her analgesia; the tablets had been left on her bed table. She helped Amy to take her tablets and rapidly proceeded to get her out of bed, Amy sounded distraught, she shouted "*leave me alone*", eventually she was transferred to her chair. The nurse later explained that it was difficult to wash Amy this morning as you need to be polite and kind when looking after her. This morning the nurse said she felt 'excited' because she was so busy. The nurse described the experience as horrible and acknowledged that Amy did not enjoy her wash.

Amy seemed to find mealtimes uncomfortable, as she was given her lunch one day she said to the nurse "*I'll pay for it but I can't eat it, let the foreigners have it*". I encouraged Amy to eat her lunch, she told me it was foul. She asked if she should dish out my lunch. She moved the food around her plate and then carefully tipped it all into the dregs in her coffee mug. The nurse came to clear the plates and commented that the 'soup' looked absolutely horrible. Amy replied "*the cat wouldn't eat it"*. A registered nurse noticed that Amy seemed to find the huge plates of food that were put in front of her rather daunting. This nurse observed that Amy

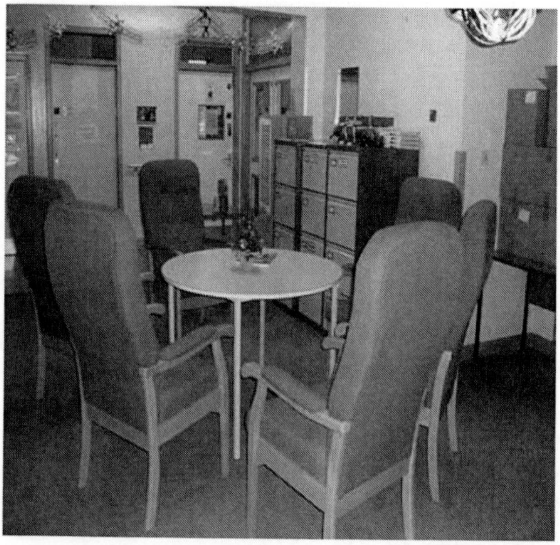

had lost a lot of weight and found that she was more inclined to eat when "*I got her a bowl or a small plate and I put little* things *on a plate and 'cos she'll eat it with her fingers*". This approach was not followed by all staff. A nursing assistant took some porridge into Amy, she stood some distance from her and said "*sugar and milk?*" Amy replied "*I didn't ask for porridge this morning*", the nurse tutted. She added sugar and milk and put the dish on Amy's bed table. She barked at Amy to sit up. The nurse returned and shoved some toast on the table. Several minutes later she reappeared and buttered the toast without comment. Amy ate a minute bit of her breakfast and it was soon removed largely uneaten without comment. Amy's diet seemed to consist mainly of the chocolate and biscuits that her husband brought in and the frequent cups of tea she was given by both nursing and domestic staff.

Amy clearly enjoyed company, she was a great talker, much of the content of her speech, particularly when she was more agitated concerned religion and she seemed fearful of divine retribution. Amy tried to offer words of wisdom to staff "*learn to love your life by leading your life, life will teach you a lesson*". This statement was completely ignored. The nursing staff got Amy to spend long periods each day sitting at the nurses' station to provide Amy with some company and also give the other patients in the bay some peace and quiet.

Amy's husband mentioned the decision to allow her to sit at the nurses' station "*I find that* very *kind, very* kind *of them to let her do that, I think that, you know, for, for a busy ward, I think that's* kind". Whilst Amy sat at the nurses' station staff of all disciplines talked to her. Although Amy enjoyed having company she sometimes seemed to find the level of activity overwhelming. She disliked noise, one morning as she sat at the nurses' station the telephone rang virtually constantly, Amy said angrily "*stop it, horrible thing isn't it*". She listened to what is going on around her. As she was sitting by the telephone a nurse rushed to answer it, her manner was abrupt. Amy looked at me and commented "*someone's for the high jump*". She became visibly upset if she thought there was any conflict on the ward, as two nurses talked in the corridor outside her bay Amy said "*I do wish they wouldn't stop arguing, would stop arguing I mean*", she laughed gently realising her error.

On occasion some of Amy's retained abilities became clear. When reading a magazine she commented on an article about a character in a television programme who was going to die shortly. Amy was obviously familiar with this series, her husband also mentioned it. Ironically the character in question had developed Alzheimer's disease, Amy's husband said "*I thought <u>oh no</u> he's got it as well, I don't want to be reminded about that damn thing*". Amy was saddened at the thought of the imminent death of this character despite the fact that many staff had told her it was not real. Amy told the nursing staff that she wrote poetry, she had some of her work with her. A nurse gave Amy a plain piece of paper and a pen "*what shall I write?*", "*anything you want to ... anything you want to*", "*what shall I write?*", "*write about today, write about your husband, we don't know him as well as you do*", "*I should hope not*", they both laughed, "*I can't be bothered*" says Amy, the nurse went off. Amy let me read some of her work, she had written some astonishingly insightful poems about being in hospital. She said "*I've got an extraordinarily imaginable mind or so I've been told*".

The senior nurse explained that her aim when caring for Amy was to "*kind of make the most of the, you know, the skills that she has got, which are still there, it's about trying to value that*". Others seemed not to notice what Amy had to offer. This was evident when Amy was sitting with me at the nurses' station. A nursing assistant started to tell me about a project she had done about dementia. Amy worked hard to join in the conversation so I had one person talking in each ear and neither of them was going to give way. They both talked ceaselessly and ignored what the other was saying. Amy seemed to want to belong to the staff group. She talked about the disorganisation on the ward, she said "*look at the state of this*" as she began to tidy the nurses' station yet again. As she finished the tidying Amy noticed a nursing assistant wandering around the desk clearly looking for something. Amy said "*what are you looking for dear, 'cos I've been here most of the morning*" the nurse replied brusquely "*you won't know where it is Amy*". Amy didn't reply, the look of absolute hurt on her face was clear to see. This pattern was repeated on many occasions. Amy was regularly given a reminiscence book or some old photographs to look at, few staff engaged in any discussion about these pictures and she was left to thumb through them alone.

As Amy lived her day to day existence on the ward plans were being made for her discharge. Amy's husband was virtually unable to think about her care on the ward. He struggled considerably when I asked about her care. He evaded the question and quickly noticed when I asked it again. He finally answered it briefly saying "*I think she's getting as much care as she would if she was private, I don't see they can do any more*". Although his words were positive they were said with an overtone of absolute resignation. He talked about how difficult Amy could be to care for and alluded to her verbal and physical aggression towards staff. There was an implicit suggestion that staff were doing their best in caring for someone who frequently did not appreciate their efforts. Amy's husband seemed to be embarrassed by her behaviour and to feel some sense of responsibility for it. The impression was that he felt she received the care that she deserved. He seemed wholly preoccupied with her discharge plans, particularly the financial implications of any decisions that were made.

During various discussions amongst the multi-disciplinary team it was thought that Amy's husband was very unlikely to be able to cope with her at home any more. His health was deteriorating and Amy was becoming more and more reliant on home care and respite care. Amy's community social worker had indicated that there were problems with home care and that night cover could not be provided. Amy's husband had been providing a high level of direct care for her whilst they were at home. He talked about the burden of this and the detrimental effect it was having on his well being. He described his absolute exhaustion as her disturbed sleep pattern gradually worsened. He seemed enormously relieved to abdicate responsibility for her direct care whilst Amy was in hospital.

The ward doctor talked to Amy's husband about the possibility of residential care. Her husband recounted this conversation saying "*she'll never recover sufficiently for me to look after her not in, that's what the doctor said, he advised me to get her into a home, two doctors, my doctor and the ward doctor. I don't want her to start thinking about coming home* **cos she's not**, *it's impossible*".

Amy's husband seemed to derive comfort and validation from the fact that the decision was doctor driven. His overwhelming concern seemed to be about finances, "*I'll have to have some sort of financial assessment presumably, let's hope they're not too hard on us*". Having made the decision that Amy should go into a home her husband gradually receded from the story. He visited her less frequently as his own condition declined.

As soon as the decision to look for a residential placement was agreed Amy was referred to a hospital social work care manager. At this stage Amy's daughter arrived on the scene. She was a lady who lived many miles away and cared for her disabled husband. She planned to stay for a week to sort everything out. She met with the nursing staff and forcefully expressed her dissatisfaction with some aspects of Amy's care, particularly the state of her clothes. She told the nurse that the ward was a "*stinking place*". Amy's daughter visited her solicitor and arranged power of attorney. She then met with the care manager who contacted the brokerage service for details of available placements. The daughter visited these homes and deemed them unsuitable. She rang round many homes locally and visited them until she found one that met her requirements which included a Christian ethos and accessibility for Amy's husband. She arranged for the home manager to visit Amy and he agreed to her transfer. Initially social services refused to fund the home that had been chosen. After much fraught negotiation a compromise was agreed which involved the payment of top up fees. Amy's daughter returned to her own home and several days later Amy was taken by ambulance to her new home, she seemed unaware of what was happening. Two days later she returned to hospital having fallen and fractured her other hip.

Ben's Narrative

Introduction

Ben was admitted as an emergency with a chest infection and inability to cope at home. His stay in hospital lasted for three and a half weeks and ended with his transfer to a residential home.

The Person

Ben was a ninety three year old man who had been admitted primarily because he was no longer able to cope at home. His package of care to support him at home had broken down due to his increasingly challenging behaviour. He also had a chest infection. He had had several previous admissions the last being approximately five months before. His most recent mini mental examination score was 1. Ben lived in his own house and had been receiving home care three times a day, seven days a week, to attend to his personal hygiene, nutrition and medication needs. Ben's only family was his daughter who lived many miles away. She had a child of her own who had special needs and required considerable care. This made it difficult for her to visit Ben and her visits were very infrequent.

The first time I met Ben he was sitting in an armchair by his bed in a six bedded bay on Freshwater Ward. He was wearing hospital pyjamas with the logo of the laundry service emblazoned across them, the top was green and the trousers bright orange. With his pyjamas Ben was wearing dark socks and black lace up shoes, an incongruous looking outfit. He was wearing large, very dirty glasses. Ben was sitting staring into space; he seemed totally detached from his surroundings. He gave an immediate impression of being a quiet, private man. Ben had a bed table in front of him with a drink and some tissues on it. Beside him was a Zimmer frame. Ben's speech was virtually inaudible and he spoke only when conversation was initiated by others. He was able to tell me very little about himself but as time passed he did reveal a little about himself. He told me that he used to teach Divinity. One of the few possessions that Ben had was a copy of Psalm 23 which his daughter had sent him. He recited it fluently and said that he looked forward to putting it up on his wall at home.

During our conversations it became clear that Ben was thinking about the future and what it might hold for him. He said to me *"don't know what's happening to me .... do I stay here forever? .... people never look and they never speak, the doctors and that they come in, there's a reason for it but it's not very satisfying"*. When Ben talked about the time he had spent on Freshwater he described things being very dark, he didn't know exactly what but knew it was black. He said "*not exactly happy is life you know*". After a long pause Ben spoke again, *suddenly his face crumples he talks about being brave and unpleasant, someone being angry. "I don't know, I'm not sure about it here", his face crumples again.* Later he described his experiences further *"what happens, nothing much, but you don't expect much, no reference to the so called doctor"*. I asked Ben if the ward was a good place to be, he told me "*it's horrible sometimes, the feeling's horrible, for one thing they change their ideas"*. I asked if it was difficult when people changed their ideas, Ben responded *"yes, it's a bit horrifying some of these things are"*. Ben appeared to spend some time sitting and thinking about his future. When we first met he talked about going home but gradually over the weeks this talk diminished and he seemed to lose sight of this goal.

Ben's capacity to meet his own activity of daily living needs was severely curtailed by both his dementia and his acute health problems. Ben was able to eat and drink independently; he did need to be prompted. Physically, he was able to wash himself but did not do this unless he was guided through each stage of the process. He was consistently incontinent of urine and occasionally incontinent of faeces. Ben walked with the aid of a Zimmer frame, he had a very unsteady gait and had fallen both before and during this admission. He had no ability to take his medication as prescribed. His sleep pattern was severely disrupted and he spent much of the night awake. He communicated with difficulty especially when he was approached suddenly and with too many choices at once. When given sufficient time he was sometimes able to communicate thoughtful ideas that gave some insight into what he was thinking.

The Cultural Context

Ben was in a bay with five other men all of whom looked old, frail and unwell. The room felt small, gloomy and rather cramped. The view out of the window was of other hospital buildings. The four walls of the bay seemed to be the limit of the patients' horizons. Ben had very few possessions with him. He used hospital wash things, the clothes in which he was admitted remained in his locker other than his shoes. There was an absolute lack of interaction between patients in the bay, they simply did not speak to each other. The bay was a hive of activity in the mornings as patients were helped to have a wash. Much of the therapy and medical care was delivered in the morning and the bay was visited by a group of phlebotomists. At the end of the bustle of activity in the morning the patients had lunch. After this there was a quiet time and the bay often remained peaceful for the rest of the day as few patients received many visitors.

The Plan

The plan for Ben's care was to treat his chest infection and assist him to meet his day to day activity of daily living needs. A major element of Ben's care was to expedite his discharge to a suitable setting. His chest infection responded quickly to a course of antibiotics and after a week he was declared medically fit for discharge.

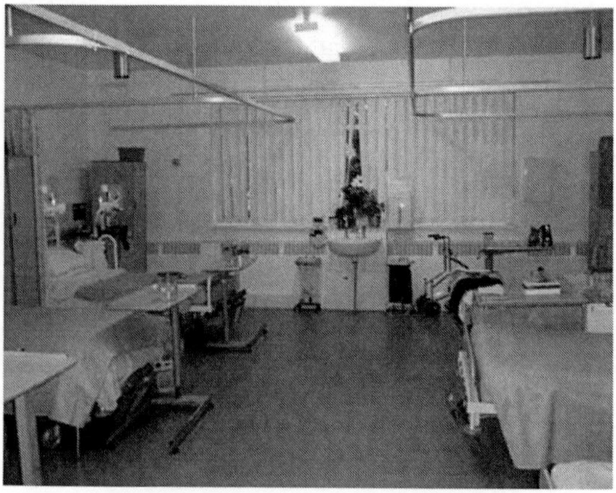

The Enactment of the Plan

On admission Ben was unkempt and unshaven, his clothes smelt strongly of urine. A nursing assistant gave Ben a bath soon after his arrival on the ward. *"I'd say once he'd had a bath and a hair wash, his nails had been done, his feet had been soaked, he had proper shoes and socks on, and clothes, the jumper with the 'kerchief ... he looked dapper, he did look dapper though. He looked lovely and when he smiled it sort of reached his eyes as well, he was, it was a true smile he was giving you".*

Ben was helped to wash each morning. A nursing assistant gathered up Ben's wash things and some clean pyjamas, she issued a list of short instructions which Ben complied with. After a few minutes a registered nurse went behind the curtains and asked if he could take over Ben's wash so the nursing assistant could go to coffee. The nurse reported bluntly that she had *"done the bottom half but not the top"*. Neither of them talked to Ben. As the registered nurse continued to wash Ben another nursing assistant and a student nurse entered the bay and walked in behind

Ben's curtains. The registered nurse sent them off with a list of jobs to do in another bay. A few moments later the student nurse returned, the nursing assistant then reappeared. Both went behind Ben's curtains with no warning. The patient in the next bed pulled back Ben's curtains to see what was going on. The nursing assistant told him very sharply to stop looking. Throughout his wash Ben and the nurse both spoke but didn't actually respond to each other. *"You're very good at doing that"* said Ben referring to the nurse tying his shoelaces, the nurse responded *"I'll just clean your glasses"*. When Ben had been washed the nurse tidied up the area, checked Ben was warm enough and gave him a drink. Ben looked clean and tidy but appallingly sad and worried.

On another occasion Ben was incontinent of urine and needed to have a wash and some dry trousers. Two nursing assistants came to help him. They tutted audibly as they approached him. One commented that Ben was not 'their' patient as they were working in another bay. They gathered the necessary equipment grudgingly and pulled the curtains around Ben's bed. At first they did not communicate with him at all. They began the process giving Ben some instructions *"put your leg in, point your toes, put your foot on the floor, stand up"*. These instructions were delivered rapidly one after another *"Ben stand up tall like a soldier, stand still or you'll fall over"*. The task was performed quickly and mechanistically. Ben's incontinence became an increasing issue with the nursing staff who reported that he had passed urine into his supper and into a clinical waste bag. One recounted with amusement the fact that Ben dismantled the radiator in the bay during the night and passed urine into it. One morning the curtains were partially around Ben's bed. I noticed he had a cardboard urinal in his hand. A moment or two later he emerged from the curtains with his trousers soaked in urine, he walked through a small puddle on the floor. He leant on the linen skip which just started to move. A nursing assistant quickly stopped him and told him he needed to move back and sit in his chair. She guided him firmly and told him to sit down. She mopped up the puddle and then told Ben to stay in his chair until she came to help him wash. Ben said he was cold and she put a blanket around his knees. A little later a therapy assistant came into the bay and looked behind Ben's curtains, she asked if he was alright, she picked his blanket up off the floor and noticed his pyjamas were wet. She spoke to the nursing assistant who said to her that Ben missed the bottle and it went everywhere. She said "*I drew the short straw this morning"*, it was clear that she was finding the shift hard going. Ben was rearranging his bedclothes. The nurse went in to help him wash. She stripped all his bedclothes and put them in the linen skip. He said "*I'm not really used to this"* she didn't respond. She asked him to lift his bottom off the chair which he did. She left his bed space and returned with a matching set of pyjamas. She asked him to take off his pyjamas and gave him further short instructions which he complied with. She started to wash him. She spoke a little more gently, she said to him "*hang on*", he said "*hang on's not my name"*, the nurse grunted in response. It seemed that his incontinence was also a cause of concern to Ben as he communicated during one conversation. *He stops talking for a minute and then looks at me and says "could you just excuse me for a minute ... I need a piddle". I walk with him to the lavatory, he has a slow shuffling almost Parkinsonian gait. I tell him he's doing well walking, he says "do you really think so?" He comes back with soaking wet trousers and says he's so sorry. I tell him that the nurses will get him some dry trousers, he laughs very gently and pats my arm "thank you, you've really cheered me up". Suddenly his face creases and tears well up.*

As Ben's physical condition improved, plans for his discharge were made. Initially Ben was clear that he wanted to go home, this desire appeared to gradually diminish during his admission. This lessening of stated desire was the only active part that Ben played in the discharge process. There were several discharge meetings at which Ben was discussed. At one meeting attended by nursing staff, an occupational therapist and a care manager it was agreed that a decision needed to be made about whether or not Ben would be able to return to his own home. They agreed that Ben's case should be discussed again at a forthcoming case conference which was set up for when Ben's daughter returned from her holiday.

A case conference was booked for when all the involved parties were able to attend. The consultant, junior doctor, registered nurse and occupational therapist gathered. The occupational therapist announced that the community psychiatric nurse was not able to attend as he was on holiday. The social work care manager arrived and reported that she had just received a telephone call from Ben's daughter saying that she would not be able to attend but that she would be available by telephone. The daughter asked if Ben was attending the case conference. The doctor said that it would be too upsetting for Ben to attend as he was not able to make a decision, everyone nodded in agreement.

The meeting proceeded with each person giving their opinion about Ben's current condition and his future. The occupational therapist said that she initially felt that Ben was coping with his home circumstances but began to revise her views several days after his admission. "*The nursing staff were reporting that he was deteriorating, that he was becoming increasingly incontinent ...he'd just gone downhill and was really struggling maintaining safety on the ward let alone at home*". She reassessed him and found that his condition had deteriorated to the point that she thought it would distress him to repeat his cognitive assessments. She stated that his community psychiatric nurse had reviewed Ben and that he had "always *been adamant that the patient went home, and then when the CPN came in and reviewed him and said that he'd gone downhill considerably, and I knew then that my sort of inkling had been confirmed and that he wasn't coping as well as he had been when he was at home*". After extensive discussion the care manager summarised that Ben needed residential care for safety reasons. The doctor stated that this decision was made for "*more than safety reasons, it is a matter of acceptable risk*". Having concluded that Ben needed residential care the staff discussed his particular requirements. On a previous admission a member of staff had found that Ben enjoyed painting. This appeared to be the only 'personal' fact that was known about Ben. This notion was taken by other staff as being paramount in planning Ben's future care. When selecting a residential home one senior member of staff stated "*we tried to make sure that in the alternative solution there was as much, for as many of the issues that Ben had always felt were important went with him which was about having a nice view and being able to paint*". The idea was followed by a colleague "*that's when I said he would need to go somewhere that would allow him to paint because that was something that was obviously really important to him*". I noticed that in all the conversations I had with Ben he never mentioned painting and yet it seemed to have become his defining feature in the minds of some staff.

At the end of the case conference the doctor telephoned Ben's daughter, the doctor broke the news of the decision gently expecting the daughter to say that she wanted Ben to return home. The daughter said she had already been looking at homes near where she lived. They had a brief conversation in which the doctor justified the decision, the doctor then suggested that the daughter discussed placements with the care manger. The doctor closed by saying that there was a limit on how long Ben could stay in hospital awaiting placement.

The question of how the decision to seek placement should be communicated to Ben was discussed. The doctor reported that Ben was still saying that he wanted to go home from time to time. Today he asked very crossly on the ward round "*when am I going home?*", the doctor sidestepped the question. The occupational therapist and care manager suggested strongly that Ben should be informed, the occupational therapist stated "*we need to keep him in the loop, needs to know what is going on, it is him*". They agreed to go and talk to Ben and plant the idea that he will be moving on. They agreed with the doctor that at this stage they would put it in terms of a temporary move to be nearer his daughter. Ben seemed unmoved by the news he was given.

His daughter worked closely with the care manager to find a suitable residential home. A week later she found a home that would accept Ben. His daughter visited Ben with the care manager and told him a little about the home, she let the care manager do most of the talking.

Ben was transferred to a residential home a week after the case conference. A week later the home manager rang the ward to complain that Ben had had a difficult transition, he was extremely disturbed and having frequent aggressive outbursts. The manager thought he would have to move to another home as they could not manage him.

Eileen's Narrative

Introduction

Eileen was admitted to hospital from home. She had just returned to her home following a brief stay in respite care where her condition had deteriorated rapidly. Eileen remained on the ward for eight weeks until she moved to a residential placement.

The Person

Eileen lived in a bungalow with her husband who was her main carer. She had been diagnosed with dementia several years ago. Her condition had gradually deteriorated over the years but since being in respite care her decline had been dramatic. On admission Eileen's mini mental state examination score was 0. She attempted to communicate verbally but mostly only made incomprehensible sounds, occasionally she managed to articulate her thoughts. Eileen looked considerably younger that her eighty four years.

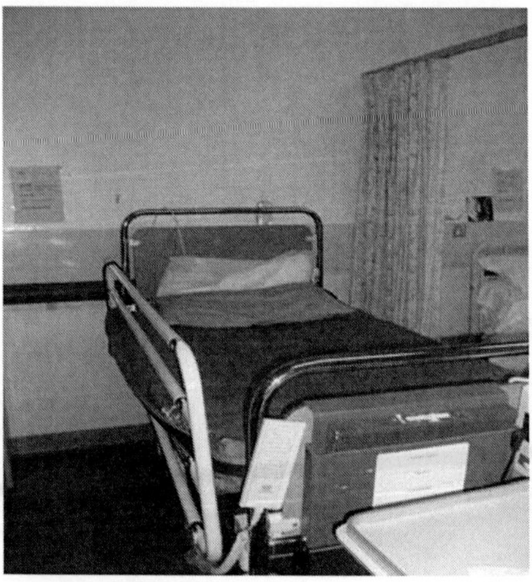

She had thick brown hair which was clearly regularly cared for, her skin was clear with few wrinkles. Her eyes were bright and alert much of the time, Eileen rarely made eye contact. Eileen always wore two ornate rings which looked slightly bizarre with her gaudy pink hospital nightdress. Prior to her admission Eileen's husband described her as being able to walk a few steps with assistance although he did acknowledge that it had been getting gradually more difficult for her to get out of the chair. On admission to hospital Eileen was totally immobile. She had gross leg oedema and a large pressure sore on one heel and was physically very weak. She needed to be prompted frequently to eat and drink and often needed assistance. Eileen was doubly incontinent as she had been for some time at home.

The Cultural Context

Eileen was nursed in a four bedded bay on Ventnor ward. Her bed space was very much her own as her husband had bought in a number of her own possessions including clothes, toiletries, magazines and a range of drinks and chocolates. Eileen was placed by the window; she was nursed on an air bed the position of which could be adjusted automatically. The bed had integral side rails and appeared high even when lowered. Her bed looked in a perpetual state of disarray as Eileen tended to spend a lot of time tugging at and then folding the sheets and blankets. Eileen was copiously incontinent and her sheets frequently needed changing.

The three other ladies in the bay were extremely unwell and there was virtually no interaction between patients. Eileen's husband visited each day. He arrived the moment visiting was allowed and left at the last possible minute. Each day he brought in some chocolate for Eileen and often a new magazine which they sat and looked at together. The white board above Eileen's bed had comprehensive instructions about her care scrawled on it in several colours.

The Plan

On admission Eileen was diagnosed with swollen legs, possibly due to cardiac problems, a urinary tract infection and immobility. The plan was to treat the cardiac problems medically, to give antibiotics for the infection and to rehabilitate Eileen prior to her return home possibly with an increased package of care.

The Enactment of the Plan

It was clear that Eileen had quite complex medical problems. She was suffering with a cardiac arrhythmia and had become severely overloaded with fluid. These problems were treated with medication but were slow to respond. Her treatment was regularly reviewed. Her lower legs remained swollen until discharge. Her urinary infection rapidly resolved with a course of antibiotics. It was not clear why Eileen had suddenly become so immobile. It was felt that her general weakness and swollen legs were contributing factors but did not offer a full explanation. It was suggested by some of the staff that perhaps Eileen's husband had a slightly optimistic view of her previous abilities. Her husband reported that he "*was persuaded by family and a* lot of others *to have a respite*". From the way he spoke it was evident that he had come to bitterly regret this decision. When asked about the care that Eileen was now receiving her husband was initially complimentary saying "*I like this ward, the equipment, everything is* perfect *as far as I can see. I think they're wonderful"*. As Eileen's stay in hospital continued her husband became dissatisfied with some aspects of her care.

Eileen was regularly reviewed by the medical team. The doctor arrived to do his ward round. He stood at the end of Eileen's bed and said it was nice to see her, he waved, he did not wait for a response.

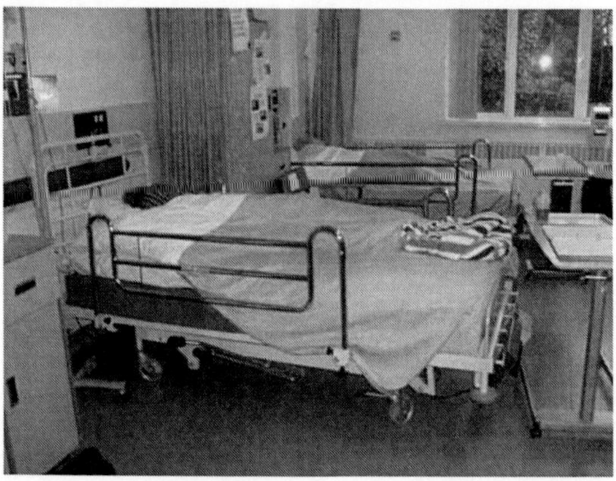

He asked the nurse about Eileen's pressure sores and inquired whether she was managing to eat and drink. The nurse responded that Eileen needed help to eat and drink, the doctor replied "*so it doesn't matter that she can't reach her drink?*", he pointed to the bed table which was some distance away. As Eileen's acute medical problems began to be controlled her care focused on trying to regain enough mobility to allow her to be cared for at home. She was assessed by a physiotherapist who concluded that Eileen had some automatic functions but that she needed to be given very short instructions. The physiotherapist saw Eileen each weekday and attempted to get her to walk. Her abilities appeared to be declining, a situation which her husband found very hard to accept. He expressed his dissatisfaction with the input of the physiotherapists saying "*she came in ten days ago and she's had one session where she's walked with the help of nurses. Since then she hasn't walked, they haven't got her up to walk despite the fact that on three days ago the doctor in my presence distinctly said to the staff nurse, she can walk tomorrow*". He continues stating "*the bank holiday has come upon us and* nothing really has happened. *The physiotherapy people are not around. I've been very concerned about that so I went to the main desk one day during this weekend and er, asked if I could talk to the physiotherapy people and they said well unfortunately they're all on bank holiday. So I am* very concerned *that they haven't walked her*". Her husband acknowledges that it is a bank holiday weekend but goes on to say "*but there's always* **something** *that* stops it *for some reason*".

He seemed to find his inability to influence Eileen's care unbearably frustrating "*I even said in the early stages give me half an hour's notice on the telephone, I'll come down and* I'll get her up, *or out of bed or whatever it is*".

The nursing staff initially tried to mobilise Eileen. They followed the instructions on the board above her bed which stated that she could walk up to thirty metres with two people or two people and a Zimmer frame. It stated that she needed a lot of help to get from sitting to standing. The nurses own assessments of Eileen's abilities were less positive in terms of her mobility. It also transpired that they sometimes found Eileen difficult to manage especially when she became aggressive. A registered nurse explained that she was waiting for three or four nurses to be available before she attempted to wash Eileen. She said that sometimes Eileen hit them, particularly when people didn't explain what they were doing and she got scared. The nurse justified having so many people saying "*might be a bit intimidating for her but it's safer for us*". Whilst she was waiting for the other staff to come and wash Eileen the nursing assistant offered her a cup of tea saying "*oh nice*". Eileen responded "*we won't get another one*", "*you will do later*" said the nurse. She then continued "yes*, you have it really, yes you do, drink your tea, you were thirsty weren't you? Staff nurse will be pleased with you, you've drunk a whole cup of tea, you are* *good*". This was all said in the type of voice that might be used when talking to a small child. A registered nurse stood by Eileen's bed and called loudly to a nursing assistant "*are you able to help us with Eileen, then we can crack on with her?*". Three nurses gathered to wash Eileen. A nursing assistant called loudly "*do you know how wet this lady is? She's saturated*". They stood around Eileen's bed and discussed catheterising her but decided she'd pull a catheter out. The registered nurse said "*shall we give her a bath? It would be easier we could hoist her into the bath chair*". A nursing assistant said in a baby voice "*you're going to have a nice bath Eileen*". The registered nurse returned "*we're going to bath you Eileen*" to which Eileen responded "*I didn't know*". The nurse said "*you didn't know, well we're going to*". The nurse went to touch Eileen who said "don't, don't". The nurse explained what she needed to do and Eileen said "*it hurts, it hurts, I hurt*". The registered nurse suddenly shouted "and up, and around". Eileen landed in the chair; she was wheeled unceremoniously to the bathroom with her nightdress just about covering her modesty. The registered nurse went into the bathroom and yelled at Eileen to stand "*and up*" and then "and down". Eileen sounded increasingly distressed. When her bath and hair wash were completed Eileen was wheeled back to her bedside. The nursing assistant called to her colleague "*are we pad and panting?*", "*yeah*" replied the registered nurse. Her pants were put on with the curtains only partly around. Despite it being a bank holiday a physiotherapist arrived to see Eileen. She went to assist with Eileen's transfer to her chair. The nurse and physiotherapist bombarded her with instructions. They were not succeeding "*come on, come on Eileen, come on, come on*", Eileen yelled out but eventually moved. A nursing assistant told Eileen that she was going to dry her hair, Eileen answered "*it's getting drier*", there was no response to this comment. This nurse recounted how pleased she was that Eileen had had a bath and that she now looked clean and cared for. She speculated about what Eileen used to be like, the nurse believed she must have been very polite because she said excuse me when she coughed during a meal. The nurse heard Eileen say 'bible' so she thought that she may have a religion. She wondered if Eileen was a teacher because she seemed like someone who was used to being in authority.

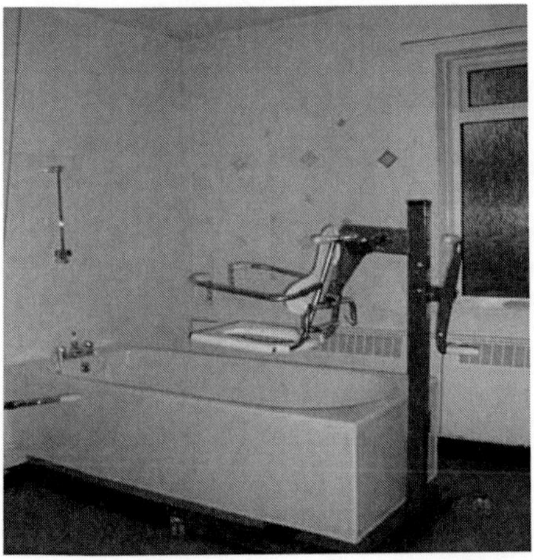

Eileen was helped to wash each day. It was an experience that regularly seemed to cause her some distress. A student nurse went to wash Eileen. She spoke to her in a normal voice. "*Will you dance with me?*", "*dance with you?*" "*I'm going to put the towel over you*". She talked quietly to Eileen and explained each bit of what she was doing. The nursing assistant joined the student behind the curtains, the student told her what she had washed already. "*I just need to give you a little wash down below*". The nurse said "*we need to lie her flat and roll her, that's what we normally do*". Eileen began to sound distressed "*no, please don't*". The nurse said "*you're wet we need to change you*", Eileen responded "*don't do it darling please, don't do that its bavvy, why are you washing your wash?*" The nurses continued washing; one said they needed to get the senior nurse to look at her heel. Eileen resisted slightly "*Eileen we need to dry you*". The nurse said "*I don't know why she's in bed*", she came out from behind the curtains and asked the registered nurse if she knew why Eileen was in bed, "*because she was falling out of the chair*". The nurse asked for help to change Eileen's sheets. The three nurses talked and giggled for a minute and then told Eileen they needed to change her bed. "*No, no, no*" she responded. They discussed the pros and cons of getting out of bed and decided to leave Eileen in bed until lunch time and then get her out and change the sheets. "*No you don't switch into there*", "*nice big puddle*" said the nursing assistant; they put an incontinence pad under Eileen's leaking heel. The wash was rapidly accomplished.

The balance between encouraging mobility and safety was becoming problematic for all involved in Eileen's care. The physiotherapist had amended her whiteboard to read 'please ↑ frequency of walks + help with initial sit to stand, try with blue belt'. The nursing staff assessed Eileen prior to each transfer, sometimes she managed with two people but she generally needed a hoist. A registered nurse acknowledged that Eileen's mobility was better with her husband's guidance. Eileen did not like being hoisted. A nursing assistant arrived at Eileen's bedside with a hoist *"we're just going to put you back into bed*" she said in a baby voice, "*pop your hands across your chest"*. They put a sling behind Eileen and moved the hoist into place, "*give yourself a cuddle darling*", the nurses moved quickly, "*oh this hurts*" said Eileen. The nurses laughed quietly amongst themselves although this seemed unrelated to Eileen, "*oh deary dear oh dear*" she said. Eileen's husband seemed unsurprised that she didn't like the hoist "*I can understand that because it's a frightening looking thing, like a small fork lift truck"*. He expressed some frustration about the fact that the nursing staff seemed to be using the hoist more and more and not working on Eileen's mobility. He explained "here *if she resists and even wants to bite them or whatever then they just back away, they say they're not* allowed *to do this or not allowed to do that. I can understand that but I feel that in the old fashioned days the sister and all the nurses would just have got hold of her firmly and done what they had to do like I have to do at home, but now they're frightened of being sued or whatever*". He said that he had found that there had been a "*resistance* to getting a grip of things" and "*that they've got this attitude is quite annoying in everything they do*". He went on to recognise other aspects of care "*otherwise I think they're wonderful. It's not a nice job or an easy job*". On occasion Eileen attempted to voice her own feelings. Whilst being washed Eileen became overtly distressed as she struggled to say "*it's very hard now*" she looked sad "*domey, domey, domey, dome, grope the grope, it's very hard, it's terrible*". This utterance was completely ignored. Eileen's attempts to communicate gradually diminished.

The uncertainty about Eileen's future was discussed at a multi-disciplinary team meeting attended by medical, nursing and therapy staff. The plan of Eileen's care appeared vague, several staff reported on conversations they had had with her husband, each offered a slightly different interpretation. Her husband appeared quite clear about his thoughts "if she can walk again, *even with me just holding her then I can continue to look after her. If that's not going to be possible then I don't see* quite *how I can manage*". The occupational therapist suggested that there was a need to have a clear pathway for Eileen's care as her husband and the staff needed to know what they were aiming for. She said that at the moment it was not clear whether they were aiming for mobility or safe hoist transfers. The physiotherapist said that Eileen's mobility was now as good as it was going to get but that it had been suggested to her husband that it may improve once she is back in her own home. Eileen's husband had told some staff that he could only manage Eileen at home if she was mobile, others stated that he wanted her home regardless. He had voiced concerns about residential care "*then of course the last option is for her to go into a nursing home which I am hoping won't happen for two reasons, one is the expense of it and the other is that ..... I, I've experienced being at home on my own and it's not very nice [voice cracks]*". The conclusion of the multi-disciplinary team meeting was that they should aim to discharge Eileen home with a big package of care and a hoist. The nursing and therapy staff felt that Eileen's husband was unrealistic about her scope for recovery but that he should be left with some hope.

The occupational therapist planned to assess Eileen's transfers and complete a site visit to her home. Following these assessments and discussions with her husband it was concluded that Eileen needed too high a level of care to return home. Eileen was referred to a social worker who found a vacancy at a suitable residential home. Eileen's husband did not want her to go to this home. He found one he preferred and that was nearer to their home but at present this home had no capacity to take Eileen. Eileen was rapidly transferred to the first home on the agreement that she would move to her husband's preferred location as soon as a vacancy arose.

Dora's Narrative

Introduction

Dora arrived in hospital as an emergency admission from her residential home. She had a urinary tract infection as a result of which she had become very agitated and volatile. The carers in her home had become unable to cope with Dora's behaviour. She spent five weeks on the ward prior to transfer to a specialist older people's psychiatric unit.

The Person

Dora was a person who was very alone in the world, a fact which she seemed to feel keenly. She had been living in a residential home for two years. She had a daughter with whom she had no contact and an old neighbour who visited her once whilst she was in hospital. Dora was a very communicative person, she particularly enjoyed talking to men and would always mention if a doctor or clergyman had visited her. She was remarkably accurate in knowing who she had seen. Dora talked a lot about her family; her husband had died many years ago. She regularly said that he had been a good Catholic, the church was a common topic of conversation for her.

Dora was ninety two years old. It was unclear when she had been diagnosed with Alzheimer's disease. Dora's latest mini mental state examination score was 0. This was not congruent with her obvious insight into much of what was going on around her. She was a slim lady with a mass of curly white hair, faded blue eyes and a set of slightly loose dentures. Dora wore her own clothes when she first came into hospital but after a short time seemed to lose the desire to get dressed. She was mobile with a zimmer frame and walked up and down the ward corridor particularly when she was feeling unsettled.

The Cultural Context

Dora was cared for in a side room on Ventnor ward. The furniture had been moved around to meet her needs. The bed was against the wall as she preferred this. Dora mostly sat in an armchair at the doorway of the room so that she could see what was happening on the ward. She didn't like sitting in the room as it was quite dark and the only view was of other parts of the hospital building. She had a television but said that she wasn't much interested in watching it. Dora had quite a few of her own belongings with her including multiple tubes of denture cleaner which she frequently rearranged. She had one get well card which she kept on her bed table, she was unsure who had sent it to her but she looked at it and admired it frequently. Dora had a small collection of her own clothes.

Dora watched the work of the ward and sometimes commented on what she saw. "*The nurse and that do come round, they get a bit browned off with it, you can tell they do*" she said "*they take on a load of like nurses, see 'em once, you don't see 'em no more*". Dora avidly watched a lady who was in the bay opposite her room. As the nurses struggled with the lady Dora commented "*gotta put them somewhere haven't they?*" She told me the lady "*kicked up*"yesterday as well. Dora said she wouldn't like to be a nurse as it tires you. She said she had worked as a nurse in the past. She commented on the care she saw now "*they don't do it properly now, nah [fiercely], don't do it like they done it years ago. They don't care, they don't care if they do it or if they don't do it, they don't do it, sometimes it's terrible. I don't know how they get away with it*". Dora sometimes seemed to find the ward disturbing. She disliked interactions that she believed were unfriendly. She commented about a relatively peaceful ward round "*just before lunch there was a going on about something, I don't know what it was. I wasn't involved in it but they were quarrelling*". She said later "*always someone quarrelling, arguing, you'll never win like that*".

The Plan

Dora was initially admitted with a urinary tract infection. The plan was to treat the infection and for Dora to return to her residential home.

The Enactment of the Plan

On admission Dora was disturbed and agitated. She was unable to settle on the ward and spent much time walking up and down the corridor banging her zimmer frame loudly on the floor and shouting. Her behaviour deteriorated in the latter part of each day. On occasion she attempted to barricade herself into her side room. If approached by staff she swore vociferously and attempted to bite them. Dora was treated with a course of oral antibiotics, this was successful in managing her infection. Her behaviour calmed slightly but she remained feisty. As soon as her infection resolved Dora was declared medically fit for discharge. The nursing staff telephoned the home to plan her transfer. The home informed the staff that they were not willing for Dora to return as the carers had threatened to walk out if she came back as they could not tolerate or manage her behaviour. The home had a mixture of general and elderly mentally ill (EMI) places. The ward staff suggested that Dora could move to one of the EMI places but the home refused to have Dora back under any circumstances. This decision effectively rendered Dora homeless. The multi- disciplinary team (MDT) decided that Dora should move to an alternative EMI placement as soon as a vacancy arose. The allocated social worker agreed to seek an appropriate placement.

Whilst awaiting placement Dora remained on the ward. She continued to be agitated and aggressive on occasion. Dora said that she was very fed up and didn't know what to do, she wanted to go home to her own place and stay there. She said she didn't much like being in hospital "*it gets you down, it do, it really gets yer*", "*oh I don't know I'm sure, just before lunch I felt terrible, nobody come to you and said to you what's the matter or nothing ... they didn't care, so long as they come in and you see 'em, you see 'em and they see you, that's all that matters*". Dora regularly expressed concern about not knowing what was going to happen to her "*you don't know where they're going to put yer, you're never,* every day *it's change which is wrong*".

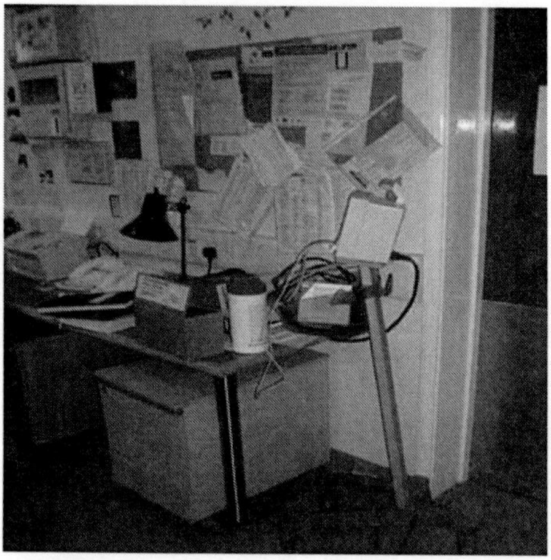

One morning I arrived on the ward to find Dora sitting at the nurses' station. She told me she was very fed up, she had been there since seven o'clock. She looked up at the clock and said it was eight o'clock now. She said that no-one told her what to do "*it's awful isn't it?*" She had a quick look at a medical textbook and then said she had to go down to the shopping centre to get the bus. Two nursing assistants talked about Dora expressing empathy with her situation. They were unclear about whether anyone had spoken to her about a plan, they said that one of the things that Dora often voiced was that she didn't know what was going to happen. They agreed that they would feel frightened if they didn't know what was happening to them. They felt that this underlying fear may contribute to some of Dora's challenging behaviour. One said "*how can you be* warm *with people when you don't know what's going to happen to you*?"

The nursing assistants who regularly cared for Dora said they had got to know her and that she felt safe with them. They talked about how they provided care that minimised Dora's agitation. One nurse explained that she just gave the care that Dora would tolerate. If she refused a wash at a particular time the nurse would not push the issue as this would "*just wind Dora up and increase her aggression*". The nurse said she would just return to Dora later and try again. She was clear that she felt under no pressure from registered nurses to give care that Dora would not agree to.

Dora's aggressive outbursts continued at differing levels throughout her stay, the way in which these were managed varied among staff. One morning Dora threatened to throw her breakfast at a nursing assistant, the nurse spoke calmly to Dora saying gently "*no, don't do that*". Dora put the bowl down and ate her cereal. Although the nurse sounded calm she

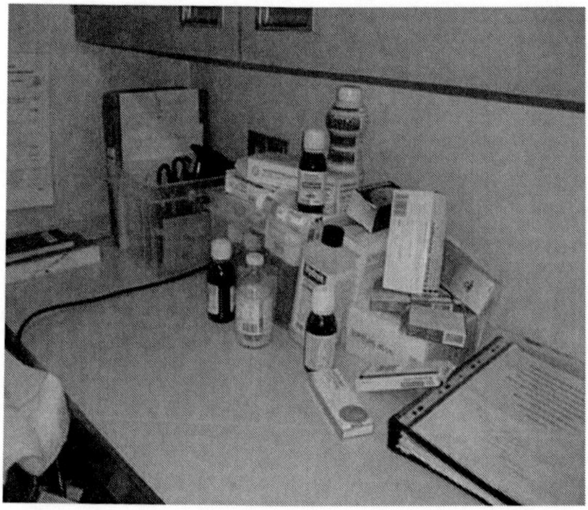

looked anxious, her colleague stood close behind Dora seemingly to protect the nurse if Dora did become more aggressive. The situation was quickly and effectively diffused. When talking to the nursing assistants they were clear that Dora's behaviour did not concern them. One nurse said that she didn't feel much when Dora was aggressive. Her colleagues said that they were used to aggression and that it didn't frighten them, one stated "*you just cope don't you?*" The permanent nursing staff on the ward had a clear strategy for managing Dora's outbursts "*if she wants to go a certain way and she's wandering, she's* wandering *and you're not going to stop her, she will bite, she will shake with anger*". The nurse said that when this happened they left Dora alone.

Dora decided it was time to go downstairs. A nursing assistant said over Dora "*oh she's up to that again*". Dora became a little agitated, the nurse remained calm and gentle. Dora got more cross and said she was going home. The nurse tried to guide her towards her room but she got more cross and banged the Zimmer frame. She was left to walk to the end of the ward, she called out "*where have I got to go? Where are you?*" She called out "*yoohoo*" the domestic answered and she went up to Dora who asked her to take her downstairs. She said she couldn't and offered her a cup of tea. Dora starts to shout how terrible it was. Dora wandered down the ward and met another nursing assistant who suggested she had a wash and a cup of tea. Dora shouted that she wanted to get downstairs. The nurse walked away for a moment and then returned to offer Dora a cup of tea. Dora said she wanted to go downstairs and have a wash. The nurse said she could give her a wash. Dora started to shout "*leave me alone, this is terrible, it's wicked to treat people like it*". The nurse guided Dora back to her room. Dora complained she needed to go to the lavatory; she had been to each lavatory in turn over the last hour or so.

The nurse mentioned this to the senior nurse who offered Dora some medicine for her bowels; they stood in the corridor and helped Dora to take her medication. Dora headed for the staff lavatory. She said "*it's terrible here, they're not doing what they're meant to do*". The senior nurse spoke to another nurse about sorting Dora's bowels with an enema or suppositories as she thought the discomfort was agitating her. The nurse reported back that she had just retrieved some net knickers from the staff loo, there was also a bowel motion so no need for an enema. Dora walked up and down the ward peacefully and unhindered. Eventually a nurse brought Dora back to her room, she shouted "*they don't care, I don't know what to do, my legs and my back they're terrible*".

The nursing staff expressed sadness at Dora's situation. They strove to maintain some sort of normality for her. They were very aware of her disrupted sleep pattern saying "*we try, we try and keep her awake during the day and get her into a proper sleep pattern again*". They likened Dora's disrupted sleep to how they felt when working night duty and suggested that this may contribute to her agitation. The nursing staff felt that Dora was very bored on the ward "*she needs a job"*. They had enabled her to do some tidying at the nurses' station but thought she would be much better in a home where she could be involved in more consistent activity. As her stay progressed Dora became more subdued, as she went to the bathroom one morning I note *Dora stops in her journey, she looks utterly exhausted*. Dora said she felt tired and funny this morning, she was not sure what kind of funny it was but said that you often do feel funny in the morning at her age.

Dora's days passed in a haze of uncertainty for her, she frequently voiced her concerns about her future. She was regularly reviewed on the medical ward rounds although she was not convinced of this saying "*and the doctor do come round when he think he will, it's terrible really*". The senior doctor went into Dora's room and said good morning to her, they shook hands. He told her that she looked well and said it was nice to see her. He exited before Dora had spoken. On hearing the news that Dora was now homeless the doctor was not happy. He discussed Dora with the senior nurse; he was keen to increase her antipsychotic medication to try to control her behaviour. The nurse indicated that Dora had previously become drowsy with this medication so they agreed to restart it at a reduced dose. The doctor asked about Dora's psychiatric care, the nurse reported that the community psychiatric nurse (CPN) had stated that she did not need to see Dora whilst she was an in-patient. The doctor was incensed by this information stating that it "*beggars belief"*. He described Dora as "*a wandering dement who is aggressive and difficult*". He said she needed to be transferred to a psychiatric in-patient unit as she had no physical health problems and needed a review of her psychiatric medication. The nurse asked the doctor if he would refer Dora to the psychiatric team, he refused stating that it was a management problem. At the next MDT meeting it was clear that no progress had been made with transferring Dora's care. The doctor restated that it was a management problem. A discharge co-ordinator offered to ring the matron of the EMI ward to try and expedite transfer. The doctor stated that Dora was not safe here and that the staff were not safe looking after her, she needed to be "*shifted*". During the next ward round the doctor explained Dora's case to a medical student. He said that Dora was admitted from a rest home where she had been aggressive and hitting staff. She had become delirious due to a UTI and it was appropriate that she was in hospital. Now she was physically recovered and needed psychiatric assessment, he said it was not acceptable that the psychiatrists seemed not to want to take over her care so they could 'fiddle' with her complex medication needs. The discharge co-ordinator spoke to the psychiatrist's secretary who said she wasn't sure that they want a 'social' admission. After more than a week of prevaricating about who was responsible for referring Dora to the psychiatric team the doctor eventually decided to make the referral himself. He telephoned the psychiatrist who visited Dora the following day and agreed that she should be transferred for psychiatric in-patient assessment prior to long term placement. A bed became available two days later and Dora was transferred. She had no preparation for this move as no-one had told her the plan.

Discussion

This discussion draws together individual stories that have been captured during data collection. Although each person had their own unique story there were commonalities across a number of experiences. Findings are set within the context of existing literature and the broader social and political milieu.

At present exceptionally little is known about the experience of people with dementia in acute hospitals. Literature about carers in this setting is also relatively sparse. Data indicates that older people with dementia found being in hospital a difficult experience. Their days were long, punctuated mainly by brief interludes in which essential activities were completed. Those who were able to articulate their thoughts generally described their admission in relatively negative terms. Observation demonstrated that other participants found the delivery of care stressful and traumatic on occasions. On the whole, care was delivered according to ward routine with little attention being paid to the desires of individuals.

Attempts by patients to communicate were not always supported and were, relatively frequently, totally ignored. Lack of recognition by staff of these participants as people with their own biographies and range of human needs had a major impact on their perception of hospitalisation. These findings are considered in relation to the general literature concerning the care of people with dementia and the small body of work that has investigated the experiences of people with dementia in institutional settings.

In order to set this work within the current context of dementia care, a brief review of current approaches to care is provided. General literature broadly divides dementia care into two camps "old culture" and "new culture". The two cultures are briefly explored and the extent to which each was experienced by the participants is discussed below. "Old culture" is based very much on the biomedical model with an underlying philosophy of "no cure, no hope". This negative mindset and assumption of futility in caring for people with dementia is congruent with wider societal attitudes. The society in which we live tends to view old age negatively and place a premium on high levels of cognitive function (Post 1995). Therefore people who are both older and have impaired cognition can become stigmatised (Goffman 1974) and, at the extreme be categorised as non-people (Dewing 1999). Belief that people with dementia are "empty shells" (Moore and Hollett 2003) with no capacity to participate in their care typifies the "old culture" philosophy.

Kitwood and Benson's seminal work (1995) heralded the development of the "new culture" of dementia care. It was Kitwood's belief that the individual's experience of dementia could not be explained by neuropathological changes alone. He argued that the experience is influenced by a combination of neuropathology and external influences. Kitwood stated that the approach that other people have towards the person with dementia has a major impact on the person's experience of the condition. He describes negative interactions with others as malignant social psychology (MSP), he delineates seventeen different elements of MSP. This type of interaction gradually undermines the individual. Kitwood (1997a) is clear that the term malignant does not imply that those delivering care are bad, he stresses that much care is delivered kindly and with good intention. The malign element is a result of our cultural heritage rather than any ill intent on the part of individuals.

Preserving personhood is the focus of the "new culture" of dementia care. Personhood is defined as:

> "a standing or status that is bestowed on one person by others, in the context of relationship and social being. It implies recognition, respect and

trust. Both the according of personhood and the failure to do so, have consequences that are empirically testable" (Kitwood 1997a:8).

Whilst Kitwood is clear that it is possible to test the extent to which actions of others impact on the personhood of individuals it is suggested that in practice this effect is difficult to discern with absolute certainty. The speed with which some patients move through acute hospitals and the number of staff with whom they come into contact would make such judgements complex and potentially unreliable.

Whilst it is acknowledged that measurement of this preservation of personhood is challenging, it may be suggested that care that is based on person-centred models should enable the personhood of individuals to be protected and possibly enhanced. Packer (2000a) states that person-centred care has long been embraced in the philosophy of dementia care. However this author provides a realistic perspective on the extent to which the philosophy is actually applied to practice. Packer (2000b) notes the growth industry in education and publications that espouse person-centred care but questions the extent to which this alters processes of care in the long term. It is acknowledged that, whilst the concept of person-centred care has been present for many years, it continues to lack a cohesive and consistent definition (Packer 2000b). It is considered that provision of truly person centred care, in whatever way it is defined, is likely to require considerable investment from everyone involved. It may also be a provocative undertaking (Packer 2000a).

Although an absolute definition of person-centred care remains elusive there are a wide range of models relating to the concept. Three of these that are particularly relevant to caring for people with dementia include positive person work Kitwood (1997a), communicative care (Vittoria 1998) and person-focused care (Cheston and Bender 2003). These models each take a slightly different approach but all attest to the centrality of the need to know the person, the necessity of communication that acknowledges the emotional or felt meaning and the requirement to work with rather than for people.

The extent to which the participants' experiences mirrored "old culture" and "new culture", person-centred care is explored in more detail below. Data are rich in examples of ways in which personhood is preserved and undermined. A range of examples of MSP are summarised in table 3-2. As can be seen it is difficult to separate each element and on occasion several different types of MSP can be seen within a brief interaction.

Table 3-2: Examples of Malignant Social Psychology

Element(s) of MSP	Example
Treachery Invalidation	*A very young NA tries to humour her by saying that she is here on holiday. Phyllis does not accept this at all and says Roy, her husband, will be waiting for her.*
Disempowerment	*She asks if he can shave himself, he says he can. She says "are you sure? I don't want you to cut yourself". The NA proceeds to shave Ben.*
Infantalisation	"*I've made it into soldiers for you*" referring to Hilda's breakfast.
Intimidation Imposition Accusation Disparagement	*The NA starts to give out lunches in the bay. He goes over to Walter and asks him if he wants lunch. Another NA comes in to help get Walter out of bed. She asks him if he is going to sit up in bed or sit out in his chair for lunch. They pull the curtains round the bed and start to get Walter into his chair. They bombard him with instructions, "sit up, sit yourself up, no, no". It seems that Walter would prefer to stay in bed "you can't do that, look what you've done in the bed". It appears that Walter has been incontinent. They tell him to sit in his chair and eat his lunch. He does not look comfortable or settled, they tell him to sit in his chair and eat his lunch and they will "clean him up afterwards". To add to the humiliation the curtains are pulled back and the bed stripped and remade in the middle of the bay.*
Labelling	The "only social" label that is frequently applied to patients who did not have any acute care needs.
Stigmatisation	*The SN says "we'll start these two when I get back" pointing at Eileen and a very poorly lady in the next bed*
Ignoring Banishment	*An NA sits down by me and starts to talk about a project she did on dementia. Amy works hard to join the conversation so I have one person talking in each ear. They both talk incessantly and ignore what the other is saying.*
Outpacing	*They give him some instructions "put your leg in, point your toes, put your foot on the floor, stand up", these instructions come in quick succession and it sounds as though Ben is struggling to comply "Ben stand up tall like a soldier,* **stand still** *or you'll fall over".*
Objectification Disruption	*The doctor gets to Walter and says "hello, home on Wednesday for you". Walter doesn't respond. The doctor looks a little more closely at Walter and removes his glasses without comment, he says "umm .... ptosis here" he turns to the junior doctors and asks what are the most common causes of ptosis in the elderly. He then replaces Walter's*

	glasses slightly askew and moves onto the next patient. Walter straightens his glasses and carries on drinking his tea.
Withholding	*She walks with Amy and her Zimmer frame to the bathroom and starts to talk to her, Amy says 'if only it didn't hurt so much' the NA completely ignores this. Amy limps a little further towards the bathroom.*
Withholding	*People are still wandering up and down outside Tom's room talking, they seem to be disturbing him much more now. Tom gets momentarily agitated and tries to get out of bed..... someone shouts "Pat there's a phone call", Tom answers "yes okay", he is left alone in his distress.*
Mockery	*She [the NA] starts to take out the contents [of the locker] mostly hospital mugs and cup holders and very few of Hilda's own possessions. She says to the lady in the next bed "I think we like hoarding" they both laugh.*
Disempowerment Intimidation Outpacing Objectification Imposition Disparagement	*The NA goes to Anthony and stands at the end of his bed "shall we give you a wash now?" He doesn't respond. The two NA's collect the equipment for his wash and close the curtains* "right *Anthony let's give you a nice wash then, then we'll* try *and sit you out in the chair". There is something in the NA's tone that makes her sound as though she is not looking forward to this procedure. A SN goes behind the curtains, the three nurses talk about what needs to be done on the ward. "Can you wash your face Anthony? That's better, that's it. Let's wash your body my darling, let's wash your arms, relax,* **relax***" says the bank NA. "Wait, wait, let's get the soap off" says the other. They give instructions one after another in quick succession. "Right, coming to me, rolling to me love alright". The interaction is only functional. "Come to me, come to me, Anthony,* calm down, *just relax, bend this leg, keep the other one straight, you'll be on the floor if you go on like that, stop fighting Anthony", they bombard him with instructions. The NA leaves to get a continence pad "I wish he wouldn't do that he makes it twice as hard for us" she says on her return. She barks "roll to the other NA, relax these legs, roll, roll, just roll to the other NA, don't fight. Anthony turn your head, this way to me,* ***roll***". *She sighs loudly "you're stiff as a poker, just keep your arms still". The NA goes to get the hoist "just relax your knees sweetie, just relax, right we're going up now" as they raise the hoist. "Right lift your feet up marvellous".*

Infantalisation Objectification	*The student nurse opened the conversation with Walter saying "shall we go and have a bath now? That will wake us up". This question was followed by Walter being taken to the bathroom. The student nurse takes him to the bathroom. She holds his hand but walks an arm's length ahead of him and doesn't interact at all. It looks as though she is taking her pet for a walk.*
Infantalisation Withholding	*A student nurse comes into the bay and starts to do the menus for that evening and breakfast and lunch for the next day. The choice on the menu is vast. She goes through every option with a man with a visual impairment. When she gets to Walter she offers him a jam sandwich for breakfast, no choice really, then fish fingers for supper, she selects whatever he is going to have with the fish fingers.* In other periods of observation when Walter was given a choice when completing his menu he did not opt for jam sandwiches and fish fingers. He still had capacity to select food the food he enjoyed.
Infantalisation Objectification	*A SN comes into Tom's room with his lunch. She tells him it is time for lunch, he doesn't seem to register anything. She tries to prop him up with pillows. She takes the lid off his meal tray, it is mince with mashed potato and carrots, she mashes it all together with a fork. She asks Tom to open his mouth, he doesn't respond. The SN has not told him what he has for lunch. Tom only opens his mouth when the fork is actually touching his lower lip, it looks as though it is an automatic response. He has four mouthfuls of the mixture, between mouthfuls the nurse completes bits of Tom's paperwork, he seems to have some difficulty swallowing and I can see quite a lot of food left in his mouth. The SN moves on to his pudding, apple and custard, she gives him three spoonfuls interspersed with orange juice and then stops. Throughout the meal the nurse keeps up a constant conversation / questioning "is it alright?", "are you alright?" "open your mouth". He doesn't respond. She completes the food and fluid charts.*
Disparagement	Walter was known to have been a pharmacist; he was still able to talk lucidly about this work. This did not have any impact on the nurse who was administering his intravenous medication. She said to Walter by way of explanation "*let's sort this wire out then, I'm going to pop some water in, lift your arm up then*".
Outpacing	*The nurse comes into the bay with the drug trolley; initially he looks at Walter's drug chart and moves on without waking him. When Walter wakes and mumbles the nurse goes back to him and asks him how he is feeling, Walter mumbles and the*

	nurse says "not so good?" Walter says yes and the nurse asks specific questions "are you uncomfortable? Do you have pain? Do you feel sick?" The questions are delivered so rapidly that Walter doesn't have a chance to formulate an answer. The conversation finishes and the nurse moves back to the patient in the next bed.
Ignoring Mockery	*Walter is dozing in his chair. His drip runs out so the nurse comes to change the bag. She says hello to him and then can't get the pump to work, the nurse says she has locked the pump as "Walt was trying to help yesterday" she giggles a little.*

The examples above indicate the great prevalence with which MSP occurs in practice. It is, of course, relatively easy to identify snapshots of MSP. Identification of discrete examples of person-centred care is more difficult. This may be because, in dementia care, we have been conditioned to see and hear the negative. Equally those that work in a person-centred mode may do this consistently making it more difficult to capture specific incidents. However there were examples of care being delivered from a person-centred perspective in which staff and patients were seen to connect with each other; these were often very brief episodes. Examples of this type of care are outlined below:

The nurse walks up to Tom and makes eye contact, she speaks to him in a normal but deliberate tone and says hello. She asks him clearly if he is alright, she asks the question very clearly and then leaves an almost uncomfortably long pause to allow Tom to answer, he says "yes". She waits for a moment and asks Tom if he is comfortable, he takes her hand and kisses it gently, she smiles but says nothing.

The nursing assistant helps Hilda with her menu. She gives her one menu at a time and gives her time to read them and make her choices, the nurse ticks these off. Hilda has a very clear view on what she likes to eat. They chat about filling in the menus and how boring it is reading them out time after time, they both laugh, the SNA gives Hilda her full attention for a moment.

Walter returns from x-ray in a wheelchair. He is met by the therapy assistant who stops the porter at the door of the bay. She asks Walter if he would like to walk to the window of the bay. He stands up and starts to move, he say's "let me just get clear of the thing behind me" referring to the wheelchair footrest. He starts to walk slightly unsteadily towards the window but tries to turn towards his bed. The assistant asks him to keep going to the window which he does. She asks if he can see what the builders are doing outside, he says no. I ask if he can see without his glasses, he says no. The assistant helps Walter to walk back towards his bed; he says he needs to go to the toilet and just starts to go. The assistant takes him to the toilet; she then gets him clean pants and trousers. She makes absolutely no fuss and just puts the soiled clothes in a bag in his locker. She then looks for his glasses and cleans them, she bends down to talk to Walter and asks him if he wears his glasses all the time or just for reading. He says he wears them all the time and she puts them on for him.

What was absolutely clear during data collection was that much of the care appeared to be delivered with kindness and no deliberate negative intent. Staff seemed to focus on ensuring that patients were kept clean and dry and had adequate food and drinks. Although this approach could largely be considered "kind" in that the staff thought that they were doing their best for patients, it enabled staff to ignore the uniqueness of individuals. This idea is in keeping with some of the literature on care delivery. Whilst kindness is an important factor in care delivery it is stated by Ashworth and Ashworth (2003) that caring with kindness does not equate to affording the individual respect. These authors argue powerfully that there is a need for staff to recognise that each individual has their own unique lifeworld, they suggest that such recognition would enable staff to act respectfully. Ashworth and Ashworth (2003) acknowledge that there is still a lot of work to be done to humanise the way in which older people with dementia are viewed. This thought was clearly illustrated in a number of interactions between staff and patients.

Instances such as ignoring the communication of patients or not allowing them to undertake tasks of which they are capable have a detrimental effect on their well being. The assertion of Killick (2004) that an individual's failure to connect with another may lead the person with dementia withdrawing into themselves and reducing their efforts to communicate due to the frustration of not being listened to was seen in a number of the participants. Equally some participants were seen to give up attempting to undertake certain tasks. As Faulkner (2001) suggests disempowering patients in a single task appeared to have a cumulative effect to the point where they did not retain any desire or ability to self care. The experience of participants indicates that the care that they received was far from being person-centred. Their care was primarily based on ensuring that their physical needs were met. There was relatively little evidence of staff getting to know, or developing relationships with, patients.

When considering relationships between people with dementia and staff, Kitwood (1997a) discusses the work of Buber. It is suggested by Buber (1937) that there are two alternative ways of being in the world, he describes the notions of I-It and I-Thou. When relating to another, I-It implies coolness, objectivity and engagement without commitment whereas I-Thou requires real involvement and therefore an element of personal risk taking. Data suggests that there is still currency in Kitwood's (1997a) assertion that the I-It mode of relating in health care is so common that it is often taken as normal. There were exceptions to this thought and examples of staff moving, albeit temporarily, to the I-Thou mode. It was rare to witness spontaneous conversation between people with dementia and staff. Generally interactions were limited to those related to functional activities.

This idea is congruent with the findings of Norman (2006) who proposes that nursing activity involving people with dementia is clearly divided into either practical or emotional work. Practical aspects involve minimal collaboration with relationships being those of provider and receiver of care. Emotional care was characterised by a higher level of collaboration, some negotiation and some prioritisation of patients' needs. Norman (2006) does not elaborate on the extent to which each type of care was delivered but from the extracts of data that are provided it is possible to deduce that functional care dominated. In this study there were few episodes of communication that moved beyond that which allowed physical care to be delivered. On occasion communication moved into the realms of I-Thou. Patients and staff conversed in a way that allowed them to achieve a level of interconnectedness, a state which McCormack (2001a) describes as being a relationship of equals which is situated in a framework of negotiation. These brief encounters in which there was mutual respect gave apparent pleasure to both parties. This approach evoked and reassured the selfhood of participants. In these brief moments of authentic relationship the patients appeared to experience a fleeting nourishment of their personhood. Personhood is discussed further in the section related to the current state of practice.

Literature concerning the new culture of dementia care, with its focus on preservation of personhood and person-centred care continues to grow. Evidence about the experiences of older people with dementia in institutional settings remains small. A very limited number of studies have sought the views of patients and residents in a range of facilities. The definitive finding that is common to this study and the literature is that people with dementia are able to actively engage in research. The extent to which current research can be compared is limited as the settings were relatively diverse. There were similarities between this study and the work of Norman (2003a) which also investigated patients' experiences in acute hospitals. This author attests to the notion that people with dementia are treated differently, as a stigmatised "they" (Goffman 1974). Norman (2003a) observed that patients, who might or might not have a confirmed diagnosis of dementia but who showed signs of cognitive impairment, were quickly labelled by staff and subsequently treated in a different manner to other patients. In common with this study Norman also observed that patients' attempts to communicate were often misinterpreted or disregarded. These patients equally expressed concerns about the lack of information they had about plans for their care.

Other studies that have inquired about residents' experiences have been conducted in specialist mental health or dementia care facilities. In small scale studies Barnett (2000) and Train et al (2005) investigated the views of people in long term care environments. These residents appeared to value the security of being in a familiar environment. This comfort was not experienced by a group of veterans who expressed a sense of uncertainty and bewilderment as they struggled to understand why they were unable to leave the locked unit in which they resided (Moore et al 2003). Brief descriptions of the units suggest that those studied by Barnett (2000) and Train et al (2005) were more homely than the veterans unit. It is notable that Norman (2006) suggests that the patient participants in her acute hospital study construed the ward as a living environment. This perception is contrary to the findings of this study in which the participants were aware that the hospital was not their "home" and therefore they felt some anxiety about what would happen to them next.

Train et al (2005) asked twenty-one residents in ten long stay hospital wards and homes about their experiences of care. A number of these residents commented about the staff being rough when delivering care. Although the participants in this study did not directly articulate concerns about rough handling, their responses to care indicated that when they were not informed of what was going to happen next or were manhandled they became distressed. An issue that was raised by a number of residents in the study of Train et al (2005) was that of choice. Some residents reported feeling confined to the home, others yearned for very simple choices such as being able to have a drink when they wanted one. Participants in this study raised few issues of choice despite the fact that this was routinely denied to them. It may be suggested that their level of uncertainty about what was happening to them was such that they were willing to tolerate the lack of opportunity to make choices.

These findings present rather a bleak picture of the experiences of patients. They describe their time in hospital in quite negative terms and some express particular concerns about perceived arguments and ill feeling on the wards. Several patients felt that they did not know what was planned for their future. It was evident that the care that was delivered tended to focus on physical activities rather than the holistic approach that is advocated by the proponents of person centredness. Most care appeared to be delivered with kindness but this did not stop the niggling erosion of personhood through the inadvertent use of malignant social psychology. The experience of being in an acute hospital seemed to have the effect of slowly but surely diminishing the person.

Data demonstrated that, in common with people with dementia, their carers often found hospitalisation a difficult experience. A total of seven carers were involved in this study. Three were husbands of patients, one son, two daughters and one friend. There is a moderate body of knowledge about lay carers' experiences of the care received by people with dementia in in-patient facilities. Most of the literature relates to care in residential or mental health settings rather than acute hospitals.

In this study ways in which carers discussed care was wholly unexpected. They tended to provide very broad statements including "*well they're marvellous people here, you can't fault them at all whatsoever ..... they are,* they're terrific". I had believed that carers would express much more powerful feelings about the finer points of how day to day care was delivered. I had also anticipated some debate about topical issues that have been highlighted regularly in the media such as poor nutritional intake and the use of tranquilising medication (Guardian 1999, 2006, Daily Mail 2006). Both anecdotal evidence and the literature support the idea that carers often have very definite views about the care that is delivered. An example of this includes the work of Hodkinson (2004) who writes with conviction about the care her mother received during admission for planned surgery. Hodkinson cites the lack of understanding and communication, both between staff and with her mother, as the major factors that led to suboptimal care.

Carers appeared to struggle or to be reluctant to express their thoughts on quality of care. It is possible to speculate on a number of reasons for this. Ways in which participants were recruited to the study allowed ward staff to filter out those whom they felt were unsuitable or difficult, I was aware that some more vocal carers were not invited to take part. Those carers who were involved may have been reluctant to articulate their thoughts candidly whilst their relatives were still in-patients in the belief that any negative comment may impact on future care. The three husbands provided very general statements about care. Their broadly positive thoughts may simply be attributed to the fact that they genuinely felt that their wives were receiving satisfactory care. Equally it was notable that they all expressed some gratitude that the burden of being responsible for day to day care had temporarily been lifted from them. This release, even if only short term, may have been sufficient to encourage the carers to take a very uncritical stance. The concept of deserving, or of having a right to, a certain level of care may also have influenced their thoughts. As a group of older people they may have been more accepting of the care offered and have more limited expectations than younger generations (Bytheway 1995). Periods of observation suggested that the husbands felt some sense of responsibility for the ways in which their wives behaved. When they displayed socially unacceptable behaviour the husbands' embarrassment was palpable. Together these factors may have rendered the carers particularly reluctant to express any concerns about quality of care.

Carers spoke of their experiences of providing care to their relatives; some described it purely in terms of burden whilst others acknowledged a sense of satisfaction. The burden of care is the focus of much of the research involving the carers of people with dementia (Cheston and Bender 2003). This burden may include feelings of physical and emotional overload, anger, frustration, dissatisfaction and guilt (Schofield et al 1998, Broe et al 1999). Although caregiver burden is well documented it is also noted that many carers derive enormous satisfaction from their caring role (Jeon et al 2005). Whilst caring for people with dementia can be seen as both satisfying and demanding (Pickard et al 2000) the carers in this study, with one exception, were older people who reported becoming increasingly frail themselves; this led to caregiving becoming an increasing strain.

The extent to which carers wished to be involved in the process of caring in hospital varied greatly. Husbands appeared broadly content to step back from the caring role, they seemed relieved to allow others to take over their responsibilities. In principle Eileen's husband was willing to relinquish his role as direct care giver, in practice he found this extremely difficult. It is suggested by Andren and Elmstahl (2005) that whilst family care givers experience both positive and negative reactions to caregiving one of the satisfying aspects is providing best care. Eileen's husband rapidly became dissatisfied with aspects of her care which he clearly felt he could do better. This type of discontent with the performance of others is noted by Redfern et al (2002) who found that disruptions to usual routines were likely to increase care giver stress. Eileen's husband experienced great frustration and forcefully expressed his dissatisfaction when staff appeared not to listen to, or act on, his advice about the best ways of caring for his wife.

Investigations have been conducted into the extent to which carers are involved in care delivery in in-patient settings. In a small study in a psychiatric inpatient unit for older people Walker and Dewar (2001) found that the majority of carers expressed dissatisfaction with their level of involvement. This was attributed to two main causes, hospital systems and processes and relationships between staff and carers. Staff on the ward where Eileen was nursed certainly had a routine they preferred to follow. Hughes (1984) suggests that a desire to control their own time and protect their routine can result in nurses dismissing carers' demands. However, this ward did not appear to have such an entrenched routine that this would be the case. It would appear that communication became strained and that Eileen's husband may have been implicitly critical of the nursing staff about their lack of ability to get her to walk as he did at home. The major issue effecting Eileen's husband appeared to be the lack of communication that is reported as being so prevalent between carers and staff (Simpson et al 1995, Gilmour 2002, Walker and Dewar 2001).

Involvement of lay carers in care delivery can be an area of contention. Allen (2000) suggests that it may be difficult for carers to negotiate an active role in a hospital environment that is alien to them and which tends to favour service providers. In this study it appeared that carers at each end of the spectrum of care delivery were generally satisfied with their experience. Doris's carer was absolutely clear that she intended to continue with her usual role. She communicated this expectation to staff as soon as she arrived on the ward and it was accepted particularly by nursing staff:

> *"The first day I came in they sort of said visiting time's not 'til,* I said I've come in to help, to help you, *I wash and do everything else here, one of the girls or a couple of the girls help me if she's being Doris, otherwise I do exactly the same here, I don't mind cos I don't like leaving her you see".*

Doris's carer reported that the nurses welcomed her with open arms and told her to get on with it "*but they do help me*". The relationship she forged with nursing staff was strong and they readily accepted her input into care. It is notable that the medical staff were slightly more circumspect about her input:

> *The carer tells the NA's she doesn't think Doris is very well today, she sounds a bit chesty. The carer stops one of the SN's and tells her that Doris's breathing does not sound so good, she is worried because Doris had a chest infection last week. The carer says that Doris should be having some oxygen but that she won't tolerate it. The SN says that the doctors will be round soon. The carer refers to them by their first names. The doctors arrive to do the ward round; the carer says that Doris is not breathing so well and perhaps she needs some more antibiotics. The doctors say probably not at the moment, they have a very brief conversation. The carer tries to engage them further by asking more questions, they answer tersely and move on. They do not listen to Doris's chest. The carer is not happy but acknowledges that she cannot force the doctors to do anything.*

This observation was somewhat at odds to the carer's assertion about the doctors "*they tell me everything, they're very good because they know I'm with her all the time*". Doris's carer became quite troubled when she felt that her expertise was not being recognised. This was evidenced again in an interaction with an occupational therapist in which she was advised to leave Doris on the commode if she resisted being moved:

> *"It's alright saying you can't force them to do this, that and the other, but it comes to a point where, where it's dangerous. Like this morning and the occupational therapist came and she just said leave her on the commode and I thought if she falls off the commode and whacks her head what are you supposed to do then?.... I said to one of the girls did she know she's got dementia, I wasn't impressed".*

This carer had the advantage of some familiarity with the hospital and its systems through a previous admission with Doris. She also had tremendous force of personality. She was welcomed by staff who willingly provided assistance with care whenever requested. This experience was totally different to that reported by Warner and Wexler (1998) who found that many carers of people in hospital were simply left to get on with it. It is likely that the clarity with which Doris's carer expressed her needs played a pivotal role in her partnership working with the nursing staff. At the other end of the spectrum several relatives were content to take no part in care delivery. These two approaches appeared to be acceptable to staff, possibly because the wishes of the carers were clear and unchanging. Staff evidently categorised these carers, particularly the carer of Doris, as a "saint" (Cheston and Bender 2003). They regularly commented on her devotion to duty.

Staff were clearly appreciative of the input from Doris's carer. Relationships between staff and Eileen's husband appeared much more strained. As suggested previously, communication was not effective and Eileen's husband felt that his expertise was not recognised. This can cause enormous frustration to carers (Hodkinson 2004). It is suggested by Allen (2000) that staff may view getting to know patients and their needs through their lay carers as undermining their professional role. In this case the lack of consistency in advice and the way in which it was delivered was more pertinent. Poor communication and lack of clarity about levels of involvement in care giving appeared to lead to Eileen's husband being cast in the role of "sinner" (Cheston and Bender 2003). This stereotyping resulted in a further reduction in communication as he became more discontent with the care and staff became more cautious about approaching him.

Plans for the future occupied a considerable amount of the carers time and thought. This was particularly the case for the three carers who eventually came to the conclusion that they would have to move their relative to a long term residential placement. As is so often the case, this decision was precipitated by the health crisis that had required hospital admission (Wright 1998). The choice to seek residential placement was a cause of great anguish, in different ways, to each of the carers involved.

Transition to residential care is a major life event (Centre for Policy on Ageing 1996). Victor (1992) suggests that entry is sometimes regarded by carers as the final sign of failure. This idea certainly appeared congruent with the regrets that were expressed by the carers. It is very common for admission to a residential home to be "expert driven" (McAuley et al 1997) with doctors often taking the lead role (McAuley et al 1997, Brown 1998). The decision to admit each of these patients to residential care was heavily influenced by the multi-disciplinary team. Carers all appeared to experience ambivalent emotional reactions to their decisions (Dellesega and Nolan 1997), these included both relief and guilt (Lewycka 1998). In the case of Amy's husband, his abdication from involvement in selecting a home may have been a part of the process of gradual detachment from his wife (Jones and Martinson 1992). Carers of Eileen and Ben remained fully engaged in each step of the journey.

The Audit Commission (1997) propose that the decision to seek residential care is sometimes made more difficult because alternatives are not explored, often because there are few genuine choices. In these instances the hospital team invested considerable time and energy exploring alternatives to residential care. In reality potential plans were often thwarted by limitations of finance and staff availability. Brindle and

Holmes (2005) suggest that it is vitally important that future care needs should be based on ethics rather than expediency. Whilst each decision was ethically sound and agreed by both carers and the multi-disciplinary team, it may be suggested that the pressure to vacate hospital beds (Lundh et al 2000) added some time pressures to the carers. Each carer was supported by a member of the social work team. However, as noted by Lundh et al (2000), it took an assertive and persistent person to influence the process of selecting a residential home.

Carers found the act of telling the person that they were moving to residential care extremely painful to the extent that Ben's daughter chose to enlist the help of the social worker. This phenomenon is also seen in the study of Lundh et al (2000) in which carers spoke of their experiences of moving family members into residential care. The emotional turmoil of the move to residential care was compounded by the concerns some carers expressed about the financial implication of such a move. Financial burdens of care in old age have been debated extensively in the press and media but, as yet, little empirical research has been completed.

A complex picture was painted by carers. It was striking how circumspect they were when commenting about the care received by their relatives and friends. They were mainly complimentary about the care given however they spoke in very general terms and tended not to articulate fully the thoughts that underpinned their opinions. Possible reasons for the paucity of data concerning care are examined. The extent to which carers wished to, and felt able to, contribute to care in hospital varied. It was evident that it took some confidence and determination to continue in this role. It appears that the major barriers included the hospital routine and the lack of effective communication between staff and carers. Although carers appeared reluctant to criticise staff it was clear that some resented the lack of acknowledgement of their expertise. Although the burden of day to day care had, on the whole, been lifted the carers remained central to care as they concentrated on the difficult decisions and arrangements that had to be made in relation to the future care of their relatives. In theory they were supported to make these decisions and assisted to make the necessary arrangements. In practice there was a powerful impression that, despite acknowledging this support, the carers felt very much alone in planning the future for their relatives and themselves.

The Current State of Practice

This section reflects on the current state of practice as observed; it embraces the thoughts of staff about the care they deliver to people with dementia. Staff involved in the study included registered and non-registered individuals from a range of disciplines including nursing, allied health professions, social work and medicine. Eighty-five staff agreed to participate in the research although in reality a small minority were not actively involved as they were never present during the periods of observation. Composition of the staff participant group is presented in table 3-3.

Staff Group	Number of Participants
Registered nurses	25
Non-registered nursing staff	33
Registered allied health professionals	9
Non-registered allied health professional staff	3
Social work staff	2
Medical staff	13

Table 3-1: Composition of Staff Participant Group

A total of twelve interviews were completed with staff with each discipline being represented. Data were analysed to elucidate the ethnographic "what" and "how". This section is divided into three themes which have been derived from the data: philosophies of caring for people with dementia, the value that staff attach to their work and the ability of staff to provide care. Findings are considered in the context of current literature.

Philosophies of Caring for People with Dementia

Data suggest that many staff had clear personal philosophies that they felt influenced the way in which they delivered care to people with dementia. These philosophies were, to some extent, based on intrinsic beliefs and personal experience rather than on any specific knowledge or education. People with dementia were clearly viewed as being different to other patients. Staff seemed particularly prone to labelling these individuals, labels took several different forms but were powerful and pervasive.

When asked about the way in which they cared for people with dementia several staff struggled to articulate their thoughts. Staff that provided direct care tended to suggest that they delivered care in the way they would like their families to be cared for. One nursing assistant stated:

> *"I think you've got to um,* respect *them, I think, you know and maybe treat them how you would like, or your relative. Imagine that was your gran there that you've known all your life, you know I sort of, sort of treat people how you would like to be treated I think".*

This thought was reiterated by another nursing assistant "*you try to give every patient the care that you'd want your relative to have I think*". Similar ideas were expressed by a registered nurse

> *"it's mainly, how maybe it's a gut feeling of how, maybe I feel that if it's my family how would I want to look after them, if it's* my *god forbid any of* my *family members how I'd feel that I'd like the nurse to look after them. I'd want to be treated with respect. I would like them to be cared for kindly I suppose".*

Senior staff tended to use more abstract terminology which appeared to be derived from their training. One social worker described her approach as "*we're looking at* person-centred". The idea that these patients were individuals with their own unique biography and history which may influence their thoughts on care was alluded to by a colleague who stated:

> *"you have to think of them in the context of their life as well. I think thinking about their history gives you a lot of respect for that person and makes them become a person and not just a patient".*

Some of the staff who delivered direct care felt that it would be useful to know more about people's biographies and their lives beyond hospital. This was expressed by one nursing assistant "*yeah, it would be nice to see what they're like at home*". However this seemed to be a distant thought rather something that may be enacted in practice. The idea was positively rejected by one nursing assistant who stated that she preferred not to know about the person prior to their admission "*because you don't have any pre .... ideas of what, what they* should *be like or anything*".

Whilst staff had developed personal philosophies about caring for people with dementia, it was evident that their thoughts had also been influenced by the culture in which they were working. One example of such cultural influence was the tendency to label patients. The most frequently mentioned label was that of the patient who was "only social".

Others that were regularly used were applied to patients who were deemed to be "sweet" or "difficult".

One belief that emerged on each ward was the concept of the patient who was "only social". It seemed that for patients with dementia there was a delicate balance of whether their acute physical illness outweighed their dementia. If so, dementia appeared to be temporarily forgotten. For example in a ward handover five patients were known to have a diagnosis of dementia but, this was only mentioned in relation to the one person who did not have an acute illness. In meetings, patients who had dementia tended to be talked of quite dismissively, for example Anthony was described as *"assessment done, awaiting vacancy"* and Hilda as *"just awaiting placement"*. Patients who had been categorised as "only social" tended to be placed at the bottom of the hierarchy on the wards. It was observed that these patients, especially if they were relatively independent in terms of personal care, could spend hours and hours being totally overlooked by staff.

The label of "sweet" was attached to patients who were consistently undemanding on both the time and emotions of staff. They tended to be compliant, gentle and grateful for the care they were given. Hilda was such a patient, she was described as "*a cheerful little thing*" who was "*happy in her own little world*". Those patients who were not so biddable were at risk of being defined as "difficult". Once a patient had exhibited "difficult" behaviour it appeared that they were labelled and that the way in which staff interacted with them subtly altered. Ben quickly gained the label of being "difficult". One registered nurse described an incident in which Ben unexpectedly hit her, he lashed out once but did not cause serious damage. The nurse explained that the incident had shocked her but claimed that it had made no difference to the way in which she cared for Ben. She seemed to contradict herself as she went on to say *"I'm at arm's length, I'm <u>not</u> going to go too close to him"*. This finding is comparable with that of a small scale study by Nolan (2007) who discovered that nurses felt safer and more able to engage in participatory care with patients who did not exhibit any aggressive behaviour. Belief that Ben was physically aggressive had clearly permeated the thoughts of staff from other disciplines. A social worker explained:

> *"I was told by everybody that the individuals wishes was to return home and respecting that wish and when I went down to see the person they seemed to be always like sleeping and I don't think it's a good idea to wake somebody up and start asking these quite* difficult *questions, and we'd also had, um, a sort of concern that when this person's woken can become, um, physically and verbally aggressive".*

As far as I could ascertain Ben had one single incident when he hit a member of staff; however this appeared to be the social workers evidence on which she based her decision not to speak to him. This idea would support the concept that if a patient is perceived as aggressive the social distance between them and practitioners rapidly increases (Burgener et al 1992).

Use of labels is noted in the work of Norman (2006) who found that staff were inclined to categorise patients as either positive and acceptable, in which case they were viewed as a whole. These individuals tended to be compliant and relatively independent. The alternative label was negative and unacceptable. These patients were reduced to their parts and tended not to be acknowledged as people. These labels have clear parallels with those of "sweet" and "difficult". The difference in the findings involves the extent to which labels were attributed. Norman (2006) observed inconsistencies and variations over time and between nurses, whereas in this study labels tended to stick and gradually permeate the staff group.

Staff articulated a clear set of beliefs about caring for people with dementia. Some of these were based on the idea that care should be delivered as they would expect for their own families, others appeared to be more rooted in learnt theory. There appeared to be little correlation between espoused beliefs and actions in practice. Much of the care appeared to be delivered with kind intention but there was a powerful tendency to label and thus depersonalise patients. A person with dementia being labelled is a well known phenomenon. Participants in this study already carried the labels of being older and cognitively impaired which are so often applied at societal level (Rodeheaver and Datan 1988, Adams and Bartlett 2003). Once admitted to hospital they were often labelled further. Whilst Adams and Bartlett (2003) suggest that being endowed with a label can sometimes be of benefit in terms of opening up areas of service provision, in this case the opposite appeared to happen. Attribution of labels seemed to enable staff to recast these patients as the "empty shell" (Moore and Hollett 2003) or "fragments of humanity" (Keane 1994) rather than as real people with their own preferences about the care they wished to receive. A number of interactions indicated that staff had mentally moved these patients from the category of person-as-individual, a person who is capable of a relationship, to person-as-other, someone who is incapable of a relationship (Malloy and Hadjistavropoulos 2004) and therefore they become merely objects of care. At the extreme, some staff appeared to believe that the objects of care had ceased to have feelings as their cognitive function had declined Dewing (2001).

These findings demonstrate the extent to which the current state of practice is congruent with that documented in the literature. Individual thoughts about how care should be delivered varied. It was evident that a number of staff adhered to the often held view that patients with dementia are non-people (Ashburner et al 2004), equally other staff did not. There was clear evidence that patients were labelled and that the effect of such labelling was almost entirely negative.

The Value That Staff Attach to Their Work

Staff suggested that caring for people with dementia in an acute hospital was viewed by others, and possibly themselves, as relatively unskilled and less prestigious than the work of other specialties. Staff questioned whether an acute hospital was an appropriate setting in which to care for people with dementia.

Conversations with staff demonstrated that many of them felt they had no particular skill in caring for people with dementia. They often reported that they just did the work that needed to be done. A small number of staff alluded to the idea that caring for older people demands specialist skills. One nurse talked about her choice to work with older people:

> *"they're multiple pathologies aren't they? They've got so many different things wrong with them that one thing can compound another. It's a difficult and very delicate balancing act".*

This nurse went on to talk about the effect that inter-current physical illness had on dementia and the complexities of caring for people with multiple problems. A therapist expressed similar views on the challenges of caring for people with dementia and acute health problems saying "*it becomes a lot more complex*". Few other staff alluded to their individual skills although the strength of the combined experience and knowledge of the multi-disciplinary team was a source of pride to the registered staff.

Although staff claimed little special knowledge they demonstrated a considerable level of expertise on many occasions, for example:

> *Two physio assistants come and ask Anthony if he would like a walk. They bring a standing hoist and ask Anthony to sit forward so they can put the sling down his back. He doesn't respond so one explains that he needs to hold her hands and lean forward. Again he doesn't respond, she tries once more but agrees with her colleague that it is better to leave him today. They seem to have an intuitive feeling and stop before Anthony becomes too frustrated. They explain that they will*

come back tomorrow as they are not here this afternoon. They tell me that they can 'feel' that today is not going to be successful and that it is better to stop now rather than upset him.

Whilst this example may initially appear to be relatively trivial it demonstrates the ability of these assistants to engage in brief but meaningful interaction with Anthony in which they were mindful of his verbal and non-verbal communication. In this short episode of genuine understanding between himself and the assistants Anthony appeared to experience a fleeting nourishment of his personhood. This interaction and other similar encounters were striking in that they appeared to be valued by patients but they seemed to be imbued with ordinariness by the staff involved who were often unable to recognise or articulate the skills that they were using.

Many staff, particularly nurses, appeared to view their work as routine and mundane. On one occasion I asked some nurses about how they organised their work and how they delivered care. Initially the staff looked at me as though I was asking strange questions the answers to which should be quite obvious. In answer they generally agreed that they helped self-caring people first and then moved on to more dependent patients. This habitual approach was put somewhat more bluntly by a registered nurse who organised her work in a comparable way when she asked her colleagues loudly "*is that it with the singles then?*" meaning had all the relatively independent patients had a wash. This nurse went on to talk about "*doing the heavies*" after they had taken their morning break. Staff offered no real justification as to why they adopted this approach to organising care. The question of how they delivered care seemed to perplex this staff group even more. Their responses included "*we look after these people the way* we *think they should be looked after*". A more simplistic reply was offered by one individual who stated that she delivered care as she did because "*that's how we do it .... we treat them all the same*".

The concept that dementia care is seen as occupying a relatively low position in the hierarchy of acute care may be a reflection of the way in which society as a whole tends to view this condition. At a societal level dementia remains low on the agenda (Means et al 2002). Rate of change is slow although there are some signs that this situation is beginning to change with the publication of documents such as the National Service Framework for Older People (DoH 2001b), Everybody's Business (CSIP 2005), Dementia: Supporting People with Dementia and their Carers in Health and Social Care (NICE 2006), Dementia UK: The Full Report

(Alzheimer's Society 2007) and Improving Services and Support for People with Dementia (National Audit Office 2007). People with dementia tend to be viewed as relatively unimportant (Herskovits 1995). As a society we are often fearful of dementia (Kitwood 1997a) with some suggesting that this can be attributed to our concern about potential disruption of social order by people considered to be a risk to others (Moon 2000). On an individual level people frequently dread the thought of becoming old and infirm themselves.

These societal attitudes to people with dementia appear to permeate views relating to health care for this group. The apparent lack of pride that the staff felt about the care they delivered and the expert knowledge they had acquired may be attributable to a number of causes. Longstanding lack of political interest in dementia and the low status offered to people with dementia and front line paid workers is noted by Innes (2002) and Means et al (2002). As stated previously, political interest in dementia care is beginning to develop but the impact of this remains at best variable. Caring for older people is traditionally viewed as the poor relation of health care. Gerontological nursing is not seen as an attractive career option (HAS 2000) although paradoxically it is an area in which nurses can make a real difference (Nolan and Tolson 2000). Marshall (1999) proposes that staff in the field have low status although this assertion is not justified. It is suggested by Dewing (1999), Normann et al (1999) and Stokes (2000) that older people continue to be viewed negatively by the multi-disciplinary team. In the field of dementia care Ashburner et al (2004) describe the traditional approach as being task-focused, depersonalised and mundane. Nolan and Tolson (2000) point to the "heavy" images and stereotypes with which dementia care is currently labelled. Given that staff, to some extent, live within this culture it seems hardly surprising that they do not express great pride in their work. It may be that staff are genuinely unaware of the tacit knowledge that they have acquired in practice, or they do not recognise their learning as it has no formal basis. The idea of not appreciating their own expertise was discerned by Allan (2002) in a study that mainly involved non-registered staff. Allan found that many of these staff were highly skilled but found it extremely difficult to articulate what they did. It is notable that even experienced researchers cannot always pinpoint these skills with Westlund et al (1990 cited Allan 2002:20) saying that good care staff had a "certain something".

Societal concerns about dementia are reflected and possibly magnified in acute hospitals. It is well documented that these environments are not well placed to provide care for people with dementia (Hodkinson 2004,

Dewing 2001). In a study involving seven registered nurses, Nolan (2007) discovered that acute care environments were viewed as having a major detrimental impact on the ability of these nurses to provide good care; they particularly cited issues of safety and overstimulation. It is well documented that the ability of people with dementia to cope with environmental stressors is compromised (Erikson and Saveman 2002) and that acute care settings can overstimulate individuals. As one of Nolan's (2007:420) participants stated the environment "triggers the confused patient and it makes them more anxious, more worked up". Attitudes of staff towards people with dementia can be negative. Pritchard and Dewing (2001) state that these patients are often perceived as relatively unimportant or unworthy. It is suggested by Marshall (1999) that staff simply do not have time to care for this group and resent having to do so. Marshall (1999) summarises this idea in a quote from staff in an acute hospital "they should not really be here". It may be suggested that a senior member of medical staff in this study had similar thoughts when saying:

> *"these patients just have very minimal contact with anybody while they're in hospital which is why we would all argue that it's, you know, it's* not *a good place for them to be".*

However whilst staff acknowledged that an acute hospital was not an ideal place to care for people with dementia, the feeling of staff towards patients seemed to be of resignation and sadness rather than resentment.

Data suggest that staff in this study do not value highly their contribution to the care of people with dementia. They tend to view themselves as the poor relations of health care. This phenomenon is well recognised within care organisations and tends to reflect societal attitudes towards people with dementia and those who provide their care. A number of staff suggested that an acute hospital was not a suitable environment for a person with dementia. However, this thought was framed in terms of the harm it may do to the individuals rather than on any resentment on the part of staff.

The Ability of Staff to Provide Care

The extent to which staff felt able to provide care to people with dementia was influenced by their preparation for this role. It became evident that staff felt a great sense of uncertainty about some aspects of care, particularly those involving higher level psychosocial skills. The tendency of staff to focus care on essential physical needs was marked. It may be suggested that this strategy was used to avoid the more challenging situations which generated feelings of uncertainty. Focus on physical care also allowed staff to maintain a safe distance from people with dementia and thus avoid high levels of emotional engagement (Ashburner et al 2004).

Degrees to which staff felt that they had been prepared to care for people with dementia varied considerably. Non-registered staff who delivered most direct care appeared to have had least preparation. When asked about what she had been taught a nursing assistant responded "*they teach you a bit about to stand back*". This participant went on to explain that the only education she had received was during a session about managing violence and aggression. Another nursing assistant explained that she had attended an induction programme prior to working on an older peoples unit "*I had a two week course but nothing was to do with dementia patients, there was nothing at all*". Registered nursing staff also felt that they had little preparation, some had received no specific education, others had actively sought opportunities. One registered nurse had attended a single dementia study day locally which she thought was "*marvellous, absolutely amazing but it's very difficult to apply those principles to an acute medical ward*". Social work and occupational therapy staff believed that their training had embraced dementia care, these participants all talked with ease about the major concepts of new culture dementia care such as personhood, person-centred and holistic care.

The concept that staff working in acute care settings are not well prepared to work with people with dementia is not new. This lack of education is alluded to by Aveyard (2001) who states that evidence suggests many people providing care in the acute environment have limited specialist education. Burgess and Page (2003) support this idea stating that acute health care staff frequently lack an adequate understanding of the needs of this group. It is debateable if this lack of preparation would be tolerated in other specialities, as Packer (2000a) suggests many staff find it unacceptable to work in areas of care for which they have had little or no education. Most staff in this study had received minimal or no education about how to care for people with dementia. The exception to this was the occupational therapy and social work staff all of whom stated that dementia care was an integral part of their initial training. Whilst these staff spoke with more confidence about some of the concepts of dementia care such as personhood and person-centred care there was no consistently discernable difference in the care they provided in practice.

Staff, particularly nursing and therapy assistants, were very aware of their lack of specific education. A number of them voiced concerns about their poor knowledge and expressed a desire to learn more. These individuals clearly articulated their wish to care for people with dementia as well as they could. Virtually all direct care was delivered by non-registered staff, predominantly nursing assistants. The focus of most care was firmly embedded in ensuring that a patient's physical needs were met:

> *The bank NA is sitting in the bay writing her Kardexes. I ask her if she has been looking after Walter this morning, she says that she gave him a wash at his bedside, he was very drowsy and she demonstrates how his head kept dropping quite dramatically. She says it was a "nightmare" trying to shave him and I get the impression that she is not satisfied with the result. She tells me that she got all his day clothes out of his locker but that she knew he couldn't cope with getting dressed "so I just put him in pyjamas".*

The description that this nursing assistant gave of caring for Walter and the way in which this was said made it very clear that she did not feel satisfied with the result of her work as Walter did not look the way she wished him to. Desire for patients to look as though they had been cared for was seen again on the day that Hilda was discharged to the residential home. She was helped to have a bath and her hair was washed. She was dressed in a clean set of relatively matching clothes:

> *Hilda returns from the bathroom with wet hair. The NA finds a hair brush and hair dryer and starts to dry Hilda's hair, Hilda raises her eyebrows to me. I would guess that she is a lady to whom a blow dry is anathema.*

The nursing assistant was insistent that Hilda should look nice, as though she had been cared for when she arrived at the home.

Delivery of day to day care focused very much on ensuring that the fundamental physical needs of patients were met. There are a number of possible explanations for this approach to care. At an organisational level in acute care there is an ongoing pressure to achieve rapid, efficient treatment and throughput (Archibald 2003). The culture of the organisation also put a premium on physical care, possibly because it is clearly observable and also amenable to measurement or audit unlike psychosocial care. This approach puts people with dementia at a double disadvantage in that their psychosocial needs tend to be neglected and they are often not able to conform to the ethos of acute care settings (Archibald 2003). A further factor which influences care delivery is that staff who were providing direct care had been trained in the art of physical care and were therefore confident and comfortable working in this mode.

To the outsider the organisational focus on efficient physical care could be likened to a description by Collopy et al (1999) of the total institution with the batch processing of people in which individuality is subsumed in the routine work of the organisation. It may be suggested that concentration on physical care was a method of compensating for lack of expertise and therefore staff strived to give the best care they knew how within the familiar "bed and body" framework (Gubrium 1975). As part of the effort to be caring, staff had a tendency to take over tasks if patients did not complete them rapidly. This phenomenon is noted by Hansebo and Kihlgren (2001) in video recorded interactions between patients and staff. This approach has the effect of disempowering patients and causes a decline in other abilities, thus patients gradually become more dependent (Wells and Dawson 2000, Faulkner 2001). This in turn leads to "excess disability" (Brody 1971) in which there is a discrepancy between functional capacity and the extent of the actual impairment. So whilst staff are striving to care they may be compounding the patients problems.

Staff appeared relatively at ease in meeting the physical care needs of patients. Care that fell outside this boundary seemed to cause more concern and often led to feelings of uncertainty. The issues that unsettled staff tended to involve either communication with patients or incidents when patients displayed overt emotion.

Both medical and nursing staff struggled during interactions with Hilda, particularly when the subject arose of her moving to residential care. In one conversation a senior doctor tried to explain to Hilda that she would not be able to return to her own home.

The doctor seems reluctant to be too blunt; the junior doctors look on and make 'sad' faces. They all seem uncomfortable and at a loss as to what to do.

Sometime after this encounter a registered nurse came to talk to Hilda:

The SN explains that she came into hospital because she was found wandering in the street and she didn't know where she lived. Hilda says "I didn't know that", she seems a little unsure if this is true from the doubtful expression on her face. Hilda repeats that she wants to go back to London, the SN says that we are not in London now, Hilda says

"I know". She says that Hilda has lived locally for many years. She asks where Hilda lives now, Hilda says she can't remember, a flicker of sadness crosses her face. The SN turns to me and says "I don't know what to say next" I nod but keep quiet. The conversation proceeds with the SN trying to offer rational explanations but Hilda has a reasonable answer for each point. The SN says that the manager of the home came to visit Hilda last week, Hilda cannot remember this. The SN tells Hilda that she must have liked him because she looked happy enough afterwards. The SN turns to me again and says "I think we're going round in circles here", again I just nod. She says to Hilda that she has to go now as she has other work to do. Hilda says okay. She stops crying a minute or two later but still looks incredibly sad. She gets up and folds her clothes with a huge amount of care and precision, she puts them in a neat pile on her bed.

These conversations were evidently difficult for both Hilda and the staff involved. The major dilemma for staff appeared to be the fact that they wanted to tell Hilda the truth but equally they were very aware that each time they did this she became incredibly distressed.

Episodes in which patients became "difficult" also appeared to cause staff some discomfort:

Phyllis suddenly gets very cross saying to an NA that she wants to go home. A very young NA tries to humour her by saying that she is here on holiday, Phyllis does not accept this at all and says Roy, her husband, will be waiting for her. She says she has a husband at home waiting for his supper. The NA looks very uncomfortable, she smiles at me and looks very embarrassed and unsure what to do. Phyllis is determined to go home, the young NA tries to distract her but she gets more cross. The NA leads her out of the bay to the safety of a group of colleagues at the nurses' station. The physio talks briefly to Phyllis and then moves on to see another patient. Phyllis is walked around by various members of staff. Phyllis gets as far as the end nurses' station. The SN gets her to sit down and tries to explain that she needs to stay in hospital until her plaster is off. This seems to agitate Phyllis more and she is verbally extremely cross and bordering on aggressive. The SN persists in trying to explain but it is not helping. Phyllis stands up and says she is going home.

Uncertainty about how they should manage, or respond to, some situations was evident. For example a nursing student was unsure if she should take any action when Walter was eating his breakfast.

Walter picks up the croissant and starts to eat, he looks like he is enjoying it. He keeps eating it until it is finished. Then he starts on the cold porridge which he eats with determination. The St/N notices, she pulls a face at me but lets him carry on eating.

This apparent embarrassment was echoed as a registered nurse helped Doris to take some medication.

The nurse helps Doris to take her medication. She is patient and encourages Doris with each tablet. Suddenly Doris picks up her orange juice and throws it over her bed and drug chart, the nurse laughs gently.

Care delivered to people with dementia focused largely on ensuring that their essential physical needs were met. This activity seemed to be driven by the desire of staff to meet certain standards rather than the needs of individual patients. Care involving a deeper level of communication, or episodes in which patients displayed overt emotion, generated feelings of uncertainty in some staff. A number of staff had adopted the habit identified by Ashworth and Ashworth (2003) of routinely dismissing what patients were saying. This may represent the value that staff attribute to patients or may be a tactic to avoid episodes of conflict or aggression. It may be suggested that this withdrawal by staff was counterproductive. Cohen-Mansfield and Werner (1995) and Harborne and Solly (1996) propose that patients exhibit challenging behaviour in an attempt to gain some attention. Therefore ignoring a patient's attempts to communicate in whatever form is likely to set up a vicious circle of aggression and ignoring. The result of such treatment can lead to patients retreating into themselves as a protective measure or as a result of their frustration at the failure to connect with others (Killick 2004). It was notable that staff who communicated effectively with patients used an adapted version of their usual style of communication. They tended to speak normally but present one question or idea at a time ensuring that they left time for a response before moving on. Staff who achieved less effective communication used a "special voice" that was high and patronising, they did not appear to expect a response from the patients. This group of staff appeared to believe there was a "right" way of communicating. This concept lent weight to the idea that they thought of people with dementia as different or lesser mortals.

It appeared that actions taken by patients to communicate their feelings and needs were interpreted by staff as being difficult (Hodkinson 2004). Patients who exhibited more overtly "difficult" behaviour tended to be avoided. This reaction has been noted by Hallberg (1990) who suggests that people who are seen as disruptive receive less care and attention and that the care they do receive tends to be more task-orientated and lacking social input. It is possible that this type of withdrawal from patients is influenced by exaggerated fear and feelings of embarrassment and worry if interactions do not go well. It is noted by Ashworth and Ashworth (2003) that in exchanges with people with dementia, health care staff tend to routinely dismiss their attempts at communication in order to avoid episodes of conflict and aggression.

A lack of certainty about working with people with dementia was observed on a number of occasions. In many situations this appeared to lead staff to provide only essential physical care and avoid more meaningful interaction for fear of "setting them off" and precipitating a difficult and potentially embarrassing situation. A number of staff reported that they felt poorly prepared to care for people with dementia. Their lack of education led to provision of care that tended to focus on physical rather than more holistic care. Staff expressed strong feelings of uncertainty about caring for this group and it is suggested that this uncertainty underpinned many of the actions that undermined the personhood of people with dementia.

Overall findings of this study present a very sad picture of the care of people with dementia in the acute hospital setting. Patients have relatively negative feelings about being in hospital and may find the environment noisy and stressful. They express concerns about the lack of information they are given regarding plans for their care. Care delivered focuses on physical needs and is not always tailored to the requirements of individuals. Those patients that are physically fairly independent may spend long hours alone with little company or stimulation. Carers were relatively uncritical of the service although this finding may have been influenced by the design of the study. Their desire and ability to have some input into the care of their relative was at times hindered by poor communication and by organisational barriers. Several carers experienced major concerns about plans for the future for both themselves and their relatives. They acknowledged the support that they were given by hospital staff but continued to feel very alone in their quest to ensure the provision of ongoing care. Staff, on the whole, attempted to deliver the best care they could given their acknowledged lack of education and the constraints of the organisation within which they were working. Care was predominantly focused on physical needs. Generally it appeared to be delivered with kind intent but was plagued with episodes of malignant social psychology which gradually undermined the personhood of patients.

When reflecting on this rather bleak picture, it would be easy to simply attribute blame. This would most usually be focused on staff for not routinely achieving the highest standards of care. This approach would be unjust and also counterproductive. A review of the reasons for some care being suboptimal may be more valuable. Findings of this study suggest that the following issues inhibit the development and application of the new culture of dementia care:

- At a societal level people with dementia are frequently considered to be second class citizens, this belief is reflected and even magnified in the acute hospital setting.
- The current health care system is performance dominated and therefore inimical to truly person-centred care for people with dementia.
- There is a tension between trying to provide care for acutely ill people with physical health needs and people with dementia who might or might not have acute health problems.
- Staff are working in environments that do not necessarily value their individual contribution or make them feel well supported.
- Staff are frequently ill prepared to care for people with dementia. This tends to draw them towards working within the "bed and body" framework (Gubrium 1975) and away from the more emotionally engaged, holistic, person-centred approaches to care.

It is evident that some of these issues need to be addressed at high levels. To some extent care of older people with dementia is rising up the political agenda with the realisation that this issue will continue to grow as the population ages. This change should, in time, filter down through National Health Service organisations to the areas where care is delivered. Accepting that a cultural change will take many years to achieve, there is a need to consider ways in which care can be improved from the "bottom up". Such improvement would seem to hinge on the immediate environments in which staff are working and on meeting their development needs. It is suggested by Packer (2000a) that education is a valuable tool but that used in isolation it is not sufficient to change practice. Although Packer does not justify this statement, it does appear reasonable. The environment in which staff work is also critical to their capacity to provide new culture dementia care. One of the consequences of working in a large institution is that staff may feel their individual contributions are negated (Menzies Lyth 1988, Kitwood 1997a). Nolan et al (2002) stress the importance of ensuring that staff feel well supported and that their contribution to care is valued.

The findings of this study suggest that a single approach to practice development is unlikely to effect any real change. The concept of developing dementia care practice in acute hospitals is considered by Norman (2006). This author suggests that there is a need for targeted practice development. Norman (2006) has developed a resource package that is intended to enable staff to enter into two way relationships and thus improve patients' experiences of hospitalisation. Whilst this method has some validity it does raise the question of how staff can be assisted to move to a point where they realise the value in developing two-way relationships. Reasons why staff do not engage in such relationships are largely unknown. It may be suggested that working in the I-It mode (Buber 1937) which is so common in health care (Kitwood 1997a), is simply a mechanism used by staff to protect themselves from some of the experiences that may be encountered when working in a person centred way. As Packer (2000a) suggests person-centred care is demanding and challenging for both staff and patients, staff may prefer not to risk entering this arena. An alternative explanation is that staff, for whatever reason, become "switched off" when caring for people with dementia and function on an automatic level in which only the required physical care is delivered with scant attention paid to the individual.

Whilst Norman's (2006) resource package is undoubtedly valuable, it is suggested that the provision of such tools and education alone is not sufficient to change practice. The idea that a multifaceted approach is required is supported by Packer (2000a). This author summarises her ideas for improving dementia care in an adaptation of Kitwood's equation of dementia: dementia care worker = training + personality + biography + physical and mental health + social psychology at home and work. This equation, whilst laudable, is perhaps difficult to relate to staff who have been in post for many years. It is suggested that there is a need to find ways in which to engage such staff and motivate them to reflect on their own practice, bringing to the fore the need to recognise the uniqueness of each individual. It is felt that traditional approaches to education are unlikely to result in a change in mindset and a realisation that care can be delivered differently. It is suggested that there is a need to engage with staff on an emotional and cognitive level to really effect a change in practice. This chapter analyses the ethnographic "what" and "how" of the data. In order to develop practice it is essential that the ethnographic "why" is also considered. This analysis is undertaken in chapter four in preparation for the practice development part of the thesis.

Conclusion

The aim of this study was to explore the experiences of patients, lay carers and health and social care staff of the care received by older people with dementia in the acute hospital setting. The purpose of the study was to generate new knowledge and insight that can be used to influence practice.

Experiences of acute hospital care are presented from the perspectives of patients, lay carers and health and social care staff. These sections include extracts of data that are discussed in relation to current literature and set within the wider social and political context. This approach has allowed the newly developed knowledge to be demonstrably grounded in the data.

The pictures illustrated in the chapter are complex. Patients found the episodes of being in hospital difficult and at times uncomfortable. They described the experience in broadly negative terms, expressing particular concern about perceived arguments and about their lack of knowledge concerning plans for their future care. Responses of patients to some of the care indicated that it was detrimental to their personhood. During the course of observation patients were seen to gradually diminish as their individuality was lost amongst the efforts of staff to meet their physical care needs. At present there is virtually no literature relating to the views of older people with dementia about their care in acute hospitals. Words and actions of participants indicate that their experience needs to be improved and are congruent with the idea that the time has come to embrace the new culture of dementia care in acute hospital settings.

Carers had great difficulty in commenting in any detail about the care received by their family or friends. They were generally uncritical of the care except in cases where they felt, often justifiably, that their expertise exceeded that of the staff but that, despite this, staff did not take sufficient notice of their advice. The extent to which carers wanted to be involved in care was variable but some found an acceptable level difficult to achieve. Plans for the future, particularly in terms of residential care and financial issues, caused great concerns to some carers. Thoughts they expressed were in line with previous research. The exception to this was their apparent reluctance to discuss their thoughts on quality of care in any detail.

Experiences of staff covered a broad spectrum. They often had clear ideas about the standard of care that should be delivered but this was more often based on personal philosophy than any other knowledge. There was a marked tendency to label patients and to use this as a basis for judging what care would be given. Many staff felt ill prepared to care for people with dementia. Even those that had built up a repertoire of skills through experience were slow to recognise or express any pride in their expertise. Most interactions were based purely on meeting physical care needs. Psychosocial needs, in particular, issues of communication and "difficult" patients evoked great feeling of uncertainty in staff. Staff consistently avoided engaging with patients on an emotional level and recognising them as individuals with unique lifeworlds and needs. It appeared that staff were often working in a "switched off" mode.

In essence the data portrays a sobering picture of the experiences of patients, lay carers and health and social care staff of the care received by older people with dementia in the acute hospital setting. This chapter broadly presents the "what" and "how" of this ethnography. The "why" is presented in chapter four together with a practice development project that is intended to address some of the issues that have been identified.

CHAPTER FOUR

PRACTICE DEVELOPMENT

Introduction

In this chapter, analysis of the data continues. The "why" element of ethnographic analysis (Katz 2001) is considered in some detail. This explanation of what was found to be currently "going on" in practice areas is used to set the scene for practice development and guide further activity. Ways are examined in which this research study may be used to effect a change in practice. This is a vital component of the work as the purpose of this research was to generate findings which would be valuable in influencing improvements in care for older people with dementia in acute hospitals. A range of potential frameworks for influencing practice are considered, including the use of dissemination, education and practice development. Use of dissemination in changing practice is investigated. The main focus is on non-traditional approaches, in particular ethnodrama and research based drama, and story telling and evocative writing. These methods were selected primarily for their congruence with the ethnographic underpinnings of the research study. Literature concerning the use of education to enable staff to provide a higher standard of care for patients with dementia is reviewed. The philosophy of practice development is considered and how it may be applied to this. A model of practice development, which is linked with the ethnographic approach to the study, is proposed. Implementation of the initial stages of this model is discussed. Subsequent stages of the model are described including potential evaluation of its effectiveness.

Background

It is recognised that this study is just one of many new qualitative studies that are produced each year. It is estimated by Mulrow and Cook (1998) that over two million articles are published annually in over twenty thousand health related journals. Despite this burgeoning number of publications there is little evidence that research findings are applied in practice (Waddell 2002). The danger is that this study will join the wealth of work that is completed but then sits on a shelf having brought about little or no change in practice (Finfgeld 2003, Troman 2001). It may be argued that as this work is being completed as part of a Doctor of Professional Practice programme, with an inbuilt expectation of practice development, it stands a better than average chance of being influential. It is recognised that qualitative research, if done well, is worth disseminating (Keen and Todres 2006). This thought is taken a step further by Gray et al (2000) who are convinced that researchers have a responsibility to ensure that their work makes a difference in the everyday world. This sentiment is echoed by Richardson (1994), Mienczakowski (1997) and Denzin (1997). It is acknowledged that there is a growing call for research to be applied in practice but there are indications this has yet to be achieved.

Traditionally the success of academic research has been assessed using narrow criteria including output of published, peer reviewed articles, bibliometrics and citation counts (Davies et al 2005). This approach pays little attention to the concept that researchers should aim to offer some "return on investment" (Wooding et al 2004), which may be judged through the impact that the research has on practice. The relative inability of research to influence practice is not new. However, the issue is becoming more frequently recognised, particularly with the notion of evidence-based practice becoming so prominent.

A vast amount of literature is now available that does not appear to be assisting practitioners to change practice. Indeed, as Waddell (2002) suggests, the sheer volume available may be daunting and possibly inaccessible to those providing direct care. It is evident that some steps have been taken in an attempt to make research findings more readily available. There are an increasing number of systematic reviews which synthesise the findings of a range of studies, these include papers published from central sources such as the Cochrane Collaboration. Another approach to enabling practitioners to apply research in practice has been the production of clinical guidelines. These summarise best research and make recommendations for practice. Despite the profusion of guidelines there is little evidence they have any impact on practice (Cabana et al 1999). It could be argued that this position has changed in more recent years with the production of guidelines from the National Institute of Health and Clinical Excellence which practitioners are advised to follow. It is suggested by Waddell (2002) that summarising research findings and production of guidelines may be helpful to practitioners but this alone is not sufficient. This author points to the need for more active dissemination approaches such as audit and feedback. It remains clear that at present little is known about which dissemination techniques work best with which decision makers in which settings (Lomas 1997).

Regardless of the uncertainty of how research can be best used to influence practice Nutley et al's (2002) assertion that there is a need to address the gap between what we know and what we do remains valid. There are a range of frameworks that may be considered to contribute to changing practice. Frameworks that will be explored in more detail are dissemination, education and practice development. To set this in context and to assist in identifying the most appropriate methods of using this study to change practice the ethnographic "why" is considered in a review of what was found to be "going on" in the practice areas involved in the research.

The Ethnographic "Why"

Findings of this research portray a complex picture of care received by patients with dementia in an acute hospital. Patients described the experience in largely negative terms. Their responses to some of the care implied that it was detrimental and observations indicated that the patients' personhood gradually diminished as staff attempted to meet their physical care needs. Carers found it difficult to articulate their thoughts about care. They were generally uncritical except in cases where they felt their expertise was disregarded by staff. A number of carers experienced problems in negotiating an acceptable level of involvement in their partners' care. Staff tended to have clear ideas about standards of care that should be delivered. This was frequently based on personal philosophy and beliefs rather than on the wishes of patients. Staff reported that they felt ill prepared to care for people with dementia; they tended not to recognise or appreciate skills they had developed in practice. Psychosocial needs of these patients evoked great feelings of uncertainty in staff.

In essence, the findings reveal a sobering picture of the experiences of patients, lay carers and health and social care staff of the care received by older people with dementia. A common response to the findings would be to simply attribute blame, usually to staff, for not providing the highest standard of care. This would seem unjust given that the majority of staff appeared to be working relentlessly to deliver what they believed to be appropriate care. A more fruitful approach may be to consider further analysis of why the situation was as it was in order to elucidate the actions that would need to occur to effect a change in practice.

As discussed in chapter three, staff working in wards where the research was conducted had a clear concept of the care that they were trying to provide. The philosophy of care held by staff tended to be based on care that they would like their families or themselves to receive in similar circumstances. Many staff struggled to articulate their philosophy further than this.

Care that was observed appeared to reflect the accepted ideal within contemporary health care. That is, it could be deemed to be efficient, effective and productive (Malloy and Hadjistavropoulos 2004). Care that was provided was set firmly within the "bed and body" framework (Gubrium 1975) with little attention paid to the psychological, spiritual, emotional or social needs of patients. Delivery of care was seen to be highly routinised with patients expected to fit in with the work of the organisation rather than the patients being viewed as valued users of services provided by the organisation.

The extent to which care was mechanised and patients' own needs and desires were subsumed to ensure that the organisation ran effectively was shocking. Despite having practiced as a registered nurse for over twenty years, I did not feel that I had previously witnessed care that was so influenced by the needs of the organisation rather than those of individual patients. It is debateable whether I have genuinely not worked in this type of culture or perhaps more disturbingly had become desensitised, as many of the practitioners I observed, to such an approach. It is possible that becoming a participant observer, slightly removed from the everyday work of the wards, allowed me to view care through a new and alarming lens.

Care that I observed with its focus on efficiently meeting physical needs could be likened to Goffman's (1961) description of the experiences of people residing in total institutions. Goffman (1961:11) describes total institutions as places where a number of individuals, removed from wider society for a significant time "together lead an enclosed, formally administered round of life". Collopy et al (1991:8) elaborate on this description when discussing the experiences of residents in nursing homes. These authors suggest that "daily life in the institution is tightly scheduled and is organised around "batch processing" of inmates or residents," (Collopy et al1991:8). This description has great resonance with what I observed, particularly in terms of the extent to which people with dementia were expected to comply with activities such as bathing early in the mornings regardless of their usual habits.

To enable such a "batch processing" (Collopy et al 1991:8) model of "care" to be used it may be argued that there is a need for staff to be able to view patients with dementia as "others" or not complete and worthy human beings. It appears that in this case the process of stigmatisation and labelling may have been used to allow staff to categorise patients as "others" and not deserving of the treatment provided to those who were cognitively uncompromised. Goffman (1961) suggests that the process of stigmatising individuals in some way operates as an effective method of social control but, more than that, it allows people to be stripped of their former identity and their humanity. It may be considered that for people with dementia the process of stigmatisation is well advanced before they enter the acute hospital. As Kitwood and Benson (1995) state, dementia is often viewed as the steady erosion of personality and identity to the point where no "person" remains. If staff believe this concept of dementia and then additionally label these patients as "sweet", "difficult" or "only social", it is not wholly surprising that care is constructed for non-humans. This allows the central tenets of privacy and respect to become superfluous and "care" to be impersonal and unthinking (Malacrida 2005).

Goffman's (1961) description of the total institution provides a stark analysis of the way in which one group of human beings, given the opportunity, will treat another usually weaker and more vulnerable group. Whilst some parallels may be seen between the total institution and care that was observed in this research, it is felt that this link does not explore in sufficient detail why "care" is as it is. There is clearly a need to explore in more detail what is actually "going on" in practice and to develop an understanding of what influences the behaviours observed.

There are a range of potential explanations about the care observed in this study. I have chosen to focus on two concepts that are particularly resonant with the findings of the study. Firstly empathy, or rather the evident lack of empathy, displayed by many staff. A review of empathy offers a greater understanding of the actions of individual practitioners. The second concept is that of Bourdieu's (1977) Theory of Practice which provides a broader focus on the culture of the organisation. This theory links closely with the concept of empathy and demonstrates how "non-empathic" behaviour may be passed from one practitioner to another.

Empathy is a concept that has been well documented in the literature although much of the writing tends to focus on empathy in relation to doctors rather than other health care professions. It is suggested by Hart (1999) that empathy has many shades of meaning. However there are some common beliefs about the concept, these include the idea that it involves "feeling into" another's world (Hart 1999). Empathy is generally considered to embrace both cognitive and affective domains; there is a need to comprehend another person's experience and feelings (Hojat et al 2002) and a capacity to enter into these feelings (Hojat et al 2001).

It could be argued that Balint 1964 (cited Evans 2003) was instrumental in bringing the concept of empathy to the fore in health care. Balint pioneered the idea of the therapeutic value of practitioners themselves proposing that the

> "ability to listen is a new skill … in learning to listen to patients the doctor begins to listen to himself …. [which requires] a limited though considerable change in personality"(Balint 1964 cited Evans 2003:11).

The value of empathy in health care is recognised by many, its merits are seen as including

- Being a base for moral development (Hoffman 1990, Olsen 1997)
- Possibly being the trait that makes us most human (Azar 1997)
- Contributing to good attitudes towards elderly patients (Bagshaw and Adams 1986)
- Being a basis for better therapeutic relationships (Bertakis et al 1991, Livinson and Roter 1995, Hart 1999)
- Possibly mediating stereotyping of minorities (Vescio et al 2003)
- Benefiting patients (Howie et al 1999, Hojat et al 2002)
- Embracing emotional as well as intellectual engagement and therefore helping practitioners to see the patient from a more holistic viewpoint (Halpern 2003)
- Potentially increasing adherence to care recommendations (Vermeire et al 2001, Roter et al 1998)
- Potentially increasing staff satisfaction (Suchman et al 1993)
- Enabling the practitioner – patient relationship to move from I-It to I-Thou mode (Hart 1999)

Empathy is clearly seen as a positive attribute in health care practitioners and one that I frequently saw subsumed in depersonalised, mechanised methods of care. There is some evidence that empathy is a trait that is often compromised during training. A range of research indicates that empathy declines during medical training (Diseker and Michielutte 1981, Bellini et al 2002, Hojat et al 2002, Bellini and Shea 2005). This research all focused on entrants to the medical profession, however it is suggested that some of the findings, possibly to a lesser extent, are likely to be applicable to other groups of health care staff. A number of explanations are postulated for this decrease in empathy. In medical education it is suggested that students are socialised into a state of "detached concern" (MacLeod 2000). They are taught a point of view and a technical language that allows them to think of patients and disease in a completely different way to lay people. It is argued that this type of socialisation is substantially different from that of other health care staff which perhaps teaches a more holistic view of patients. It is suggested that other staff, in particular nurses, tend not to lose their empathy during pre-registration education but rather this loss largely occurs as staff work in practice on a day to day basis. Reasons for this may be two fold. Firstly, as Kitwood (1997a) states, it is part of the human condition for us to fear being old and having a cognitive impairment. Exposure to this reality on a daily basis is likely to lead to staff building a protective shell around themselves which precludes having real empathy with patients. This idea is supported by Salinsky and Sackin (2000) who suggest that staff may have a range of defences that are built up over time through a combination of personal and professional circumstances. These authors describe this defence as being a state of having an "illusion" of professional self that remains unaffected by human emotions. Salinsky and Sackin (2000) argue that this state is unsustainable and practitioners needs to recognise that their professional persona is merely a specialised part of their personal self. An alternative or possibly additional explanation is that reduction in empathy may be attributed to staff entering the health care habitus on a permanent basis. This idea is explored in more detail in the next section.

Whilst empathy is seen as an essential component of high quality patient care, the extent to which it can be developed is debateable. It is suggested by LaMonica et al (1987) and Kirk and Thomas (1982) that empathy is a personality trait that cannot be taught easily. Equally Goldstein and Goedhart (1973) and LaMonica et al (1976) argue that empathy can be improved through targeted education. This thought is supported by Steplen and Baernstein (2006) who conducted a literature review of educational interventions to increase empathy in medical students. Whilst acknowledging the limitations of their work, these authors conclude that empathy can be measurably enhanced using a range of interventional strategies, feedback on performance and reflection. It is emphasised by Beach et al (2004) that to achieve real empathy there is a need to mean and not just act, a similar philosophy to McCormack's (2003) call for authenticity in relationships. It is recognised that increasing empathy is likely to involve considerable "emotional labor" (Larson and Yao 2005) and high levels of motivation (Evans 2003). I believe the investment needed to develop or rekindle empathy in staff would be worthwhile as a lack of empathy compromises the provision of person-centred care as has been demonstrated in the findings of this study. Whilst a lack of empathy in individuals offers some explanation for the care delivered, it is evident that there is also a need to consider the culture in which staff are working.

Bourdieu's (1977) Theory of Practice has been used to illuminate why care was as it was and what was "going on" in practice from a broader perspective. Bourdieu offers a more sensitive and sophisticated way of analysing the actions of practitioners and patients than is possible when attributing their behaviour simply to being an integral part of a total institution or linking behaviour with a lack of empathy. Bourdieu's model moves away from the notion that people can be defined by social class membership and offers instead a much more complex explanation of individuals occupying positions in a multi-dimensional social space. Three key concepts are encompassed in this model: practice, field and habitus.

Key concepts of Bourdieu's model will be explored in more detail in relation to this study. Practice may be described as social interaction of everyday life (Jenkins 2002). It is suggested by Bourdieu (1977) that every group of people who view themselves collectively have theories about the world and their place in it. These ideas are constructed in and through participating in everyday life. These constructs are not merely theoretical; they are concerned with doing as much as knowing. Jenkins (2002) states that people develop acquiring and learning a range of practical cultural competencies including social identity. The fact that people have grown within a culture makes it difficult for them to see social reality as anything more than "the way things are" (Jenkins 2002:70). It is therefore argued that many people, for much of the time, take themselves and their worlds for granted. This concept was seen on many occasions when I asked staff about the care that they delivered. When they stopped to think, they would often answer "that's the way we do it" demonstrating little obvious underpinning thought. At a simple level this was also illustrated by a conversation I had with two nursing assistants. When I asked how they organised their workload, they looked at me as though it was an extraordinary question the answer to which was so obvious that the question should never have been asked. They slowly explained that self-caring patients were attended to before more dependent patients. Variations within this were only seen if patients had an early appointment or if they had been incontinent. No heed was paid to individual choice.

Bourdieu (1977) explains the field as being a system of social positions, these are structured internally in light of power relationships and are constructed according to underlying principles that dictate practices and experiences within that field. The field could be described as a social milieu where individuals struggle to secure specific resources (Jenkins 2002), it is a space where conflict and competition occur. It is not a static arena but rather a series of structures and activities which relate to people in the field each of whom is capable of producing effects on it (Rhynas

2005). Fields in this study can be defined as the three individual wards that participated.

Each field comprises a structured system of social positions in which people may strive to gain dominance (Jenkins 2002). Ability of players within the field to gain dominant positions is influenced by their access to, and possession of, four types of capital: economic, social, cultural and symbolic (Bourdieu and Wacquant 1992). In this study the construction of the field was influenced by the patients, lay carers and staff who were present at any given time. Throughout the study it was evident that the field changed as it was influenced by the behaviour of, and relationships between, key players. The extent to which patients and staff were in possession of capital varied although it was always clear that patients were at a disadvantage.

Ways in which staff interacted with patients could increase their capital in very small, but significant, ways which allowed them to be recognised as functioning members of the culture. Economic capital was inevitably weighted in favour of staff although occasionally they took actions that enabled patients to gain minute amounts. Evidence of this was seen when one patient was unable to buy her daily newspaper from the mobile vendor as the ward was closed due to infection. One of the nurses asked me if I could go to the shop for the patient, the nurse handed the patient her purse so she could give me the money. This small act acknowledged the importance to the patient of getting her newspaper and recognised her ability to manage her own money even if in a very minor way. This allowed the patient an element of economic capital. Despite small gains to the patients in terms of economic capital it could be suggested that staff are in a more powerful position as they are in paid employment whilst many patients had virtually no economic status or even access to money whilst in hospital.

Social capital is measured in terms of valued relationships with others. It may be argued that staff, whilst not necessarily having valued relationships in the work setting, did as a minimum have some sense of belonging to a group. Patients reported feelings of loneliness and many did not have meaningful relationships with others. Relationships between staff and patients rarely appeared to have depth and meaning. An example of this was seen in a conversation between two nursing assistants. They talked about the way that two patients with dementia were behaving the previous day; one nurse said "I'm convinced they've worn themselves out …. up all day …. up all night honestly, I felt like Barbara Woodhouse 'sit'". This was said with no animosity at all. Although this conversation conveyed no ill intent it does very clearly demonstrate the way in which these nursing assistants interpreted the position of patients within the culture.

Cultural capital is based on legitimate knowledge. Once again staff are in a dominant position as, although many felt that their knowledge is limited, they did have the advantage of knowing about routines and expected plans of care. Patients were rarely privy to this type of information and often showed their distress about not knowing what was going to happen to them.

Symbolic capital refers to the value attached to a person by others. It could be suggested that this type of capital is limited for both staff and patients. Staff reported that they felt undervalued as they worked in a speciality that was perceived as being afforded little prestige by other areas. Equally patients fell at the bottom of the hierarchy at both macro and micro levels. Within individual ward settings the staff had greater symbolic capital simply in terms of being employed to deliver care.

Bourdieu's (1977) third concept is that of habitus which is a set of practices that are shared by a group of people within a field and which provides guidance on appropriate behaviour for everyday situations (Lumme-Sandt and Virtanen 2002). It is suggested by Rhynas (2005:182) that habitus is "embodied reality that is often unquestioned because of its inherent nature". Habitus may be developed as the behaviour of others in the field is imitated and a process of iterative learning occurs (Lane 2000). It is concerned with how people, in light of incorporated knowledge and thoughts, act, think and place themselves in given situations (Sidenvall 1999). The major influence on habitus is experience rather than deliberate teaching. The development of habitus inclines people to act in certain ways and provides the basis for the generation of practices. The fact that the development of habitus is largely subconscious can be problematic. Jenkins (2002) suggests that the power of habitus derives from the thoughtlessness of habit and habitual action rather than from consciously learned rules and principles.

In practice there were many examples of the way in which habitus had developed within individual wards. Some of these could be seen as almost insignificant, for example a nursing assistant came to take Hilda's lunch plates away, Hilda asked her to take her cup and glass away as well, the nurse said to Hilda "no, we don't take them now", she offered no other explanation. Hilda looked really disappointed. I asked her if she was a neat and tidy person, she smiled widely and said "yes". This small incident demonstrates the extent to which the habitus of staff dominates that of patients which may be wholly neglected.

Data from this study indicate that staff have a well defined habitus. Despite the fact that very few had received any education about dementia care many had developed ways of working and interacting with people with dementia that represented a cultural norm. These behaviours appeared to have become integrated into their practice although as Lumme-Sandt and Virtanen (2002:289) suggest it is likely that staff functioned within a set of rules of which they were not consciously aware, a situation which these authors describe as "knowing without knowing". Whilst staff maintained their habitus it could be argued that patients rapidly lost theirs. Each one of the activities that they would automatically engage in was gradually eroded. This notion was demonstrated by Sidenvall (1999) in a study of mealtimes in an older peoples rehabilitation unit in which care was predominantly task rather than patient-orientated. The result was that staff effectively maintained their habitus whilst patients rapidly lost theirs as they were denied any opportunity to manage their mealtimes in their usual way.

Bourdieu (1984:101) brings together his three concepts in a perceived interaction which he expresses as [(habitus) (capital)] + field = practice. Reflection on this research indicates that staff retain their habitus whilst patients tend to lose theirs. Staff have a greater share of capital. It is clear that any struggle for capital is an unequal one and that staff effectively maintain dominance in virtually every respect. This dominance allowed staff to routinely occupy higher social positions within the field. These factors, in combination, undoubtedly influence the practice, of everyday life on the wards. This idea is acknowledged by Sidenvall (1999:321) who suggests that it allows for the development of a "special institutional culture" in which staff have a leading position and patients are subordinated. It is argued by Parker (2005) that this situation is perpetuated as the system is internalised by individuals, this is then reflected back on the world.

Whilst Bourdieu (1977) provides a useful tool to analyse some of the factors that influence the way in which care is delivered to people with dementia in acute hospitals it does not acknowledge the possibility of change or challenge to the current position (Morgan 1999). Parker (2005) argues cogently that Bourdieu's model does not account for the paradigm shift that has occurred in dementia care over the last two decades. It could be argued that whilst there has been a shift in thinking from a biomedical to a psychosocial person-centred base, there has not been a parallel shift in action. Key points from this study that have been identified using Bourdieu's model are that:

- Staff appear to be “switched off”, often working in an automatic, “non-thinking” mode.
- There is little evidence that staff view patients as individuals with their own unique lifeworlds.
- The power relationships between patients and staff are weighted heavily in favour of staff.
- The habitus is deeply ingrained with new staff rapidly being socialised into the cultural norms, this reflects Sidenvall’s (1999:321) “special institutional culture”.
- Staff tend not to question the way in which they deliver care accepting instead that it is “the way things are” (Jenkins 2002:70).
- Staff, on the whole, appear to have little empathy with patients with dementia

This analysis supports the concept that the paradigm shift from “old culture” to “new culture” care has yet to occur in practice. Analysis suggests that education alone is unlikely to effect a real change in practice. The current state of what is “going on” in practice indicates that there is a need to consider approaches to practice development that will engage staff on an emotional level. This will enable them to examine their own beliefs and behaviour and how this impacts on the people with dementia for whom they are providing care. To an extent, this idea is supported by Parker (2005:261) who asserts that there is a need for “training at a deep and reflective level in which the new culture of dementia care becomes part of daily practice rather than a distant ideal”. It may be argued that Parker’s reference to training offers a rather narrow approach to development. In order to achieve a broad perspective, the value of dissemination, traditional education and practice development are considered as tools to support improving practice.

Methods of Developing Practice

This section considers using dissemination, traditional education and practice development as tools to support improving practice. A review of how the most valuable elements of these tools have been amalgamated in a model of practice development is provided. Implementation of the initial stages of this model is then explored.

Dissemination

Dissemination, defined as the spreading of knowledge, is viewed in different ways according to the standpoint of the researcher. For academic researchers it is likely to be seen as an essential component of their activity, both on a professional and institutional level. It may be argued that for practice-based researchers dissemination sits much lower on the agenda and may, in reality, never occur. Whilst dissemination is recognised as being vital, it may be considered that alone it is unlikely to have any real impact on practice. Traditional methods of dissemination are particularly limited in their ability to develop practice. The fact that dissemination is often seen as an adjunct to the research process rather than an integral part of the project (Dahlberg 2006) may limit the amount of thought it receives. Traditional dissemination tends to be focused on publication in academic journals and therefore ruled not by the research itself but more by research tradition (Dahlberg 2006). This can effectively force researchers to adjust the research to conform to existing rules to ensure acceptance for publication. In qualitative research particularly this can lead to heavily edited reports that lose essential meanings. The tendency to write in scholarly journals inevitably limits the audience and is likely to make the study less accessible to practice-based staff.

It is widely accepted that research should be used to influence practice. However, as discussed, there remains a chasm between generation of research findings and demonstrable changes in clinical practice. As Waddell (2002) notes, even the best research frequently remains unused by policy makers and practitioners. It is possible to speculate a number of reasons that could explain why research is currently having relatively little impact on practice. Current methods of dissemination tend to conform to the traditional scientific mould. A focus on "science" may be encouraged as this type of work is likely to be recognised in the research assessment exercise. The drawback to this type of dissemination is that it is liable to attract a largely academic audience (Barnes et al 2003) and to reinforce divisions between researchers and practice and action (Mullen 2003). It is possible that this focus on scientific aspects of studies is to the detriment of communicative concerns (Sells et al 2004, Todres 2004, Willis 2004). It is suggested that without effective communicative strategies researchers will continue to struggle to make any real impact on practice.

Concerns about the comparative lack of success in communicating the findings of qualitative research in such a way that they influence practice led Keen and Todres (2006) to review use of non-traditional methods of dissemination.

The major features of effective dissemination strategies are drawn together by Keen and Todres (2006:9) in an extensive literature review of non-traditional methods of dissemination, these include:

- Tailoring approaches to the audience, in terms of the content, message and medium.
- Paying attention to the source of the message.
- Enabling active discussion of research findings (Nutley et al 2002, Walter et al 2003).

It is very evident how these strategies contrast with the aims of traditional dissemination. Keen and Todres (2006) suggest that using a range of interventions offers the best chance of promoting changes in behaviour.

Literature indicates that there is a slow but steady increase in innovative methods of disseminating qualitative research that are intended to support practice development. Keen and Todres (2006) have identified a wide range of methods of dissemination, two of these that appear particularly pertinent to this study will be examined in more detail. These non-traditional approaches have been selected predominantly for their resonance with the ethnography and narrative research methods that have been used in this study. Central tenets of ethnography and narrative research include the concepts that direct, "thick" descriptions of a culture are provided often from the emic, or insider's, perspective (Geertz 1973, Fetterman 1998, Holloway and Wheeler 2002). Narratives enable the stories of individuals to be told in such a way that meaning is given to the thoughts and actions of participants (Polkinghorne 1988). Use of these research methods was congruent with my desire to ensure that participants with dementia remained central, that their voices were heard in whatever way was possible and that I was able to present a fair and authentic account of their experience of care in an acute hospital.

When considering methods of dissemination the above desires remained fundamental. I felt that use of research-based theatre and ethnodrama and evocative writing and story telling were most likely to support presenting the findings of this study in a way that was authentic, engaged an audience and could, potentially, lead to demonstrable changes in practice. These approaches will be examined and their utility assessed.

Research Based Theatre and Ethnodrama

Research-based theatre and ethnodrama are relatively new additions to the repertoire of dissemination methods in qualitative inquiry. It is suggested by Denzin (2000) that these approaches appeal to a new generation of researchers who have a commitment not just to describe the world but also to change it. At present there are only a small number of proponents of research-based drama but their enthusiasm for the approach is clear. Turner (1986:81) implicitly supports the value of dramatic performance in describing humankind as "homo performans" suggesting that the natural state of humanity is to perform. A more specific call for the use of drama is provided by Denzin (1997:94) who states that "the performance text is the single most powerful way to recover yet interrogate the meanings of lived experience".

Dramatic performance is described by Kontos and Naglie (2006) as an alternative method for translating and disseminating research which provides accessible presentations for audiences from a wide range of backgrounds. Although there are some indications that dramatic performance is being used to disseminate research findings and change practice, it is evident that progress remains slow with Gray et al (2000) reporting that only a handful of authors have attempted to present research thorough drama.

Two influential drama projects that have been extensively reported in the literature are the works "Handle with Care? Living with Metastatic Breast Cancer" (Sinding et al 2002) and "No Big Deal" a production about men living with prostate cancer (Gray 2003). "Handle with Care?" was developed from qualitative research findings. In this production people with metastatic breast cancer worked alongside a theatre company, from script writing to performance, to produce a drama that aimed to best represent the perspectives of participants in the study. It is reported by Gray et al (2000) that the theatre company found working so closely with people with metastatic disease was effective in limiting their use of artistic licence. This, arguably, would ensure that the production remained grounded in the lifeworld of the research participants. The production was intended to entertain and engage the audience rather than merely informing them. It was staged on over one hundred and fifty occasions (Gray et al 2001) to a variety of audiences and was deemed to be extremely popular with a health care practitioner audience of whom one hundred percent stated that they had enjoyed or strongly enjoyed the performance and ninety-three percent suggested that it was useful in terms of thinking about their clinical practice (Gray et al 2000).

"No Big Deal", a production about living with prostate cancer (Gray 2003), drew on a range of quotations from original research interview scripts to devise a series of vignettes that illustrated issues that had emerged from the study. In contrast to "Handle with Care" the participants in the research that underpinned "No Big Deal" were not able or prepared to go on stage. They were, however, instrumental in script development. Gray (2003) acknowledges the poignancy of having people with disease on stage but he surmises that their absence did not detract from the power of the performance. This drama was performed to a range of audiences including health care staff, patients and the public.

Gray et al (2003) studied a group of twenty-six health care professionals who attended a performance of "No Big Deal", interviewing them pre-performance and at two weeks and six months post-performance. Findings of this research lend weight to the idea that drama may be an effective tool for dissemination. Most of the participants felt that the content was accurate and reflected elements of their own practice. They spoke of the humanising effect of engaging with patients' lives on stage and the impact that this had on reducing the usual gap that exists between health staff and patients. It was suggested that this allowed them to develop insight into and empathy with the situations being experienced. Participants recognised that the drama had exposed them to a visceral encounter with patients' emotions. Gray et al (2003) state that the predominant finding from this study was the depth of intimacy and engagement with patients that was made possible through the medium of drama. These authors are realistic about limitations of this research as all the participants were volunteers and therefore likely to be more positive and open about the value of research-based drama. Gray et al (2003) are clear that drama is not a panacea and propose that to be used effectively the quality of the production must be assured, content must realistically reflect the lifeworlds of patients and staff and the style of presentation must be suited to content and health care context.

Ethnodrama as a distinct style of research-based drama has been pioneered by Mienczakowski. Ethnodrama is described by Mienczakowski (2001:468) as being about the "present moment"; it is about giving the text back to the readers and recognises that we are all co-performers in each others' lives. Mienczakowski has produced a number of ethnodramas which have involved people who are traditionally disadvantaged in health care systems. "Synching Out Loud: a Journey into Illness" was compiled from data gathered from people who had experienced psychosis. Original data from this study was reworked and fictionalised to produce a script for the drama (Mienczakowski 1995). Informants were included in the process of script development to ensure validity. Further validation was secured through informant group readings and preview performances. "Synching Out Loud" was interpreted on stage by students of theatre and nursing. This production was followed by "Busting: the Challenge of the Drought Spirit" (Mienczakowski and Morgan 1993). The project began in an urban detoxification unit. Emphasis in this production was on the use of adapted verbatim narrative. This choice was made in respect for the informants desire that their actual words should be heard by the audience. Content of the script was agreed by the informants prior to performance and the script was available to the audience following performance.

Both these works were intended to be a type of public voice ethnography that had both emancipatory and educational value (Mienczakowski 1995). This author used extensive validation processes to create a sense of vraisemblance, that is the quality of seeming to be true or likely, (Todorov 1968: cited Mienczakowski 1995). Mienczakowski places great emphasis on blurring the boundaries between policy makers, health care staff, services users and the general public. Following performances the audience were invited to contribute to a debriefing session in which ideas were discussed, interpreted and individuals were given the opportunity to respond to the presentation (Mienczakowski 2000). These types of performances are described by Mienczakowski et al (1996) as confrontational theatre in that they seek to bring about moments of catharsis in audience members. It is reported that during some performances "audience members were frequently reduced to tears" (Mienczakowski et al 1996:443).

A different concept of drama is embraced by Keady and Williams (2007) in their description of co-constructed inquiry. This research approach is built in three stages: building the set, performing the production and bringing down the curtain. Keady and Williams (2007) suggest that this approach allows the gap between researcher and participants to be bridged. It gives people, particularly those with long term conditions, an opportunity to present their subjective experience through a life-story script, a personal theory and ultimately a collective theory. This approach supports a genuine research partnership with people with long term conditions (Keady and Williams 2007). The utility of this method is illustrated in a single case study of a person with dementia (Keady et al 2007). This paper demonstrates how one individual worked with a clinical nurse specialist to co-construct her experience of living with dementia. The individual's life story proved to be a powerful influence in supporting her coping strategies. This suggests that co-construction may have implications for future research and practice.

This brief review of research-based theatre and ethnodrama indicates that these approaches have clear merit as non-traditional methods of disseminating qualitative research. These are summarised below:

- Descriptions provided by those that have used the method in practice suggest that it is a powerful and evocative tool.
- It may enable audiences to reflect on their own beliefs and possibly encourage health care practitioners to reflect on their practice.
- It may be more accessible to a wider range of audiences.
- It may encourage the sharing of experiences between lay and professional people thus increasing understanding.
- It appears to be an effective way of engaging with large numbers of people.
- It can engage the audience on an emotional level allowing an unusual depth of intimacy and engagement with patients.

However, there are some drawbacks to this method when applied to this study:

- Participants in this study would have little or no chance of validating the scripts due to their advanced dementia.
- The capacity of participants in this study to engage in co-constructed inquiry is limited due to their severe dementia and physical illness.
- Exceptionally skilled script writing would be required.
- The skill required for actors to portray people with dementia would be considerable.
- Financial outlay for this type of performance would be enormous and funding for unorthodox approaches is likely to be difficult to secure.
- The ethical basis of asking an audience to contribute to refinement of the script is dubious and may detract from the contributions that were given by original participants with such effort.
- There is a lack of evidence that this method of dissemination leads to real changes in practice.

Use of research-based theatre and ethnodrama remains a minority form of dissemination in health care. A major advantage of using such techniques in practice development is the ability of this medium to truly engage staff on an emotional level and enable them to reflect on the care that they deliver from a new perspective and thus potentially change their practice. Practical difficulties in using drama as a method of dissemination for this study have been identified. However, preliminary studies provide some evidence that it may be a powerful and evocative tool.

Evocative Writing and Story Telling

Story-telling has a long history of being a powerful tool in communication (Koch 1998). The value of stories is succinctly listed by Serrant-Green (2006) who suggests that they have a capacity to influence our future action, the ability to impact on our views of the world and the potential to encourage us to review and reflect on ourselves and others. Similar claims are made by Olofsson and Norberg (2001) who suggest that narrative can inform us about past actions and also help us to understand the meanings of such actions. This idea is echoed by Viney and Bousfield (1991) who cite the value of narrative as allowing people to create meaning in events. Serrant-Green (2006) proposes that a particularly valuable attribute of narrative is that it may facilitate access to the experiences of people that are often marginalised, overlooked, and "silenced" in a discriminatory society. This concept is reinforced by Dean (1995) and Turton (1997). It is suggested by Sedney et al (1994) and Heiney (1995) that story telling may be therapeutic. Van der Staay (1994) claims that stories can inform social policy whilst Gabriel (1995) and Yanow (1995) state that stories can be used to support change in an organisation.

Despite this long history, the concepts of evocative writing and story telling are relatively new in health care research. Although these approaches are now well accepted and increasingly visible in social science (Lieblich et al 1998, Denzin 2001) the term story telling was first added to the Cumulated Index of Nursing and Allied Health Literature in 1997. Story telling and narrative as terms are defined by Frid et al (2000) who describe story telling as a repeated rendition of a story by someone other than the narrator. It is suggested by Barnhart (1988) that entertainment is an integral part of the definition of storytelling. Frid et al (2000) define a narrative as an account of events as experienced by the narrator. Regardless of these differences, the terms story and narrative have largely been used interchangeably and synonymously in nursing work (Fagermoen 1997, Rittman et al 1997). In light of the lack of agreed definitions the tradition of flexible usage is followed in this chapter.

Bailey and Tilley (2002) suggest that stories in the health care context can move understanding beyond the biophysical domain. It is clear that the use of story telling and narratives is gaining support in health care research. However the way in which it is undertaken remains vaguely defined, as Coffey and Atkinson (1996:80) suggest "there are no formulae or recipes for the "best" way to analyse the stories we elicit and collect". Equally this sentiment may be applied to the way in which stories are presented and disseminated. Key proponents of story telling include Ellis and Bochner (2006). These authors debate the relative merits of realist and auto-ethnography. Although it is recognised that my study fits more closely with the realist genre, some of the attributes of auto-ethnography are absolutely congruent with my beliefs about dissemination. Ellis and Bochner (2006:431) argue that a realist ethnography can reduce the reader to being a "detached spectator" who may become "only a head, cut off from body and emotions". They suggest that auto-ethnography strives to get the reader "to care, to feel, to empathise and to do something, to act" (Ellis and Bochner 2006:433). This aim accurately reflects what I am trying to achieve in disseminating this work. Efforts of other researchers using narratives or story telling approaches have yielded variable results, a small range of examples from health and social care are critiqued.

Olofsson and Norberg (2001) undertook a narrative study with the intention of understanding the experiences of psychiatric patients, nurses and physicians in relation to their own and others' experiences of coercion. These authors drew on the work of a range of experts in narrative analysis to shape their work including Bruner (1990) and Riessman (1993). Findings that are presented provide some insights into the experiences of both patients and practitioners. However the paper is largely devoid of any feeling for individuals and their stories. It appears that key aspects of the interviews have been melded into distinct categories that bear little relation to the people involved and who are not recognisable in any way. It is argued that in narrative analysis confirmation or validation of trustworthiness is achieved by making the research process visible (Riessman 1993, Bailey 1996). Readers should then be able to determine for themselves whether they choose to trust the account that is being presented (Riessman 1993). Ostensibly Olofsson and Norberg (2001) have made their research process transparent and they have described their approach in some detail. However the final product feels depersonalised and makes it difficult for readers to relate to the experiences described. This paper perhaps illustrates the difficulty of trying to condense a long and complex study into a word-limited article for a scholarly journal.

A biographic, narrative, interpretive method (Chamberlayne et al 2000, Wengraf 2001, Jones 2004b) is used by Jones (2006) in his narrative concerning seven people from a "disabled"" household. Jones (2006) used a single narrative inducing question to enable participants to provide an extensive and uninterrupted account of their story. In his analysis Jones interprets the narratives of the individuals and presents parts of their stories in a way that allows the reader to develop their own understanding of, and empathy with, the protagonists. It is clear that this research is not intended to be generalised or have theories extrapolated from it. However Jones (2006) makes his contribution to knowledge absolutely clear, that it may be care givers, rather than those who are cared for who are most in need of emotional care. Narrative presented is thought provoking and undoubtedly each reader will make their own interpretation of it. Jones (2006:219) concedes that the work may rouse strong emotions in readers and justifies this by stating

> "if, by engaging with these stories through this particular lens, the reader is disturbed, even inflamed or enraged, but subsequently prodded to rethink informal care … from a new perspective, then the effort put forth here is justified".

Sells et al (2004) worked with people with severe mental illness to construct their personal narratives. Having gathered data, they described their research task as trying to organise and synthesise a chaotic collection of fragments of experience into a narrative that was coherent yet still maintained the complexity and richness of the detail that had been shared. Sells et al (2004) chose to write the stories in the first person arguing that using the third person leaves the person open to objectification if their story is told by the researcher. These authors suggest that using the third person also runs the risk of presenting stories about "types" rather than individuals. Sells et al (2004) question whether the compression of vast amounts of data into concise narratives is too neat. They go on to claim confidence in the validity of their work as the final version is an amalgamation of the interpretations of five qualitative researchers thus providing the equivalent of "inter-rater reliability". This approach to narrative development would be challenged by others who believe that a narrative is not an exact record of happenings but rather one version of events (Olofsson and Norberg 2001). It may be suggested that these researchers were trying to get the stories right. However, it is argued by Richardson and St Pierre (2005) that stories cannot be "right" but rather differently contoured and nuanced. Sells et al (2004) suggest that validity may be further enhanced by returning the stories to participants. They do not report whether this happened in their study. Bailey (1996) suggests that member checking in narrative research is of limited value as narratives are not static as the meanings of experiences constantly develop. In some respects the approach taken by Sells et al (2004) appears contrary to much of the literature around story writing and telling. However, the narratives they have provided have a real resonance and allow the reader a glimpse into the individual worlds of people with severe mental illness. These authors contend that historically this group are associated with unintelligibility or "emptiness". They suggest that this phenomena may reflect the clinicians' lack of empathy and state that a research approach that supports empathetic reflection is not only possible but an effective method of revelation.

As already demonstrated the use of narratives can be an effective method of sharing research findings, the particular value of this approach is outlined below:

- As humans are natural story tellers, this method may enable them to reflect on and understand the meanings of some of their actions.
- Evocative writing may convey new understandings of the illness experience for individuals.
- They may enhance our ability to review and reflect on ourselves and others.
- Stories may give voice to people who are traditionally silenced.
- They can crystallise events in a person's life through a particular lens (Richardson and St Pierre 2005).
- They have the potential to help us understand the diverse experiences of others and recognise similarities between these experiences and our own (Serant-Green 2006).

This summary provides a clear indication of the value of using narratives as one approach to disseminating this research. The concept that narratives allow the voices of those traditionally silenced is so pertinent to the people with dementia who were involved. The idea that narratives may encourage practitioners to understand the experiences of others and reflect on their own behaviour is central to achieving a real impact in practice. Using narratives in this work has a value in that they preserve "whole stories" in a form that has a clear relationship to the everyday lives of staff and so have the capacity to influence their approaches to care. However, the use of story telling and evocative writing remains problematic for the following reasons:

- Stories are interpretive and in turn require interpretation, this may lead to some to doubt their credibility (Ayers and Poirer 1996).
- They may be long stories that are inaccessible to those practitioners to whom they would be of most value.

- If they are to be published in scholarly journals they may have to be severely edited to meet the requirements of word limits and this may considerably reduce their power and impact.
- In much narrative work there is an implicit assumption that participants will have the ability to share their own story. In this study the idea was problematic as, although the participants appeared to have some semblance of personal narrative intact, their ability to communicate this was limited due to their dementia and often superimposed physical illness.
- This reduction in personal narrative leads to stories being recounted through my lens rather than that of the participants, although this is made explicit throughout.
- A great deal of skill is needed to write evocatively.
- There is little evidence that the production of narrative has made any real impact on practice.

It is evident that a non-traditional approach to dissemination is appropriate for this study to ensure that it genuinely impacts on practice. The value of research-based theatre and ethnodrama and evocative writing and story telling is clear. The question to be addressed now is how these methods may be harnessed to develop practice in light of the findings of this study. These ideas are expanded later in this chapter.

Education in Dementia Care

Literature relating to improving dementia care suggests that a common response to developing practice is to implement training or education programmes for staff. A brief review of health care literature reveals that there has been some progress in approaches but these generally remain within traditional educational confines. Two types of education that are particularly congruent with this study are examined, these are: confluent education and situated learning. A small range of educational materials is briefly reviewed. The impact that dementia education has on practice is explored.

It is suggested by Ortigara and Rapp (2004) that, like dementia care, education about dementia has evolved considerably over recent decades. These authors state that education about dementia was initially firmly grounded in the medical model, teaching was delivered by "experts" and focused on biomedicine. This approach was superseded by behavioural models in which staff were taught to tailor their care to match the needs of the individual with dementia. Ortigara and Rapp (2004) suggest that it was believed that adopting this type of strategy set the scene for good dementia care. These authors state that dementia education has evolved further during the last few years with a marked shift towards person-centred, relationship-based models. Principles that are central to this approach include three notions: each person with dementia is an individual with a value in their own right; that to provide best care there is a need to nurture relationships with individuals, there is a need to develop skills in seeing the world from the perspective of the patient.

Whilst Ortigara and Rapp (2004) write confidently about the evolution of education in dementia care there are hints in recent literature that these more person-focused approaches have not permeated the thoughts of all education providers. A number of recently reported education programmes continue to be based on single issues rather than adopting a whole person slant. This approach to teaching could be described as situated in the old culture in which people with dementia are problematised and seen from a negative mindset.

Landreville et al (2005) describe a training programme for managing agitation in residents in long term care. Training consists of eight hours of didactic teaching and eight hours of supervision in practice. The impression given by the authors is that the programme focuses entirely on behaviour that is perceived as negative and fails to address the needs of individuals from a holistic perspective. A further single issue study is reported by Mickus et al (2002) who describe an education intervention in which staff are taught techniques for reducing problem behaviour during bath time. The flavour of this study is behaviour management as opposed to respect for the person. Martin et al (2004) implemented education about what they describe as the highly specialised bathing interventions that are required by people with dementia living in nursing homes. Although some elements of recognition of individuality were encouraged in this programme, the feeling remains of a task that must be performed rather than an activity in which the individual's personhood may be respected and even enhanced.

These studies provide some indication that even quite contemporary education has not yet fully embraced the concepts of new culture dementia care (Kitwood 1997a). Equally, others have recognised the need to provide person-focused, relationship-centred education that is tailored to the needs of learners. Alternative methods for delivering education have gradually evolved over a number of years. In parallel with this change there has been a growing realisation that educating staff in isolation will not lead to sustainable improvements in care. It is recognised by Lintern et al (2000) and Packer (2000b) that training alone will not change practice. Although these thoughts are not fully justified, it would appear from observation and experience that they have considerable credence.

Other authors concur with the idea that training will not produce changes in practice. Moniz-Cooke et al (1998) state that whilst education may produce some changes initially, staff tend to revert quickly to prior ways of working. In order to overcome this issue it is suggested by Lintern et al (2000) that whatever training is put in place must be congruent with the aims and objectives of the organisation and that managers must be committed to the endeavour. Engagement of managers is taken a step further by Mueller-Hergl (2003) who insists that managers demonstrate their commitment to cultural change before their staff can attend training.

Requirement for consistency between the beliefs and values of the organisation and training that is provided is vital in enabling staff to change practice. Ballard et al (2001) argue that when current practice is criticised but no alternatives appear to be available staff are likely to exit education feeling demoralised and deskilled. James et al (2003) state that giving learners information that is incompatible with the belief systems of the organisation in which they are working can be counterproductive. This idea is supported by Mueller-Hergl (2003) who suggests that if an organisation is not ready for change there is a likelihood that staff will become increasingly disillusioned and leave their employment.

Current approaches to dementia education appear to be moving from traditional didactic methods to a more experiential stance which embraces the needs of adult learners. Didactic approaches are rejected by both Innes (2000) and James et al (2003) on the grounds that they are highly unlikely to effect real change. James et al (2003) also cautions against the tendency of these styles to draw attention to problems in staff performance which can negatively impact on the learning experience. Use of teaching methods which are specifically aimed at adult learners is increasingly advocated.

An experiential, person centred approach is promoted by Ross (2005). Although the aim of the course was to provide staff with an "arsenal of skills and resources to deal with … challenging and difficult behaviour" (Ross 2005:41) this perhaps belies the trainers' underlying mindset. The value of experiential learning is considered to include an increased capacity for the learner to understand the person with dementia at a deeper level (Wood 2002, Beckett 2001). It is also thought to meet the needs of present day adult learners who are accustomed to visual interaction (Kemeny et al 2006) and who may lack confidence in engaging with traditional methods of education (Bova and Kroth 2001, Cohen et al 2001). Whilst some authors are enthusiastic about the use of experiential learning it may be argued that it is extremely difficult to recreate the experience of dementia in others. Use of this technique is questioned by Becker (1998) who states that unless skilfully facilitated it may create anxiety that limits learning and unintentionally supports negative attitudes.

Realisation that dispassionate, factual teaching is not advantageous is recognised by Bell and Troxel (2003a). These authors explain how education being provided to a group of carers in a residential setting had ceased to be effective. Participants were bored and appeared to learn little from the sessions. The authors chose to implement a more interactive style in which the teaching was tangibly linked to the participants' everyday work and in which the experiences of residents were seen in the light of them being whole people. The aim was to keep the session simple and to ensure that staff left with the intention of completing an agreed follow-up activity that would impact on care. The change in style is reported to have led to significantly more interactive sessions in which the staff were fully engaged. A person-centred approach to education is also advocated by Boettcher et al (2004a) who describe a programme which aims to enable staff to view patients as human beings rather than as objects for whom tasks need to be completed.

There are two approaches to education that are, as yet, virtually unconsidered in relation to dementia, confluent education and situated learning. These methods appear to be particularly valuable in terms of being allied to the research methods used in this study and in supporting achievement of the desired outcomes.

Confluent Education

Use of confluent education in teaching staff about the care of people with dementia is not yet documented but the philosophy of this method matches closely the aims of enabling staff to deliver better care. Confluent education is an approach that deliberately integrates affective and cognitive learning. It is described by Francke and Erkens (1994:384) as a means to "integration of the learning of the head with the learning of the heart". The fundamental concept in confluent education is that it is about teaching the person rather than the subject matter (Brown 1990). It involves the structured integration of learners' thinking, feeling and actions throughout the process of education (Shapiro 1975 cited Misch and Peroquin 2005). This approach embraces the concept that empathy is a vital part of high quality patient care.

Published reports on the use of confluent education in health care are extremely rare. One article by Misch and Peloquin (2005) describes its use in the education of physical therapy students to enable them to develop empathy with their clients. Although this paper is inconclusive about the effect that confluent education had on students it does provide a clearly reasoned rationale which would suggest that such an approach should work. Misch and Peloquin (2005:45) outline the essential features of confluent education as including:

- A context or climate of two-way openness to learning.
- Awareness of the self as a legitimate object of learning.
- Subject matter that is closely related to the significant personal needs and feelings of learners.
- Experience-based learning.
- Awareness and intention to develop convergent cognitive processes integrated with other learning.
- Encouragement of the expression of feelings by both student and teacher.
- The use of feedback to refine and develop learning.
- Encouragement of diverse and imaginative thinking.
- Resubjectivisation of meanings.

It is clear that these essential features have much in common with the overall aims of this study in that the intention of confluent education is to engage learners on an emotional and intellectual level thereby enabling them to reconsider their own relationships and interactions with service users.

Situated Learning

Another educational philosophy which is particularly allied to the aims of this study is that of situated learning. The concept of situated learning emanated from the work of Lave and Wenger (1991:11) who suggested that "human minds develop in social situations". These authors propose that all learning is contextual and set within the social and physical environment. Such thoughts had considerable resonance with the embedded habitus that was discovered as a result of this research. Lave and Wenger (1991) contrasted conventional views of learning, which they describe as a process in which students internalise knowledge, with social learning which involves the whole person acting in the world. It is stated that in social learning the focus is on "person-in the-world, a member of a sociocultural community" (Lave and Wenger 1991:52). The concept of seeing learners as whole people has clear parallels with the aim of enabling them to see people with dementia as whole people. In social learning, knowing is concerned with activity by specific people in particular circumstances, as opposed to the acquisition of facts.

Principles of situated learning are described by Halse and Hage (2006) as encompassing the concepts that knowledge needs to be presented in an authentic context and that learning requires social interaction and collaboration. It is felt that the notion of authentic context can be interpreted liberally to include working alongside peers from practice in addition to learning in the practice setting. Situated learning is particularly pertinent to nursing as it recognises that becoming proficient in practice involves not only the acquisition of technical skills but also the ability to join a culture of practitioners. This idea is supported by Beck and Young (2005:188) who suggest that professional education requires the "creation of a professional habitus" which embraces a common moral and ethical code and a sense of purpose.

O'Connor (2007) appears to view situated learning as synonymous with work based learning. Despite this oversimplification the author does make some valuable points about this approach. It is suggested by Wenger (2000) that learning acquired in practice will be emancipatory, or as stated by Engestrom (2001) "expansive". O'Connor (2007) cautions that idealist notions of the benefits of situated learning should be treated with care. This author wisely notes that whilst learning in practice may be a positive experience, equally negative practices and behaviours can be transmitted with ease.

One of the key concepts of situated learning is that of the community of practice. Communities of practice are described by Seely Brown and Duguid (1991) as groups of people, often from the same organisation, who have a common sense of purpose and who have a desire to share their skills and knowledge. Wenger et al (2002) state that communities of practice share three distinctive features. They have a common goal which brings people together, members have relevant knowledge and act as a social entity and they share resources of the community as a whole.

Tolson et al (2005) investigated the value of a community of practice through setting up a virtual community of gerontological nurses in Scotland. These authors describe some of the technological issues associated with the project. Despite these issues, the nurses involved felt that the opportunity to communicate and share knowledge with likeminded colleagues across the country had been valuable in terms of enhancing their ability to describe their unique contribution to nursing and thus their ability to raise the profile of gerontological nursing as a speciality in its own right. Tolson et al (2005) concluded that the formation of a community of practice was of particular value in that it allowed nurses to share their expertise. It also encouraged recognition of strategies that had been ineffective in improving practice and so prevented them being replicated in other areas. This allowed more time to implement changes that might work. These findings concur with Wenger's (2003) assertion that membership of a community of practice can empower members, strengthen professional identity and enable clearer status to be identified. Benefits outlined are highly relevant to some of the goals of this project in that there is a real need for the nurses to recognise the value of the care they provide to patients and to become accustomed to sharing their knowledge and skills.

Whilst definitions of situated learning vary from one author, to another there are common traits that suggest that it is appropriate for this practice development. These include:

- Learners being viewed as a whole person, a concept that is congruent with the notion of personhood in dementia care.
- Recognition that learning is contextual and embedded in the world.
- A community of practice can be a powerful forum through which practitioners can share knowledge and become empowered in their practice.

Educational Materials

A brief review of the educational material available suggests that some continue to adhere mainly to the old culture of care. Several practical guides still depict people with dementia as damaged or incomplete although, as Ashworth and Ashworth (2003) suggest, the language used tends to be more polite. This negative concept can also be seen in a web-based teaching package that is currently under development. The Elderworld (2006) CD ROMs portray images of people with dementia that focus far more on disability than retained abilities. Resources that emanate from the new culture, whilst hugely valuable, tend to be slightly esoteric and of limited value to those delivering care. Dewing (2004) reviewed a number of models of person-centred care and suggests that, to be of use, these models need to be translated into everyday language. Dewing points to the need to find creative ways to move from the position where staff see person-centred care as a luxury, or something that they have never encountered to a way of working that can actually be implemented in practice. This idea perhaps lends weight to Packer's (2000a) statement that there is a growing body of evidence that training, whilst valuable, is not enough to change practice.

The Impact of Education on Practice

It is evident that a range of approaches to educating staff about the care of patients with dementia continue to be used. The extent to which these are effectively evaluated varies. Review of a small sample of studies indicates that evaluation has tended to concentrate on the participants' views of courses, self-reported changes in practice or intention to change practice. Ross (2005) reports on an educational course provided to nursing home staff, students and volunteers all of whom were involved in the care of people with dementia. Following the course, participants were asked if they would change the way they worked, affirmative answers were provided by 57%, 89% and 100% respectively. It is notable that those who were likely to provide the highest level of care for the most severely affected individuals were least likely to consider changing their practice. Lockyer et al (2005) described a course about dementia that was delivered to several groups numbering 932 physicians; the course embraced a range of teaching methods. Effectiveness of the education was judged primarily using commitment to change statements in which attendees stated their intention to change. These were supported by impact statements in which participants were invited to report self-perceived changes to their own practice. The study reports positive outcomes, however these are based purely on personal opinions. Other authors have attempted more objective measures. Bourgeois et al (2004) presented a communication skills programme to a group of non-registered staff. Evaluation was based on three observation periods, each of which lasted for five minutes pre and post training and at follow up. Improvements in communication between staff and residents are reported. It may be argued that a five minute snapshot is an extremely short time in which to judge communication. Equally it is suggested that the measure of what constitutes effective skills such as announcing care when entering the residents room, addressing the resident by name and waiting for five seconds before giving physical help could not be considered to be aspiring to truly person-centred care.

Although education clearly has a place in improving care given to people with dementia a number of pitfalls remain. In particular, literature remains equivocal about the most effective ways of delivering training to a group of staff who may have widely varying backgrounds and skills. Content of education is not yet agreed with some educators focusing on specific tasks or behaviours whilst others concentrate on promoting person-centred approaches. It is suggested that there is a need to move on a step from person-centred education to approaches that enable practitioners to develop genuine empathy with the people with dementia for whom they are caring. Whilst person-centred approaches are creditable it may be argued that they still do not engage staff on the emotional level that has been discussed in relation to the use of non-traditional methods of dissemination. It is suggested that unless teaching touches the emotions of learners they will continue to be able to exit education without any commitment to changing the care that they provide. Two relatively unused models of education are proposed as having the potential to engage staff on an emotional level. These models both appear plausible in their attempts to educate staff in ways that are concordant with the desired outcomes of this work.

It is recognised by several authors that training alone will not change care and that there is a need for organisational commitment to cultural change. Evaluation of education remains weak, mostly being based on self reported change rather than more objective measures. This brief review of education in dementia care indicates that education alone is relatively unlikely to improve care. There is therefore a need to consider more holistic approaches to change. This notion led to a review of practice development.

Practice Development

Practice development has become a common phrase in health care. It is described in broad terms by McSherry and Warr (2006:57) as an attempt to "break free from the chains of medicine, mangerialism and the hierarchy of routines" and move towards patient-focused care based on independent, accountable and autonomous decision making and practice. The exact nature of the concept remains poorly articulated (Unsworth 2000, Carradice and Round 2004). Kitson (1994) describes practice development as

> "a system whereby identified or appointed change agents work with staff to help them introduce a new activity or practice … the introduction of the development ought to be systematic and be carefully evaluated to ensure that the new practice has achieved the improvements intended".

Kitson's concept of practice development can be challenged on two counts. Firstly, the extent to which practice development is truly systematic is debateable. Secondly, the definition implies that the change agent is an external figure thus giving the impression that practice development is "done to" practitioners. This issue arises again in the work of McSherry and Warr (2006) who argue that, given that practice is now so busy and stressful, it is essential that named practice developers are introduced if organisations and teams are to be successful in modernising. It is not clear whether these authors envisage the appointment of an external practice developer or whether they are suggesting that a named person within the existing team is given specific responsibility for practice development. If it is the former this is likely to have a significant impact on the team's sense of ownership of any development work.

It is suggested by McCormack et al (1999) that practice development is often poorly regarded in health care, this may be because the outcomes of such activity are less amenable to measurement than other advances. This thought is echoed by Page (1998) who argues that the reputation of practice development suffers as it is less easy to categorise than other activities such as audit or research. McCormack et al (1999) state that, in contrast to many linear approaches to change management, practice development is "messy". This idea is supported by Bell and Proctor (1998) and Walsh (2000) who describe the process of practice development as complex and dynamic. A lack of absolute definition brings about some problems when trying to assess the impact of practice development activities. Clark and Proctor (1999) report on a collaborative practice-based research project that evolved over time as the work progressed. These authors suggest that this evolution made the project intangible. This type of flexibility may result in it being difficult to demonstrate exactly what has been achieved.

A number of authors have attempted to offer more clarity in practice development. Unsworth (2000) worked with a group of nine practitioners involved in practice development to produce a concept analysis of the term. This group articulated four critical attributes of practice development: it should lead to new ways of working which result in direct and measurable improvements in service; development should be based on specific patient need; services that are developed should be effective and should contribute to the maintenance or expansion of business. It could be argued that these attributes, whilst valuable, may be more appealing to managers than to practitioners and patients.

An alternative view of practice development is offered by Page and Hamer (2002) who suggest that it is situated at the interface of quality improvement, evidence-based practice and creativity and innovation. Emphasis in this model is on development occurring within the practice domain, the focus being on patients and an acknowledgement of the messiness and complexity of practice. This vision of practice development moves towards the definitions provided by Mallet (1997:38) who describes it as "the advancement of patient-focused care" and McCormack et al (1999:256) who state that practice development is "a continuous process of improvement towards person centred care". Centrality of person-focused care is reiterated by McSherry and Driscoll (2004) who suggest that the real value of practice development is its holistic approach and powerful drive to improve health care using the lived experiences of patients.

In order to produce a change in practice McCormack et al (1999) argue that a range of cultural values need to be considered. These authors suggest that there is a need to understand the context and culture of the organisation, there should be a commitment to user involvement, a desire for clinical and cost effectiveness, a culture that supports team development and that practice development should be practitioner owned. In a study of nurses' perceptions of practice development Garbett and McCormack (2001) found that the term was frequently associated with roles and people. People in these roles tended to be seen as "extras" with a development remit which the nurses implied was quite separate to their own work. Approximately half the respondents in this small study viewed practice development as being synonymous with training and course attendance. Cultural change was rarely considered as a concept.

A brief review of practice development confirms that the term remains relatively poorly defined. In summarising practice development McSherry and Warr (2006) suggest that it embraces engagement, empowerment, enlightenment, evaluation and evolution. Literature broadly concurs with these ideas and provides a range of key elements that are central to practice development:

- Practice development is intended to improve person-focused care (Page and Hamer 2002, McCormack and Garbett 2003, McSherry and Driscoll 2004).
- Links between practice development and education are strong through much of the literature but education does not automatically produce improvements in practice (Unsworth 2000).
- Practice development should be practitioner-owned and should empower practitioners to instigate change (Page and Hamer 2002, McSherry and Warr 2006).
- Practice development is "messy" (McCormack et al 1999, Walsh 2000).
- To be effective practice development needs to bring about cultural change (Katzenbach and Smith 1998, McCormack et al 1999).
- Methods of evaluation should be considered and agreed.

On reflection the process of practice development looks extremely daunting, particularly when related to the complex and challenging arena of dementia care in acute hospitals. It is evident that a range of strategies would be needed to produce any real change in practice.

A range of issues have been covered so far in this chapter. The practice arena has been analysed to elucidate what is currently "going on". It is recognised that research findings need to be used to influence practice. The fact that non-traditional methods of dissemination may offer a new and potentially more appropriate method of engaging with those caring for patients with dementia is explored. Use of research-based theatre and ethnodrama, and story telling and evocative writing have been investigated and their value and limitations identified. Educational approaches to changing practice are investigated, including the use of confluent education and situated learning which, to date, have been little reported in health care. Practice development as a notion is explored.

Conclusions that have been drawn so far are:

- Findings of this study need to be disseminated.
- Non-traditional methods of dissemination are appropriate with research based drama and story telling being particularly congruent with the research methods used in this study.
- Traditional approaches to education are unlikely to be helpful although some more innovative models may have value.
- Any practice development activity needs to adopt a non-critical stance and should be practitioner-owned.
- Practice development needs to be based in the real world of practitioners so that it remains contextually grounded and "real" to them.
- It should enable staff to realise their capacity to change practice
- The practice development should enable practitioners to develop or rekindle empathy.
- Methods of evaluating practice development should be agreed.

It is evident that in order to bring about a real change in practice there is a need to address the issues from several perspectives. There are a number of key strands that are essential if sustained practice development is to be achieved, these include:

- Raising the profile of the care of older people with dementia at national level.
- Raising the profile of the care of these patients at the level of individual acute Trusts.

- Supporting ward leaders to develop cultures in which the concepts of person-centred care are extended to staff and patients alike.
- Facilitating change in practitioners who deliver direct care.

The challenge is to find ways in which at least some of these ideas may be enacted in practice within the time and financial constraints that are in place. There is also a need to make recommendations for more far reaching research and practice development. Attempting to improve dementia care in acute hospitals is clearly a vast undertaking and unmanageable within the confines of this project. There is therefore a need to consider development from a realistic perspective; the initial project will focus on one older peoples unit providing acute care for people who also have dementia. Work will concentrate on beginning to change the practice of the staff who deliver most direct care to this patient group. In addition to this major strand, consideration will be given to engaging managers in the practice development process. A model of how this may be achieved is set out in the following section.

Model of Practice Development

This model of practice development has been constructed using some of the key features of changing practice that have been highlighted earlier in the chapter. It has been designed specifically for one acute hospital, the staff of which have a desire to improve the care delivered to people with dementia within the older peoples unit. Prior to developing the model I took the opportunity to send the General Manager and Matron of the unit a summary report of the research study, this included a selection of patient narratives. At a subsequent meeting the General Manager had clearly been both moved and disturbed by what she had read. She was keen to discuss the narratives and gain greater understanding of the experiences of those involved. Matron was less surprised by what she read, presumably due to her much greater exposure to day to day practice. The narratives obviously had an impact on both readers and they were eager to consider ways in which future practice may be improved. The General Manager was willing to provide the time and financial resources that were associated with this project. One early opportunistic action was for a staff member to attend a five day course on dementia care delivered by a national dementia guru. This attendance was made possible by an educator from the Alzheimer's Society who is closely linked with this project.

Following the staff member's attendance at this course I had a further meeting with Matron to discuss the project in more detail. Matron had received feedback about the course and was full of enthusiasm about changes that could be made in practice. She informed me that she now knew that people with dementia do not like the colour blue; that they like bright colours and that they do not like to use white crockery. As a result of these revelations she had decided to redecorate parts of the wards in bright colours and buy some coloured plastic picnic plates. At this point I was torn between wanting to be supportive of her enthusiasm and desire to do something and a feeling of despair at the lack of understanding of respect for individuality and personhood. On reflection I chose to try and discover the basis for these ideas. A review of literature, particularly the work of Jones et al (2006), shed light on this. Although ideas that Matron had discussed were clearly based on evidence, there seemed to be no recognition that they were concepts that needed to be considered for individuals rather than a simple solution for a complex issue.

Following our conversation I felt concerned that if Matron believed in such "quick fix" solutions she would find my proposed approach to practice development rather slow and esoteric and not in keeping with the instant changes she was keen to effect. It is notable that several weeks after our meeting these changes had not been mentioned again.

Matron, the General Manager and I discussed the model, I emphasised the need to ensure that staff had ownership of the project and that they were empowered and supported to develop practice in their clinical areas. At this stage I felt it was important to gain the commitment of the Ward Leaders as they are the group who are most likely to influence care at the point of delivery. I arranged a meeting with Matron and the Ward Leaders in which we discussed the proposed model of practice development and plans for the future. Initially we talked about the findings of my research. They had already had an opportunity to read some of the narratives and had found them moving and, in places, concerning. I took this opportunity to show this group "Ex Memoria" (Appignanesi 2006), a short DVD portraying the experiences of a person with dementia in residential care. I sought their views about the DVD and the impact they felt it may have on more junior staff.

In discussion Ward Leaders were quick and accurate in identifying deficits in the care they had viewed. When I asked if there were similarities between the DVD and the care on their wards they became more circumspect and clearly found this a challenging question to answer. Initially there was a slight feeling of defensiveness. However, on further discussion Ward Leaders began to identify some areas of commonality. They talked about the rigidity of the routine in which they work and the need to balance organisational requirements with individualised care and the need to consider all patients not only those with dementia. These issues are congruent with those highlighted by Archibald (2003) in which organisational requirements often take precedence over individual needs.

Ward Leaders recognised that care was not always to the standard they expected. I asked them about the impact they felt that "Ex Memoria" would have on more junior staff. Their initial response was "*quite shocked I think*". They then suggested that they would think "*no, we're not that bad, yes it does tell us some of the things we don't do well enough*". At this stage we talked again about some good practice that I had observed and the ways in which this could be distinguished and shared with colleagues. We went on to discuss the proposed model of practice development. Ward Leaders agreed that they would be open to some support but they were keen to utilise existing expertise and maintain ownership of the project. I assured them that these were also the aims of myself and my colleague from the Alzheimer's Society.

We discussed what the Ward Leaders would like to achieve from this practice development project, their ideas included:

- "*changing people's perceptions really .. that's what we* can *do.*"
- "*consider how frightened they might be ... and that's what we're not picking up on*".
- "*trying to listen, what are they* actually *saying ... what are they trying to say*".
- "*when a patient needs to be specialed giving the nurses the opportunity to come away from their workload .. just be with that person*".
- "*spending time with the patients*".
- "*one nurse to go to the patient not a whole* load *of people .... one person speaking quietly and calmly*".

These desired changes in practice are admirable; they demonstrate compassion and a real wish to improve care. However they hint at a slightly paternalistic mindset of working "for" rather than "with" these patients. It may be argued that these outcomes fit closely with Ashworth and Ashworth's (2003) description of care delivered with kindness but which still ultimately disempowers and depersonalises patients. I felt that the Ward Leaders still had some way to go until they fully embraced the type of care that respects and nurtures the personhood of individuals (Kitwood 1997a).

Positive outcomes that emerged from this meeting were that the Ward Leaders expressed a real commitment to working collaboratively to develop practice. It was also clear that they were willing for themselves and their staff to engage and develop on an emotional and cognitive level rather than simply seeking "quick fix" solutions. As a result of this meeting we agreed that to ensure that staff were fully involved in the project, each of the wards would be invited to nominate two members of staff who had expressed a special interest in dementia care. Nominations were invited from all occupational groups, all those received were from nursing staff from a range of grades. The course was over-subscribed but a decision was made to expand numbers slightly to accommodate most nominees. Nominated nurses were designated as "dementia champions" and agreed to be the leads for the project in their areas of practice. It was also agreed that an external facilitator from the Alzheimer's Society would be involved in the design, implementation and evaluation of the project.

A proposed model of practice development was designed and agreed with the General Manager, Matron and a facilitator from the Alzheimer's Society (figure 4-1).

Development of this model is explained below as are the ways in which it has, or will be, applied in practice. As has already been recognised, this project is a major undertaking that will require commitment, time and resources if it is to be successful. As discussed one of the first actions when designing the model was to ensure that the General Manager, Matron and Ward Leaders were supportive of the development; their commitment was readily secured. I felt at this stage that the work of convincing more junior staff of the value of this project would be considerably more challenging.

As identified in chapter three, staff involved in this study appeared to view themselves as the poor relations within the organisation as a whole. It is well recognised that the care of older people is rarely seen as a prestigious speciality in which to work. The research showed that staff were quick to devalue themselves both in relation to others in the organisation and in terms of the value they attached to their own contributions to care. They were working in a habitus which was institutionally focused and in which they did not question practice. It is hoped that the investment that is being made in this project may help to raise the profile of dementia care and allow staff to develop expertise that is recognised and valued both by themselves and by others at a wider level.

It is accepted that facilitation of change is likely to be a complex and challenging undertaking. In the first instance it is suggested by Binnie and Titchen (1999) that there is a need to win the "hearts and minds" of individuals. Ways in which this has been achieved will become clear as the stages of the model are examined. Binnie and Titchen (1999) acknowledge the necessity of staff being enabled to see the need for change and to develop a desire to change. These authors recognise that this can be a slow and frustrating process and caution against the temptation to force change. Carradice and Round (2004) state that in any attempt to produce change there is a need to be realistic about where staff are now and to avoid trying to implement exciting and innovative interventions that would move staff to the position that you would wish them to occupy. In implementing this project a range of interventions will be used as this is considered to be the most effective way of promoting changes in behaviour (Keen and Todres 2006).

These thoughts clarify that any change in practice is inevitably incremental and slow. It is suggested that one of the first actions would be to enable practitioners to reflect on the current situation. This approach is congruent with emancipatory practice development as explained by Manley and McCormack (2003). This style of development aims to improve care but it also focuses heavily on empowering practitioners to develop services and fosters the development of a transformational culture (Manley 2001). One of the outcomes of this approach is "action from enlightenment" (Manley and McCormack 2003:27). Enlightenment is a vital factor that is also alluded to by McSherry and Warr (2006). The need for enlightenment is clear as many of these practitioners appear to be operating at what Clarke and Wilcockson (2001) describe as the competent level with its associated defeatist attitude and lack of belief that the status quo can be altered. Practitioners at this level have a mindset that is located within existing structures and systems of care delivery. It is felt that staff who have expressed a special interest in dementia care may be the most receptive to changes intended to improve care.

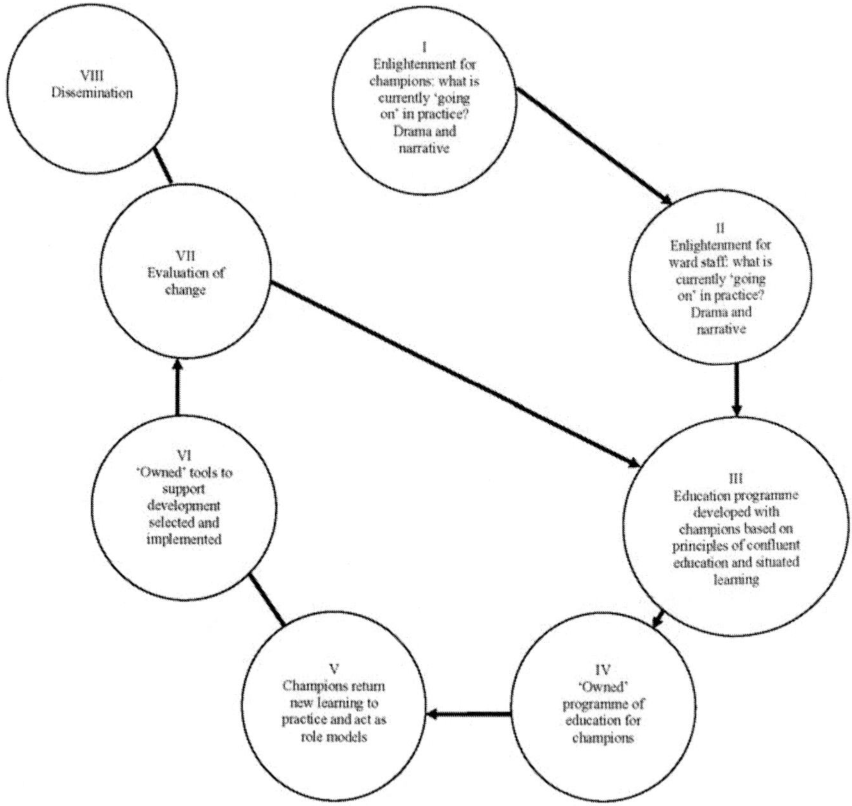

Figure 4-1: Model of Practice Development

Appointment of dementia champions who expressed a special interest in dementia care is intended to ensure that the people who are going to take this work forward have a genuine interest in, and commitment to, development. Stages of the practice development model through which champions and staff have worked, or will work, are outlined below. At each stage the intention has been to embrace the principles of confluent education and situated learning. This has been achieved by involving champions in identifying their learning needs, acknowledging the situations in which they work, treating learners as whole people, people-in-the-world, and hopefully enabling them to return to practice to influence the habitus in which they currently exist.

Implementation of the model is outlined in this section. As can be seen, the process did not follow the expected path. As it became clear that the original model was somewhat overambitious and unrealistic, the model was modified as development progressed. A draft programme was designed (table 4-1).

Workshop 1: 5th September 2007, 1.30 – 5pm Indicative content • Introductions • Feedback from research • Ex Memoria • What would you like to see change in practice? • Identification of learning needs
Workshop 2: 3rd October 2007, 9.30am – 4pm Indicative content • What is dementia? • The experiences of people with dementia • Content devised according to identified learning needs
Workshop 3: 7th November, 9.30am – 4pm Indicative content • Reflection on practice since workshop 2 • Content devised according to feedback from workshop 2 and identified learning needs
Workshop 4: 28th November 2007, 1.30 – 5pm Indicative content • Reflection on practice since workshop 3 • Content devised according to feedback from workshop 3 and identified learning needs • Evaluation

Table 4-1: Draft Dementia Workshop Programme

The development programme had a particularly inauspicious start. Organisation by the Trust was shambolic with the IT systems proving totally inadequate. Champions mostly stated that they had been "sent" on the course; they had not received any of the pre-course material and were unclear about why they were there. At this stage I was overwhelmed by frustration and disappointment, particularly in light of the amount of preparation that had occurred. I felt that this start may reflect the level of organisational commitment to the work. Despite these issues the champions, after a slow start, did appear interested and had some ideas about how practice could be changed to improve care.

Stage I: Enlightenment for Champions: What is Currently "Going On" in Practice? Drama and Narrative.

Stage one of the model involved working alongside champions to enable them to develop some insight into what is currently "going on" in practice. The purpose of this was to begin to challenge the mindset or habitus of these individuals which, as previously stated, is pervasive. Any approach to changing habitus needs to be grounded within the experiences of those delivering care. It may be argued that the first steps to change need to occur on an emotional level. Practitioners need to be enabled to recast individuals with dementia as whole people who deserve to be treated with respect and dignity. It is likely that non-traditional methods of disseminating the findings of this study would make a positive contribution to this aim.

These thoughts led back to the concept of using research-based drama and narrative to share ideas and generate new ways of envisioning practice. Having reviewed the work of others in creating dramas it is considered that the input required is simply too ambitious for this project. For this reason an alternative approach was sought.

One tool that has been developed by Appignanesi (2006) is a short film entitled "Ex Memoria". This fifteen minute DVD depicts the life of a lady with dementia living in a residential home. The film is produced in a way that focuses on this individual's view of events. It is intended to encourage viewers to consider what it is like to be an older person with dementia rather than dictating what we should think or do. Although it is set in a residential home it powerfully illustrates many of the depersonalising aspects of the care that were witnessed when observing people with dementia in an acute hospital. It may even be considered an advantage that the film is set in a residential home rather than an acute hospital as this reduces the risk that staff will interpret the DVD as intending to be critical of their current practice. As Ballard et al (2001) note, criticising staff is likely to be counter-productive when trying to enable them to improve care.

Using "Ex Memoria" is seen very much as a starting point in opening the minds of staff about the care that is currently being delivered. This type of thinking was certainly evident when the DVD was shown to Ward Leaders. Producers have devised a set of issues that may be raised following viewing; these may encourage staff to reflect on what they have seen. If managed skilfully over time staff may then be enabled to reflect on how this relates to the care they deliver. To add a more acute care focus, the narratives that have been produced as part of this study were also shared with the champions. To be most effective they were recorded on audio-tape and played to the staff group. They then had the opportunity to discuss and reflect on the content and identify how they relate to their own experiences.

The first stage of the model was intended to enable staff to really think about and reflect on the habitus which they and the patients currently inhabit. Encouraging staff to consider their current practice will inevitably be a slow process in which there is a great need to focus on both positive and negative aspects of care. Initial sessions using "Ex Memoria" and the narratives with the dementia champions yielded a range of thoughts. Feedback from the DVD and narratives was very similar to that of the ward leaders.

Champions could recognise elements that they considered unacceptable. They talked openly and honestly about the difficulties in providing best care. They noted that the organisational culture and the pressure of their workload prevented them from being able to deliver the quality of care they desired.

Stage II: Enlightenment for Ward Staff: What is Currently "Going On" in Practice? Drama and Narrative.

At this stage it was intended that champions would return to their clinical areas and replicate the sessions using drama and narratives. Champions would have received support from senior staff and Matron to deliver these sessions. It was anticipated that enabling peers to facilitate these sessions would encourage staff to engage with them rather than viewing them merely as an opportunity for senior staff to blame them for any deficits in care. During the first session with the champions it became very clear that they did not have the confidence or skill to take forward this stage of the development. Stage II was therefore postponed for further review.

Stage III: Programme Developed with Champions Based on the Principles of Confluent Education and Situated Learning

Having postponed Stage II of the development work commenced on Stage III, a programme based on the philosophies of confluent education and situated learning. Underpinning tenets of this education were very much on educare "to rear or foster" as opposed to educere "to lead forth ..." (Williams 1988:111). The intention in devising the programme of education was to empower the champions to work as equals with the educators. It was important for the educators to avoid taking on the role of "redeemer" who knows what is best and makes everything right (Mueller-Hergl 2003:9).

It is recognised that much current dementia education concentrates particularly on those delivering care within residential settings rather than in acute care. There is also a tendency for education to focus on single issues, such as behaviour management, as opposed to embracing a truly holistic, person-focused perspective. Initial stages of this project focused on enabling staff to become aware of the habitus in which they are working. This initial work also has the potential to allow staff to develop greater empathy with patients for whom they are caring. It was intended that the education should follow this approach and be firmly based in the real world in which practitioners work and aim to develop both cognitive and affective domains.

In order for education to be confluent and situated it was essential that champions and educators worked collaboratively to agree content of the education programme. One of the challenges for champions was to work with one educator, who was an expert in dementia care but not acute care, to ensure that she developed a real and shared understanding of the world in which these staff are working. For learning to be meaningful this educator needed to comprehend the challenges and issues of caring for people with dementia in an acute setting that staff face on a daily basis. To enable communicative action educators and champions worked closely together to identify specific learning needs that were relevant to care. This approach to education also had the advantage of ensuring that it remained grounded in the real world of the learners. It was also "owned" by practitioners and therefore congruent with the principles of confluent education and effective practice development.

Following discussions about the world in which they work champions appeared to feel reassured that the education embraced a sense of some of the difficulties they encountered providing high quality care to people with dementia. Throughout the sessions the educators regularly referred back to issues that had been raised by the group and thus enhanced their status as credible practitioners who understood real life issues. Champions were asked what they would like to learn. As they had received little preparation for the course, this proved to be a challenging question. Ideas they generated included:

- Stages of dementia
- Understanding the needs of people with dementia and how these may be met
- Types of dementia
- Practical steps that can be taken when caring for patients particularly when they are exhibiting challenging behaviour.

Stage IV: "Owned" Programme of Education for Champions

Following initial identification of learning needs by champions and educators subsequent sessions were planned. In reality sessions evolved over time and were adapted in light of experiences and feedback of all involved. A key aspect of learning was for champions to recognise their new knowledge and ways of thinking and consider how these may be transferred to practice.

The programme delivered was highly interactive with only brief episodes of didactic teaching. Each session included activities that enabled learners to consider their attitudes to people with dementia. They also involved a range of exercises that were intended to support them in developing, or re-engaging some empathy. Champions were able to identify many of the emotions that may be felt and were encouraged to relate their thoughts and feelings to practice. Feedback from these sessions indicated that they had a powerful impact on individuals. At each session the champions shared their experiences in practice. Some had tried new strategies for care with good effect and were keen to report on their success. This approach effectively utilised the concept of the community of practice (Wenger 1998) in which staff were able to freely share knowledge and experience. Responses from these sessions were positive; learners reported changes in the ways in which they delivered care. There appeared to be a beginning of a change of mindset in some champions in which they were more able to respect the personhood of individuals. This was demonstrated by comments such as:

- *"I got through to him"*
- *"I let her do what she wanted, gave her time to take it all in"*

Champions reported feeling more confident in practice and valued having some new strategies to use. They suggested that they had more empathy with patients through undertaking various activities. Despite their progress the champions felt daunted by the amount of change that they felt needed to happen in practice.

Stage V: Champions Return New Learning to Practice and Act as Role Models

As with Stage II, on reflection Stage V was also too ambitious. It was envisaged that as the dementia champions gradually developed expertise and confidence they could be supported and encouraged to take their new knowledge and skills into practice. In reality this sharing was only possible on a very small scale. It was evident that champions would need far more preparation before being ready to take on this role. Champions who did manage to share knowledge with colleagues reported a great sense of satisfaction that they had successfully influenced an improvement in practice, albeit on a micro level. The idea of using champions in practice was that it may begin a "bottom up" change in culture. Research suggests that the culture in which staff currently work at both organisational and ward levels does little to support them to value themselves or the people they are caring for.

Culture of the ward is critical in enabling staff to deliver person-centred care. It is well documented in the literature that it is extremely difficult to provide person-centred care in an environment in which this philosophy is not extended to patients and staff alike. Malloy and Hadjistavropoulos (2004) suggest that many health care settings remain in the bureaucratic-institutional mould and are therefore inimical to the development of authentic relationships between patients and staff. It may be argued that institutions such as acute hospitals may never be able to move totally from this model due to the nature of the service they provide. Depersonalisation that can afflict patients in large institutions is also prone to impacting on staff who may believe that their individual contributions are negated (Menzies Lyth 1988, Kitwood 1997b). It is suggested by Hirschhorn (1997) that for staff to be able to give care based on dignity and respect this must be the cultural norm of the workplace. Nolan et al (2002) concur with this thought stating that staff who feel well supported and valued contribute to maintaining a positive environment of care. The need to work within a positive culture is embraced by Packer (2000a) who is clear that in order to develop staff who will provide person-centred care these values must also be applied to staff by the organisations in which they practice. Investment in champions and the support of senior managers may go some way towards changing the culture and cultivate a realisation and appreciation of the value of all the individuals involved in care.

To date the first four stages of the model have been completed. It is acknowledged that the original model was too ambitious and optimistic. Focus of work has been on one group of dementia champions. Their evaluations of the course are almost entirely positive. Some of the personal learning and awareness identified in the evaluations indicated that the champions were beginning to develop a greater understanding of, and empathy with, patients for whom they were providing care. Feedback from champions suggests that their mindsets about people with dementia have changed and that this has influenced the care they deliver. Whilst these are self-reported changes it is evident when talking to the champions that they have gained new and more person-centred perspectives of this patient group.

Development work with the champions appears to have had a positive effect but the plan for them to take this back to practice has not been as effective as was anticipated. This finding lends weight to the assertion of McSherry and Warr (2006) who suggest that in the busy and stressful culture in which we now work it is essential to have named practice developers to drive projects forward. On reflection and discussion with the management team it has been decided that the way forward is twofold:

- To provide follow up workshops for existing champions and to ensure that their status as "experts" is secured
- To run a further series of workshops to enable a "critical mass" of staff to become engaged with dementia care.

It is believed that this approach will be most effective in bringing about the type of change in organisational culture that is needed to truly reform dementia care. It is anticipated that the original champions will be the named practice developers given their inherent enthusiasm and ownership of the project. To ensure this strategy is effective it will be vital that the champions are fully and consistently supported by senior staff within the unit. Evaluations completed by the cohort of champions will be used in planning future workshops. There will be follow up workshops for the champions, additionally there will be sessions for other staff to ensure that a "critical mass" of staff have an increased knowledge about the provision of person-centred dementia care. Subsequent stages of the model will be considered once this new undertaking is completed.

Stage VI: "Owned" Tools to Support Development Selected and Implemented

One course of action that is frequently used to improve dementia care is the adoption of new single strand innovations. Literature reveals several approaches that have been used. Three that feature most commonly are appointment of nurses with a specialist function who can be used by ward based staff to give advice about specific patients (for example Packer 2001c, Beavis 2007). Inevitably use of such experts comes at a significant financial cost. Other areas have developed dementia care pathways to guide staff through caring for this patient group for example, a collaborative pathway has been developed in Cornwall (Cornwall County Council 2007). Such work has major advantages in terms of ensuring equity, using best practice and service development (Naidoo and Bullock 2001). In addition, it can raise awareness of treatments and service that are available. Equally pathways can be seen as a "one size fits all" option and these can have a depersonalising effect on individuals. A third option that has been employed in a number of areas is the use of tools that intend to encourage staff to think about the care they deliver and find out more about patients in their care. Norman (2003b) produced a poster that highlights some important considerations when caring for people with memory problems. This is supported by an information gathering sheet which enables staff to gain a more person-focused understanding than is usually the case. Regrettably, experience indicates that adding more documentation is rarely welcomed by staff delivering care, such work tends to be seen as a further burden in an already busy schedule.

On reflection, it may be argued that the model developed for this study has some parallels with the emancipatory practice development through life-story work described by Keady et al (2005). These authors discuss a model that evolved through the integration of constructivist research into emancipatory practice development. The model identifies the need to reflect on, modify and transform practice. Work is based on a qualitative, longitudinal study using both life-story work and constructivist grounded theory. A specialist nurse from a memory clinic spent many hours with individuals with a diagnosis of early dementia listening to their stories and experiences. These narratives influenced changes in practice that were constructed from the service user experience. My goal has been similar in my desire has been to take patients' narratives back to staff to enable them to reflect on and improve their practice.

It may be argued that each of the many approaches to improving dementia care has a value. It is evident that few of them have been rigorously evaluated. It is acknowledged that such evaluation would be exceptionally difficult to achieve. In this project perhaps the most important aspect is that any tools that are used should be selected and "owned" by the staff who are going to use them. This should ensure the greatest possibility that they will be accepted, shared, piloted and evaluated. It is clear that the imposition of such tools would be unhelpful and quickly rejected by staff. The ultimate purpose of the use of any tool would be to ensure that staff develop a "clear and practised way of envisioning the personhood of the dementia sufferer" (Ashworth and Ashworth 2003:185).

As champions grow in confidence and competence it may be valuable to work with them to review some of the innovative practices and tools that have been used by others to improve dementia care. Empowering champions to choose innovations that are relevant to their practice should increase the chance that they are successfully implemented and evaluated in practice as the champions will have a greater capacity to sell the ideas to their peers and monitor uptake.

Stage VII: Evaluation of Change

As highlighted previously, evaluation of practice development can be difficult to achieve. Whilst this project appears sound and has the support of both managers and practitioners there is a need to ensure that such support remains. The drawback of much practice development activity is that it lacks absolute goals and measurable outcomes. Present systems of health care are heavily outcome driven and securing time for practitioners to think and reflect may be challenging as the value attached to such activity is inevitably low. This issue has become prevalent throughout current education systems. It is noted by Trotman (2006) who suggests that schools are now expected to demonstrate their value in terms of impact and outcomes, this leaves little space for imaginative education. Van Manen (1997) continues the concept of differing approaches to development; his thoughts are directed to research but are equally applicable to development. Van Manen (1997) argues that those with an interest in inspection and measurement are likely to find work that emanates from the human sciences lacks rigour and robustness. However this author is clear that rigorous human science can still be "'soft', 'soulful', 'subtle' and 'sensitive' in its effort to bring the range of meanings of life's phenomena to our reflective awareness" (Van Manen 1997:18). To ensure that the "hearts and minds" of managers are truly won there is a need to devise and agree methods of evaluation that are realistic but also clearly demonstrate the value of their investment. When elements of the project have been evaluated these will be used to guide further advances in practice.

A small range of evaluation methods have been selected for this work. They are based on the need to provide information that is meaningful for those funding the project but, perhaps more importantly, are congruent with the ethnographic underpinnings of this study and demonstrate observable changes in interactions between patients and staff. Evaluation methods to be used include:

- Formal evaluation of the facilitated component of the project. It is likely that this may be of most interest to managers as it will produce relatively "hard" data.
- Staff will be encouraged at each session to reflect on incidents in practice involving patients that they feel demonstrate their development of expertise or to which they would like to explore alternative approaches. Both scenarios would indicate a change in thinking and mindset.
- Champions from each ward will be asked to select and undertake a dementia related ward based project. Outcomes of each project will be evaluated individually.

Stage VIII: Dissemination

At this stage it is relatively hard to anticipate how this work will be disseminated. However methods will encompass the following philosophy:

- Dissemination is an integral part of this project. This is in keeping with the assertion of Gray et al (2000) and Denzin (1997) that researchers have a responsibility to ensure that their work makes a difference in the everyday world.
- Champions will be encouraged and supported to disseminate their work, particularly at local level, thus ensuring that they remain empowered, a central tenet of practice development (McSherry and Warr 2006).

- The work will, at an appropriate stage, be disseminated widely to ensure the best possible opportunity for the experiences of older people with dementia in acute hospitals to be improved.

It is notable that informal dissemination has already occurred as I have received a request from another group of wards to run a similar programme in their Care Group.

It is evident that this practice development was ambitious in terms of time, resources and proposed outcomes. Four stages have been completed in a modified form. There are indications that the champions have begun to re-think ways in which they envisage these patients. They have self reported changes in working practices, although these cannot be corroborated. Ways in which the champions have begun to talk about people with dementia supports the view that their mindset has genuinely changed. The project has been more difficult than anticipated largely due to the logistics of trying to get a group of staff together in a suitable venue on a regular basis. It has reinforced that practice development is a "messy" undertaking (McCormack et al 1999, Walsh 2000). Equally, it is enormously satisfying to think that this research has led to some improvements in the care for older people with dementia in one acute hospital.

Conclusion

This chapter has examined methods of improving care for people with dementia in acute hospitals. The "why" element of ethnographic analysis explored what is currently "going on" in practice. Methods by which this study may be used to change practice have been examined these included, dissemination, education and practice development. A model of practice development is proposed which draws on best practice from dissemination, education and practice development. Implementation of the model to date is discussed and future developments addressed. Implications of this model to future practice are investigated further in chapter five.

CHAPTER FIVE

INTEGRATIVE REVIEW

Introduction

Chapter five integrates the knowledge and learning that have been developed through completing the literature review, research study and practice development project to demonstrate how these elements have been synthesised to create an integrated whole. It also provides a reflection on my personal journey through the doctoral programme. The chapter begins by examining the contribution to the body of knowledge made by each of the elements. Contributions are drawn together to illustrate how the work as a whole has contributed to the knowledge about dementia care in acute hospitals. Limitations of the study are identified as are a range of opportunities for further research and practice development. Part two of the chapter maps my personal journey through the doctoral programme. Extracts from my reflective diary are used to illuminate the experience. Issues of reflexivity are discussed as is the nature of the professional doctorate and how this supports personal and professional growth.

Contribution to the Body of Knowledge

This work makes a potential contribution to the body of knowledge about the care of older people with dementia in acute hospitals. The unique feature of this work is the way in which each of the components of the study: the literature review, research study and practice development have been synthesised to produce a tangible impact for staff providing care for this group. One of the major strengths of this work has been completing the study as a professional rather than a traditional doctorate, because I have been able to produce an innovative and holistic practice development project based on a research inquiry that has potential to make a genuine impact on practice. There are two powerful threads that run through the entire thesis; these are personhood and ethnography, both of which have been fundamental to the final outcome. Individual components of the study will be explored briefly, acknowledging the contribution that each can make. Ways in which they have been integrated to make real changes in practice are discussed; reference is made to the common threads.

Literature Review

An extensive, three-part, review of the literature formed the initial focus of this study. Stage one set person-focused literature within the context of dementia research as a whole. It demonstrated a huge rise in dementia research from the mid 1990s. It was clear that the vast majority of studies were "on" rather than "with" people with dementia. Research predominantly investigated the disease process and medication. Studies that explored the views of people with dementia were very much in the minority. Phase two identified studies that had actively sought the thoughts of this group, forty-four met the inclusion criteria for review. As I considered various models for evaluating these papers it became clear that many current frameworks, whilst valuable, were not wholly appropriate. I therefore devised a set of criteria against which to judge these studies. Using these criteria the studies were graded on a scale of one to three with those at level one meeting the criteria most closely. Criteria included dementia specific areas, and the major factors I considered when reviewing these papers were ethics and respect for personhood. It became clear that there was sometimes a discrepancy between what was written and what appeared to happen in practice. I identified three papers that typified what I was trying to achieve in terms of ethical and meaningful research; they had a strong signal (Edwards et al 1998). The first review did not fully expose the difference between these papers and others. I therefore reviewed them again using a more narrative- based approach. This revealed that these researchers, whilst not necessarily writing in detail about ethics and personhood, demonstrated an exceptional ability to apply ethical principles sensitively and flexibly thus ensuring that the personhood of participants was respected. Differences in these papers were subtle and implicit, but readily recognisable in view of my desire to follow this path to an ethical and meaningful study. In completing the literature review a number of key factors in dementia research were identified:

- Dementia research continues to be dominated by the biomedical model. However there is evidence of a growing raft of work that engages "with" this group.

- Work that engages "with" people tends to focus on those in the early stages. There remains a significant gap in work involving people in the more advanced stages.
- Qualitative research methods are more congruent with person-focused dementia research.
- Whatever research method is chosen it is imperative that it is applied flexibly to meet the needs of individuals.
- Selection and recruitment processes need to protect participants from undue anxiety or coercion. However this needs to be balanced against paternalism that may erode the personhood of individuals.
- There is clear evidence that, given the right approach, people with dementia are able to communicate their thoughts and feelings.
- The skill, expertise and manner of the researcher are central to the credibility of the study.
- Underlying beliefs of the researcher are as, if not more, important than the formulaic application of ethical principles.
- There are indications that rather than feeling anxious many participants enjoy the opportunity to tell their story to an interested listener.
- There is limited evidence that current research has had a real impact on care.
- There is a need to begin to meta-synthesise findings of qualitative studies to ensure they do not go unnoticed in the vastness of this field.
- As established methods of evaluating research are not wholly appropriate for this specialised area, I have created a dementia specific set of criteria.

Research Study

The literature review provided a sound basis for planning the research study. Study aims included my determination to:

- Enable the voices of people with dementia to be heard
- Produce knowledge that would be used to influence future practice
- Set the work within the broader social and political context.

I selected critical ethnography as the research method. As the study progressed I realised that this method alone was not going to support achieving the aims of the study. I devised a redefined methodology

(Rapport et al 2004, Rapport et al 2005) which combined some of the central features of both ethnographic and narrative approaches. Using such a third position is supported by Holloway and Todres (2003). My challenge was to integrate these elements in a way that was coherent and consistent. The commentary exemplifies how this has been achieved in practice and met my goal of ensuring that the voices of the participants were heard.

Use of this redefined methodology was drawn through both data collection and analysis. Using narrative interview techniques made it possible for participants to tell their stories more fully and from the perspective of their own lifeworld. Use of combined approaches in data analysis has effectively combined the presentation of a series of patient stories with a commentary providing the ethnographic "what" and "how" of this study.

Findings of this study were not wholly unexpected. Many patients painted a bleak picture of care they received. One of the major strengths of the work was that it clearly demonstrated the extent to which they were able to contribute. Patients had mini-mental state examination (Folstein et al 1975) scores ranging from 0 – 7 indicating severe dementia; many also had superimposed physical illness. Despite this, I developed an approach to observation and conversation in which the patients were enabled to clearly express their views about care. Research involving people with severe dementia and physical illness is extremely rare. This study has shown that with the right approach they can genuinely engage in research "with" them.

Lay carers were broadly complimentary about care provided. Their concerns involved the extent to which they participated in care and their fears for the future. As discussed, it is possible that the recruitment process allowed staff to "filter out" carers who may have been more vocal. I had expected the carers to discuss topical subjects such as the use of tranquilizing medication and mealtimes but these issues were not raised.

Staff generally appeared to have good intention when delivering care. It was clear that many functioned almost entirely within the "bed and body" framework (Gubrium 1975) with which they were familiar and comfortable. Staff tended to avoid interactions which may have led to emotional encounters. This meant that patients' attempts at communication were often totally ignored thus gradually eroding their personhood. Many staff, particularly those delivering the majority of direct care, had little or no preparation to care for people with dementia. Members of two smaller occupational groups reported that dementia care was an integral part of their curriculum but this was not reflected in consistent, discernable differences in care. This finding led me to further question the value of education as the sole method of practice development.

Analysisto this point had successfully conveyed stories of participants and had addressed the ethnographic "what" and "how" (Katz 2001). However the work could still be deemed to be a good story with no practical application. To avoid this pitfall I explored the ethnographic "why" (Katz 2001), this step in analysis was essential in planning the practice development. Analysis of "why" indicated that many practitioners were largely working in a "switched off" mode. Their empathy had been subsumed in the need to fit in with the organisational culture. They were functioning in a deeply embedded habitus which went largely unchallenged. The value that staff attached to their work was poor, they described it as "only elderly care". They alluded to the idea that caring for older people was viewed by others, and possibly themselves, as relatively unskilled and less prestigious than the work of other specialties. The fact that staff described themselves in relatively negative terms, did not seem to value their work and appeared to have had little investment made in them in terms of education and development, made me question the extent to which their personhood was respected by the organisation. I felt that in order to ensure the provision of high quality care the organisation needed to invest in these staff and ensure that their personhoods were nourished. Without such investment it seemed unlikely that sustained improvements could be secured.

Practice Development

The ethnographic thread continued through the practice development with a focus on understanding the culture as a whole and finding ways in which this may be used to improve care. Thoughts of the participants with dementia directly influenced the planning of this project. A review of potential methods of improving practice revealed some clear messages. Literature indicated that education alone was unlikely to change practice and this idea was congruent with my findings. I felt strongly that any intervention should embrace the concept of nurturing the personhood of staff. Findings of this study demonstrated that there was a need to engage staff on an emotional as well as a cognitive level. Equally, I wanted to establish how essential staff were both as individuals and in influencing organisational culture. My aim was to ensure that staff were free to really think about what they do and how their behaviour and actions impact on personhood. To this end I devised a model of practice development that integrated the principles of situated learning and confluent education. This approach was intended to set the development within their lifeworld and also ensure that the staff viewed themselves as equal and valued owners of the development process. In reality the original model was overambitious. However, to date there are small but definite signs that this approach is beginning to enable staff to recast their thoughts about people with dementia and to rekindle their empathy. Champions have given some clear indications of how their new mindset has changed the way in which they deliver care. The commitment of the Trust has been demonstrated through the commissioning of two more series of workshops. It is a great achievement to have effected a change in practice and this work will be built on by all involved to secure genuine, embedded change.

Dissemination

Dissemination is key to this work. I recognised at the outset that, whilst publication in scholarly journals is important, it is unlikely to reach practitioners providing direct care. In order to reach this group a number of dissemination strategies have been used including traditional presentations, narratives and showing of "Ex Memoria". Audiences have included NHS managers, pre and post registration health care students and practitioners. Such approaches have proved powerful in enabling staff to question their practice and have been valuable in generating discussion about dementia care. I have taken opportunities to publish this work and present it at conferences to ensure dissemination at all levels. I am considering producing a DVD based on the study; this would undoubtedly be a potent way of disseminating the findings.

In summary this work has potential to contribute to the body of knowledge in the following ways:

- We now have evidence that people with dementia, even those in the more advanced stages, are able to actively engage in research. This is supported by this study and by several others including Mills (1997), Marzanski (2000) and Sabat (2002a). This research adds to this concept by demonstrating that people with advanced dementia and superimposed physical illness can also actively participate in research.
- Research "with" this group can and must be done. It needs to be flexible and sensitive to remain ethical and give participants the maximum chance of sharing their views.
- It has been established that a third position (Holloway and Todres 2003) integrating elements of ethnographic and narrative

methodologies can be used successfully to portray the experiences of people with dementia.

- Staff caring for people with dementia in acute hospitals often do not value their contribution and frequently feel ill prepared to provide care.
- Staff tend to work in an embedded habitus of which they are frequently not aware.
- The practice development model has been developed in light of the thoughts of the participants, particularly those with dementia. Relatively few studies have listened to the voices of people with dementia and tangibly used them to improve care although this approach is seen in the work of Keady et al (2005).
- There is a need to engage staff on an emotional as well as a cognitive level to enable them to change their practice.
- Use of confluent education and situated learning in developing dementia education is not documented. This innovative approach has been instrumental in the success of practice development.
- Non-traditional methods of dissemination have been effective in enabling staff to recast their thoughts about people with dementia and the care they receive.
- The combination of components of the professional doctorate have allowed me to move from a literature review, which highlighted essentials of good practice in dementia research, to an ethical and meaningful research study which integrated elements of narrative approaches in an ethnography. Findings led to the creation of a model of practice development which has been piloted and evaluated to show demonstrable changes in practice.
- This work indicates that the professional doctorate is an effective way of enabling practitioners to conduct research that has a real impact on practice.

Limitations

This study has made a potential contribution to the body of knowledge about dementia care in acute hospitals. It is recognised that it has a number of limitations as outlined below.

- The study was conducted in one acute hospital in a specialist older peoples unit. It is possible that the findings in other Trusts and units may have been different.

- Narratives presented are my interpretation of the observations, conversations and interviews. Whilst I have done my utmost to provide authentic accounts and acknowledge my influence throughout, it is possible that another researcher may have made quite different interpretations.
- Recruitment processes, whilst ethically sound, may have enabled Registered Nurses to filter out patients and carers who were considered to be "difficult".
- The fact that I spoke to the carers whilst their relatives were still in-patients may have influenced their willingness to voice their opinions fully.
- Carer participants were a particularly unrepresentative group in that most were husbands caring for their wives. This may have occurred because of the recruitment process.
- Practice development work was ambitious for such a short timescale. It needs to be more comprehensively evaluated and modified for future use.

Contribution and limitations of this study have been discussed. There are aspects of this work that are unique to the Doctor of Professional Practice programme. Whilst this study is divided into discrete chapters that are aligned to the requirements of the award, the value of the study as a whole is greater than the sum of these parts. The professional doctorate has enabled me to create a "holistic" piece of work. The notion of holism can broadly be seen from two perspectives: impact that this work has had on practice and influence it has had on me as a practitioner-researcher. This idea is congruent with Carr et al's (in press) description of the professional doctorate as amalgamating the expectation that "methodologically sound" research will be produced with the anticipation of personal and professional growth.

It is argued by Yam (2005) that traditional doctorates focus on the production of "mode one" knowledge, that is knowledge which is objective and value free. In contrast, Lee et al (2000) argue that professional doctorates enable researchers to generate "mode two" knowledge which is subjective and context bound. These authors describe such knowledge as being transdisciplinary, heterogeneous and heterarchical. They embrace its transient nature in light of the fact that it is intended to solve "real world" issues that are embedded in practice. The purpose of contributing to the solution of "real world" problems matched closely with my goals in undertaking this programme. I did not want to undertake research for its own sake; my aim was to make a tangible difference in practice. Whilst it is accepted that many traditional academics remain sceptical about professional doctorates (Ellis 2005, Yam 2005), I am in a strong position to defend my work as I am confident that it is methodologically sound and, crucially, the evaluations from the practice development indicate that the process of change has begun.

From a more personal viewpoint the professional doctorate has also been a success. The doctorate has enabled me to develop as a "scholarly professional" (Galvin and Carr 2003). I have received high quality research training; the programme has also supported me to develop into a practitioner who is still grounded in practice but who has the skills required to undertake research and implement practice development that is relevant and important to the "real world" of practice. This has allowed me to stay true to my roots as a Registered Nurse and will provide a qualification that is relevant to employment beyond the academic arena (Neuman 2005, Kuang-Hsu Chiang 2003).

The value of this work, and its limitations, have been clearly identified. Equally, the work has exposed many areas for further research and practice development. A range of opportunities is outlined below.

Recommendations for Future Research and Practice Development

It is clear that the care of people with dementia in acute hospitals remains under- investigated. In view of demographic changes and the increasing prevalence of dementia there is an urgent need to understand this subject and identify methods of improving practice. There is evidently a huge gap in knowledge and a number of areas for further work and practice development are identified below:

- This study focused on care in a specialist older peoples unit. This may imply that staff had some expertise or, as a minimum, considerable experience in caring for people with dementia. It would be valuable to conduct a similar study in a non-specialist facility.
- There is a need to explore alternative methods of enabling people with dementia to voice their thoughts. Potential approaches include co-constructed inquiry (Keady and Williams 2007), although as noted previously this may be more effective for people in the earlier stages. The use of talking mats (Murphy et al 2005) may assist people in the more advanced stages to express their views more fully.

- It may be valuable to facilitate more junior staff to undertake some life-story work with patients. This could increase their understanding and also support a more emancipatory approach to practice development. The use of co-constructed inquiry (Keady and Williams 2007) may be an effective way of enabling staff to work with people in the earlier stages.
- There are tentative indications from this study that this group may be excluded from rehabilitation services. This idea is worthy of investigation in terms of exploring potential benefit and the tendency to ration care.
- This research indicates that staff are socialised into a habitus, a "special institutional culture" (Sidenvall 1999:321). The ways in which this happens and how this practice can be changed in future are worthy of further research.
- There is a need for much greater understanding of the interface between lay carers and staff. This study, alongside those of Simpson et al (1995), Walker and Dewar (2001) and Gilmour (2002), suggests that this is not always an easy alliance. Further work needs to be undertaken to understand the dynamics and find ways to improve such relationships.
- The practice development project needs to be evaluated more fully and modified for future use. When more embedded it would be valuable to study whether it would lead to sustained changes in practice.
- Current qualitative studies tend to be "stand alone" at present which may limit their impact. To add more weight they should be metasynthesised and used more directly to influence care.

Part one of this chapter has considered the contribution to the body of knowledge and limitations of this study. It has also identified some of the distinctive features of the Doctor of Professional Practice programme. Recommendations for future research and practice development have been offered. The second part of the chapter maps my progress through the doctoral journey.

The Doctoral Journey

This section details my journey through the doctoral programme integrating both the practicalities of how the work has been completed and reflecting on my personal and professional growth during this time. To give the work some structure the years are considered sequentially although there is inevitably some overlap. Excerpts from my reflective diary are presented in italics.

The Doctor of Professional Practice programme requires the completion of four components, a systematic review, a research study, a practice development project and an integrative review which draws the work together. As the order in which the components are completed is not prescribed, I chose to work through them systematically. I needed to put some boundaries in this huge piece of work and my plan is set out in figure 5-1.

Year 1: Literature review, Research proposal, Ethics approval

↓

Year 2: Funding, Data collection, Data analysis

↓

Year 3: Practice development, Initial dissemination, Writing up

↓

Year 4: Writing up, Integrative review, Further dissemination

Figure 5-1: Plan of work

Whilst this illustration suggests that progress through the components of the programme was a simple, linear process this was not always how the experience felt. A reflection on the completion of each part is provided below.

Year One

Year one of the programme was perhaps the time of most dramatic change for me. I planned to complete the literature review and the research proposal, I also wanted to gain ethics approval for the study. It was the time at which I got to know my peer group. I quickly realised that I was going to have to devote an enormous amount of time and effort to this work.

Literature Review

Three distinct phases were included in this review. Phase one set person-focused research within the context of dementia research as a whole. This was achieved by searching cumulative reviews. Although this appears to be a straightforward undertaking, in reality it was a long and laborious process involving sifting through many thousands of potential papers. My feelings about the review waxed and waned as I worked my way through several drafts. At times it felt like a never ending task:

> 26th September 2004
> *I have worked so, so hard this weekend and still feel that I am wading through treacle although I am beginning to get a feeling for the enormity of dementia research*

Phase two involved a search for studies that sought the views of people with dementia. As I reviewed these papers I realised that the models available for review did not fully evaluate some important aspects of these studies. I therefore devised a set of criteria that allowed me to discern how research could be managed in an ethical and meaningful manner. This work progressed in phase three when three studies with particularly high signal (Edwards et al 1998) were revisited. This phase used a narrative approach which allowed me to view the papers more globally. It became clear that what set these papers apart was the way in which the research was conducted and not purely the value of the findings.

To gain more insight into the ways in which the level one researchers worked I entered into communication with Steven Sabat whose work I particularly admired for its person focus. In his response he explained his way of thinking:

> "you become someone that they can talk to because you demonstrate your desire to understand and your willingness to listen and do whatever you can to understand. You have to care about them deeply as people" (Sabat 2006).

It is precisely this type of philosophy that can be discerned in the level one papers. It is possible that this review would not be judged as valuable by proponents of the positivist paradigm as it does not follow traditional review methodology. I would challenge this idea in that my choice of approach is clearly justified and, as far as possible, transparent. Completing the literature review at an early stage was extremely useful for the following reasons:

- It convinced me that it is possible to conduct research with people with dementia that is both ethical and meaningful.
- It was invaluable in informing my submissions to the Research Ethics Committee and the Research Governance Committee.
- It added weight to my application for funding from the Alzheimer's Society.
- It reinforced that my own beliefs about people and their inherent value were compatible with undertaking research involving people with dementia.

A minor disadvantage to undertaking the review first was that it has required updating on a number of occasions. Fortunately this has been considerably less arduous than the original work. Updates have shown that person-focused dementia research is a growing area of investigation and that, arguably, researchers are building a repertoire of skills which enable them to conduct these studies in ways that are both ethical and meaningful.

Research Proposal and RA06 Initial Review

I completed the research proposal and RA06 in early 2005. Development of the research proposal involved many incarnations as I found it difficult to identify the most appropriate methodology.

Extensive discussion with my supervisors and dialogue during group supervision helped me to clarify my thinking. It was particularly valuable to be challenged by non-nurses who thought in different frameworks and encouraged me to do likewise. I identified my beliefs about, and aims for, the study. These included the concepts that the work should be set in the broader social and political context, the voices of people with dementia should be central and that the study should influence future practice.

These beliefs and aims led me to select critical interpretive ethnography as the research methodology. At this stage I felt relieved to have a plan of how I would progress the research. Equally I thought that after a year on the doctoral programme I should have achieved far more than just producing a final proposal. On reflection the completed proposal clearly showed the extent to which both my knowledge and thinking had developed over this time span. The documents were approved by the University Research Committee in February 2005, they provided useful feedback which allowed the proposal to be refined further.

Research Ethics Committee and Research Governance Approval

Gaining approval from the Research Ethics Committee proved to be a major hurdle. I felt particular pressure to get my application right as I am a member of an ethics committee. I completed the application form at a stage when on-line application had just become mandatory and the programme was still prone to errors. This was a slow process which gave me the opportunity to think through each stage to ensure ethically sound research.

I had discussed the application informally with a number of colleagues on the committee and had taken advice on making the submission rigorous. Work I had completed during the literature review was key in informing my application. My membership meant that the application had to be referred to another committee. Following submission it became evident that the committee to which I had been referred had a higher level of quantitative than qualitative expertise. The committee reviewed my application at a meeting that I was told I did not need to attend. Later I received a letter with a string of questions that I could readily have answered at the meeting. This proved quite frustrating as I had to respond in writing and wait until the next meeting the following month for further review. I chose to attend the next meeting which proved to be a sound decision. Many of the questions posed concerned qualitative research, for example the committee were keen to know the exact numbers of participants that would be recruited. They were also eager for me to devise a very precise list of questions that would be asked at interview. Opportunities to discuss and rationalise my research method reinforced to me that I had prepared the proposal thoroughly and with sufficient evidence base. Discussion was effective in resolving these issues although I was slightly surprised by the final question of “but what will you do if the patients don’t tell you the truth?” This question led to an interesting debate on the nature of truth and the fundamentally different philosophies held by myself and various committee members. Following this meeting ethical approval was granted, the site specific assessment was approved and the Research Governance Committee gave permission to proceed.

Whilst the need for rigorous ethical review is completely accepted it could be suggested that the process has become cumbersome to the extent that researchers may feel less inclined to pursue ethically challenging avenues. Ethics and research governance forms had to be completed in very precise terms and, as will be discussed later, in the course of undertaking data collection it became very evident that a sound underpinning knowledge of principalism (Wheeler 2006) and strong personal integrity were every bit as important to maintaining ethical practice as the forms that had been completed and approved.

I am hopeful that future applications for research involving people with dementia may be better understood. As a result of the Mental Capacity Act (HMSO 2005) there have been a number of changes to research involving people who may lack capacity. In order to develop a body of expertise in this area some Research Ethics Committees have been "flagged" to review such applications. It is likely that a concentration of expertise will allow committees to develop their knowledge of this area of work and increase their competence in conducting rigorous reviews that embrace some of the inherent uncertainties in this type of work.

Year one was very productive in terms of output, I successfully completed all the pieces of work I had planned. During this time I got to know my supervisors and peers and to value their diverse backgrounds and generosity in sharing their thoughts, feelings and expertise. Overall I was content with my progress through the year and felt ready to advance to the next stage.

Years Two and Three

My plan for year two was to secure funding for the research study. I then planned to complete the research process including data collection and analysis. In reality, preparation for data collection took much longer than expected particularly in relation to recruiting participants. Although data collection and analysis were iterative processes the analysis continued well beyond collection; analysis evolved throughout year three. The three aims for this time period are reviewed below.

Funding Application

I prepared several applications for funding; initially I underestimated the amount of work that would be involved in each application. Following an informal approach The Alzheimer's Society expressed an interest in funding part of this work. In order to complete my application I contacted the local branch of the Society to get their feedback on my plans. I attended a branch meeting and presented my research to an interested and challenging audience. I was not fully prepared for the strength of feeling of the members, many of whom had had relatives in hospital and had experienced less than optimal care. It was difficult and painful to listen to these experiences particularly as, until recently, I had been one of the

Senior Nurses responsible for some of the wards they were referring to. The meeting appeared to be fruitful in that it gave some members a forum in which I was able to listen to their stories. Equally they were forthcoming with further ideas for my study. It was disheartening to hear the group say that, however good my research, they doubted that practice would change. I reiterated that my aim was to produce a study that could be used to guide changes in practice. In addition to attending this meeting I also had the opportunity to meet with a particularly active and vociferous member of the Society on a number of occasions. This gentleman reviewed my proposal from the perspective of the Society and gave me many suggestions on how I could improve my chances of securing funding. After several meetings he invited me to meet his wife who had advanced dementia and lived in a local care home. I was struck by his generosity and listened with concern to his accounts of the various episodes of care that his wife had received in an acute hospital. These meetings with members of the Alzheimer's Society reinforced my belief that the study was timely and important.

My first application to the Alzheimer's Society was reviewed by in excess of eighty consumer monitors. I received written feedback from each person and this helped shape the subsequent submission. The second submission was reviewed by four consumer monitors and four professionals. After this I was invited to an interview at which I presented my research proposal and was subject to some rigorous questioning. Following this, funding was granted which was primarily used to support some of the time needed for data collection.

Throughout the funded part of the study I had regular meetings with three consumer monitors from the Alzheimer's Society, these proved valuable in terms of encouraging me to consider the research from differing perspectives. The monitors were broadly supportive although their expectations of what could be achieved with a small grant sometimes felt unrealistic and, at times, impossible. The Alzheimer's Society has maintained an interest in my work and have provided opportunities to present and publish.

The Research Process

Extensive preparation for the research study proved to be a good investment. Processes of data collection and analysis are explained in detail in chapters two, three and four. This section highlights some of the particular issues and experiences I encountered at this time.

One of the challenges I had to consider was recruitment to the study. I had designed a process which took into account best practice. However, this also had the effect of recruitment being very much in the control of registered nursing staff. Initially progress was frustratingly slow. I visited wards on an almost daily basis and encouraged staff to seek participants whilst always remaining mindful that my work was not their top priority. Recruitment did eventually get underway.

Recruitment was one of the limiting factors in this study. I was successful in gaining staff participants from a range of grades and occupational groups. A small number of staff declined to take part; this reassured me that I was not being coercive. Registered nurses started the recruitment process for patient and lay carer participants. They appeared to select any patients who met the criteria provided. A major issue was the selection of lay carer participants. I suspected that the nurses carefully filtered this group before informing them about the study. It appeared that more vocal lay carers were excluded with a result that only seven participated. As the Alzheimer's Society monitors noted, no wives were involved and this perhaps suggests a somewhat atypical selection. In retrospect I would use alternative approaches to recruiting lay carers to ensure a more representative group.

Data Collection

Following slow but ultimately successful recruitment the misgivings I had felt about actually being in the field re-emerged. Despite these concerns about returning to my previous place of work, I felt a certain excitement at having at last got to the point where I could begin data collection. The experience was not quite as I had expected as I felt distinctly ill at ease in the clinical areas. Having spent so many years in practice I suddenly felt acutely uncomfortable. I experienced a sense of physical awkwardness and a feelings of not knowing what to "physically *do* in the field" (Coffey 1999:73). These feelings continued, to a greater or lesser extent, throughout the study depending on which ward I was on and which staff were on duty. A further challenge I encountered involved my role as researcher. At the beginning of the study I invested a lot of time ensuring that staff understood why I was there and what I was doing; I was keen to present myself honestly. Whilst having a real desire to be transparent about my role I also realised that there was a need to adjust my persona to the situation:

19th August 2005

There is something in this idea – you have to be something of a chameleon – I am part humble researcher, part authoritative leader, part 'expert' and part student. There is something about adapting your behaviour as a means to an end. For example my initial presentation with the social workers was one of humble student .... please, please let me come on this visit but when they seemed to be having some concern I quickly had to adapt and become 'expert' experienced nurse to give them confidence that I would not cause any problems. The ability to vary presentation of self was clearly valuable and effective in this case.

In practice I found the change of role difficult. In particular, I had to consciously stand back on occasion and not become involved in clinical issues. The feeling of responsibility, to which I was so used, was compounded by the fact that some staff continued to seek advice and help from me. Several events tested the boundaries of research and professional roles and forced me to be flexible within reasonable limits.

Whilst some of the practicalities of data collection were complex, the emotional impact of this work proved more difficult to manage. I found myself experiencing a whole range of emotions from anger, disbelief, sadness, powerlessness, overwhelming compassion and some guilt. Some extracts from my reflective diary illustrate these emotions:

17th April 2006

This entry describes an interview with Eileen's husband:

I asked him if I could book an interview later in the week but he wanted to talk straight away. He seemed incredibly pleased that someone would listen to him, his story was heartbreaking. In the middle of the interview he burst into tears, he misses her so much and is desperate for her to come home. There were really no words to say so I just comforted him. He wanted to continue with the interview, he made that quite clear.

17th August 2005

I found myself becoming angry as a social worker recounted an episode she had encountered:

While I am talking to the social workers they tell me how difficult they sometimes find it to listen to nursing staff talking to patients, one gives the example of a patient who walked into the bay and fell over. The social worker reports that the nurse said he does it deliberately and is attention seeking. I get the impression that this is a very real concern, it is hard just to sit and listen. Sadly I can imagine it is an accurate story.

My anger and dismay following this conversation was magnified when a staff nurse described this patient as "really nasty" with seemingly little justification. I felt both sad and guilty when one lady with whom I had spent many hours was finally discharged:

2nd September 2005
I suffered very badly with Hilda going off to her home yesterday. I felt very much that I had taken what I needed from her and then abandoned her to a home which she did not want to go to. I can rationalise it by saying that Hilda got friendship and attention while she was in hospital but I still felt that I was letting her down at the last minute. I hope she will be okay.

Regardless of my initial concerns about the process of data collection I felt a sense of sadness as my time in the field came to an end:

7th September 2006
Data collection is complete now, I feel strange to be disengaging from the field, sad, the staff are not aware at all. I feel a sense of guilt, I've been totally exposed to what I thought might be happening in practice – still a sledgehammer feeling. "Emptiness" – is that it?

I found the data collection difficult on occasion and experienced a range of emotions. I consistently reflected on my observations and consciously identified my feelings which I then attempted to set aside so they did not cloud my outlook completely. I was fortunate in that I was able to debrief with friends on a regular basis. However I was left with a sense of guilt that this sometimes poor level of care was being provided on a unit for which I had until relatively recently been professionally responsible. These feelings galvanised my determination to ensure that my practice development work was effective.

Data Analysis

Processes of data collection and analysis were iterative although the analysis lasted long after the collection was completed. I started the analysis with a clear plan of what I intended to do. However as I examined and re-examined the data it became obvious that I could not follow the intended path. Originally I had assumed that I would use some form of ethnographic analysis. When I reviewed ethnographic texts it became clear that they lacked detail about the practicalities of data analysis but there was evidence of agreement on certain principles. They provided little guidance on what I actually needed to do. I began to look at more concrete methods of analysis. Initially I chose to use a well established model devised by Creswell (1998). I adapted this model to meet the needs of this study and began to apply it but as I was using it I felt that I was systematically destroying the essence of the data. I reflected on the writing of van Manen (2006:714) who suggests that researchers who are genuinely committed to qualitative inquiry should resist using methods that "hollow out our understandings and cut us off from the deeper sources of meaning". This thought drove me to search for alternative approaches. As I sought the best method of analysis I wondered if I was making life difficult for myself. I related to the assertion of Savin-Baden (2004) that it is sometimes more straightforward to adopt complicated coding strategies than it is to engage with the messiness, self critique and pain that is associated with deeper interpretation of the data. To do justice to the data I had no choice but to follow the "messy" route. I investigated the use of narrative analysis and concluded that it would be an effective way of keeping some of the patient stories intact. Literature on narrative data analysis is sparse so I simply wrote the stories of patients with whom I had spent most time. I was unsure about the quality of these tales. My peer group offered to read them. Their feedback was comprehensive and demonstrated clearly that each had interpreted the work in their own way. Some critics may cite this as a weakness of narratives however Burnard (1991) suggests that on a different day and in another situation the story may not be the same. This author proposes that such differences do not matter if it is accepted that these stories may give us an insight into some part of the human condition. The responses convinced me that this had been achieved.

One peer from an educational background with no experience of dementia wrote of her overwhelming anger at the injustice of the way that the patient was cared for. She felt that this patient was treated with a total lack of respect. Another peer who had no health care experience but had a family member with dementia wrote that her greatest feeling was of sadness as shown in an extract from her feedback:

> *The story really engaged me ... my first reflections on this study were "how sad" – sad for the loss of this lady's freedom – dignity even, and*

her tentative realisation of this, tempered by the illusion that she might be going home soon. The repetition in the story highlights the repetition of hospital life ... there is a dismissal of feelings, of autonomy – no time for real attention to engage her as a person – albeit a confused person.

This feedback convinced me of the value of these narratives, as they clearly evoked some emotional response in the readers. Their reactions had great resonance with Bleakley's (2005) assertion that qualitative studies are often labelled as "soft" but that "soft" data from narrative inquiry can often illuminate hard realities. I struggled to write the narratives, the process is recognised as challenging by Harrington (2003), an experienced journalist. This author states that story telling is actually very hard work and takes years to perfect. I am aware that I remain a novice.

Whilst acknowledging the value of narratives I was eager to analyse the data further to identify themes, commonalties and differences. The decision to go relatively "off piste" and combine methods felt slightly uncomfortable. I was aware that I was entering the "edgelands" of qualitative research (Rapport et al 2005). My decision was justified by the production of evocative writing that health and social care staff could relate to in terms of their everyday work alongside ethnographic analysis that may appeal more to those who favour a succinct, slightly less personal format.

For a short time I felt content with my data analysis but further reflection led me to consider Snow et al's (2003:183) suggestion that this ethnography could, like many others, be classed as "nice read but no theoretical implications". This thought drove me to the final stage of analysis. Katz (2001) suggests that there are three parts to good ethnographic analysis: "what", "how" and "why". I had addressed the first two parts but needed to consider the "why"; this was essential before I could progress my practice development work. This final part of analysis is discussed in more detail in the section relating to years three and four.

When I began the data collection and analysis I believed I had my research "landscape neatly arranged" (Rapport et al 2005:37). As the work progressed I found that I was gradually moving into the edgelands, a "raw and rough, sombre and menacing" place (Rapport et al 2005:37). I began to engage in thinking that I did not fully understand. I had many discussions with my supervisors which helped to shape my thinking. I reflected on and confirmed what I was trying to achieve. I also gained considerable courage from the writing of Rapport et al (2004) and Rapport et al (2005) who champion the use of redefined methodology in which there is a move away from the "recipe" approach towards an acceptance that the method will evolve as things change. I believe that my move from methodolatory (Holloway and Todres 2003) towards a more flexible approach drawing on a number of philosophies has been effective in enabling me to address the research question in this study. Use of these approaches has increased my knowledge of these research methods significantly.

The Peer Group

It was during years two and three that I felt I was diverging slightly from my peer group in terms of the way in which I was approaching this work:

5th March 2005
Today is the first day I really didn't enjoy with the group. We had to say what are our claims today. Mine were:

- *With all I have read and following many conversations I am becoming more and more convinced that this is a vital and valuable piece of research.*
- *I believe that my background as a nurse will be useful in undertaking this study but equally my decision to stand back from nursing has liberated me to think about and plan an ethically sound and personally sensitive study.*
- *I think that these claims were too concrete for the group – they are highly ethereal, highly intelligent or a little confused.*

Although we all acknowledged that we would be working on the component parts in a different order, I felt that I was the only person who was ploughing through the work chapter by chapter. I felt that perhaps this was a very dull approach and lacked the "creativity" and "organic approach" that they spoke of so often. I wondered then, and still do now, if my approach was very much influenced by my years as a general nurse in which I had to work in a methodical way and achieve goals within set timescales. As time passed I found myself fascinated by the approach of my peers; they began to talk about the idea that the doctoral qualification was not hugely important to them. They talked more about the importance of the journey and of personal growth. I struggled to understand their motivation. On reflection I think the difference was that I too attach an enormous value to the personal and professional growth I have achieved. Equally I view the "piece of paper" as a critical stepping stone that may open up opportunities to pursue a career in research and development related to dementia care.

I began year two with the intention of seeking funding and of completing data collection and analysis. I was successful in securing funding which gave me a great sense of achievement. It was also a valuable learning opportunity which will be useful to me when seeking grants in the future. My desire to complete data collection and analysis proved very ambitious. Data collection was managed within the expected timescale. The experience of collecting data through participant observation exposed me to situations and emotions that were, at times, hard to deal with. I was particularly grateful to my supervisors, peers and friends for supporting me through this time. I am sure that the emotional impact on me was an essential part of this work, without it I do not think the final product would be so "real" to practitioners. Data analysis has been a process that has taken me off in a range of different directions. The experience has been lengthy and at times unnerving; again my supervisors have been invaluable in sustaining me through my various attempts at analysis. I now feel satisfied that my analysis meets the aims outlined for this process in chapter three. I have continued to value group supervision and found that it has contributed significantly to my progress.

Years Three and Four

I entered the second half of the programme with enthusiasm. Successful completion of years one and two had been confirmed following submission of my transfer report and attendance at the transfer viva. I found the transfer viva both frightening and encouraging. My apprehension quickly disappeared as the examiners asked questions that clearly showed their interest in my work. One of my supervisors attended the viva with me and made copious notes which were essential in considering what I still needed to achieve.

At a relatively early stage I set myself a clear plan for years three and four. This included completing the practice development component, writing the integrative review, writing up the thesis and dissemination. As my work progressed I realised that I had moved quite a long way from the original plan. Data analysis had taken longer than anticipated, the process continued well into year three. I had listened to several of my colleagues and peers about taking blocks of time to write up their work. My approach had been somewhat different in that I had been writing continuously so did not have that mammoth task to contend with. The focus of my work in years three and four was therefore on practice development and dissemination. Issues of reflexivity throughout the study and the nature of the Doctor of Professional Practice programme are also discussed as, for me, they have been important factors in my experience. The final stage of this section charts the progress of the integrative review.

Practice Development

The practice development component of the doctorate was a major influence in my choice of this programme. Ironically it was also the part to which I had given least thought and which proved extremely challenging. The route to actually committing to a practice development project was tortuous. As I worked through the data and tried to ascertain what was "going on" in practice I generated a number of ideas for projects that may influence practice. The more I considered these ideas the more they seemed either overambitious or frankly dull and unlikely to spark any interest in the practitioners I wanted to reach. At this stage I was still not wholly content with my analysis. I discovered the final "why" of ethnographic analysis (Katz 2001). From the mire I began to fully recognise what was "going on" in practice. Staff were "switched off", they were working in an embedded habitus of which they were not remotely aware. Their actions were gradually eroding the personhood of patients but I was sure that most staff genuinely wanted to provide good care. The "why" revelation provided the foundation on which I could base the practice development work.

The concept that staff were providing care without thinking about the individuals they were working with, and without any apparent recognition of their own or the patients' emotions, convinced me that the practice development project needed to engage practitioners on an emotional as well as a cognitive level. If they were not able to examine their own feelings and responses and begin to understand the emotions of the people they were caring for I doubted that practice would change. It was essential that the development work was "real", something that staff could relate to in their everyday lives and so transfer to practice. I was extremely aware in planning the project that I needed to avoid any actual or implied criticism of current care as I felt this would simply demoralise or antagonise staff.

When I set up the practice development project a particular issue for me was that I was suddenly back to being reliant on others to ensure that I could complete my work on time. I chose to work in partnership with an NHS Trust and the Alzheimer's Society, undoubtedly the right thing to do in terms of the quality and sustainability of the project. However at times this partnership tested my patience as timescales slipped.

Managers within the Trust fully supported the practice development project and agreed that care needed to be improved. Practicalities of setting up and running the programme proved intensely frustrating. However, working with my colleague from the Alzheimer's Society and the nominated dementia champions was a clear success. Champions, after some initial hesitance, engaged with the programme and provided positive feedback. Evaluations indicate that the use of situated learning and confluent education have been pivotal in enabling staff to think about what they do and begin to change their approach. These are small beginnings and there is still much work to be done before changes become embedded in practice.

Dissemination

A vital element of this work was to disseminate it widely to ensure the best chance of changing practice. As discussed in chapter four, approaches to the dissemination of qualitative work are rapidly evolving and I have successfully used different approaches for a range of audiences.

In an effort to reach a wide audience I have produced some papers for publication in academic journals. I believe that I have an ethical duty to publish, particularly given the time and effort that the participants put into the study. This thought is supported by O'Neill and Duffey (2000) and Burnard (2001) who suggest that publishing is an ethical imperative as it contributes to the body of knowledge and supports development in health care. In addition to ethical concerns publishing is now a vital part of building an academic career, as Roberts and Turnbull (2002-3:12) state if "we do not publish then our work is unknown and our academic credentials are not fully established".

In writing these papers I have followed the advice of Gilgun (2005) to "loosen up" and write in a format that others want to read and will remember. Gilgun (2005:261) describes this type of writing as having "grab" and claims that "grab and good science go hand in hand". It seems that this is an ethos that has yet to permeate the thoughts of many journal editors. I have submitted a range of articles to various journals, on each occasion I have had to sacrifice some of the essence of my work in order to meet journal conventions and word limits. All but two of these articles have been rejected. In retrospect I have not managed the rejection well and have taken it too personally. I have now realised that rejection is common and that if a paper is not accepted it is often nothing to do with the intrinsic quality of the work (van Teijlingen and Hundley 2002). I have also recognised that there is a need to persevere and submit papers to other journals (Cleary and Walter 2004).

I have had the opportunity to present my work through both oral and poster presentations. This is not always an activity that I have enjoyed but, on reflection, I feel that my performance has improved significantly over time. I now feel a certain sense of pleasure that I genuinely have something to contribute. Sureness in my own knowledge has increased my confidence in presenting. I am now actively seeking further opportunities for presentation.

In addition to publications and presentations I have used some of the newer non-traditional methods of dissemination with a view to reaching and engaging with a practitioner audience. Feedback from both viewing "Ex Memoria" and listening to audio taped interactions between people with dementia and staff have been positive in that they have proved to be something that staff can readily relate to their own lifeworlds without finding them too threatening. In future it would be interesting to use the audio tapes at larger, more formal presentations and gauge their

Reflexivity

Reflexivity was central to this study but it was something with which I was not entirely comfortable. Reading the literature on this subject left me feeling distinctly uncomfortable as I discerned a high level of egocentricity in which I did not want to engage. I was sure from the outset that I wanted this study to be about the participants and not about me. Equally I acknowledged that in my role as researcher I could not, and should not, be totally invisible in the text. My reading around reflexivity suggested that there was a continuum of concepts. At one end there are those that believe that reflexivity can be self indulgent, narcissistic and tiresome (Pillow 2003). This view is supported and expanded on by Northway (2000) who suggests that reflexivity may be positively irritating to readers. At the other end of the spectrum there were those that focused more on the value of the work whilst still claiming that reflexivity is essential. For example Flood (1999:35) states "without some degree of reflexivity research is blind and without purpose".

I was clear that the narcissistic approach to reflexivity was not for me but this was not a subject I could simply ignore. I reconsidered the literature to find approaches to reflexivity that were congruent with the aims of my work and also fitted with me as a person. I identified the benefits of reflexivity including:

- It enables the values and position of the researcher to be examined (Northway 2000)
- It can open up motivations and unconscious biases (Finlay 2002b)
- It can promote honesty and transparency (Northway 2000)
- It can provide an audit trail and therefore rigour (Koch and Harrington 1998)
- It can increase the plausibility of the study (Koch and Harrington 1998)

These concepts reinforced that reflexivity was vital. The question was how to incorporate it into this study whilst ensuring that the participants remained central. This was tempered by the acknowledgment that I could not ignore my own influence on the study which needed to be made as transparent as possible in order to allow readers to make their own judgements about the work.

My aim was to integrate reflexivity throughout the study in terms of positioning myself in relation to the research and providing a clear audit trail (Koch and Harrington 1998). There are some reflexive elements that, perhaps due to their more personal nature, have not been included in the body of the work, these are discussed further here. One of the steps I took to ensure that I remained reflexive was to write a reflective diary. At the beginning I was fairly disciplined about writing and found the diary a valuable tool for recording my thoughts and feelings and clarifying my position:

29th November 2004

I have to question - why am I doing this research, for whose good? I am doing it because one of my life goals is to get a doctorate – however I have spent in excess of three years mulling over what to study. The DProf programme offered the unique/exceptional opportunity to do research and also practice development. My interest in dementia has been generated on a number of levels

- *Visiting Winnie in her nursing home and wondering what it is like for her to be there – does she know the difference between her own home, the hospital and Meadow View?*
- *What is it like to be a patient / person with dementia in hospital – or their carer? From my point of view it looks horrible – people seem to be treated in a kind of "kind but patronising" way – talked down to – treated like*

children with no recognition of their personal biography. It seems humiliating.

- *As a senior nurse I see staff of different professions and grades struggling to manage and care for people with dementia. I am sure that we should be able to do better – if we could understand a complex and dynamic situation more thoroughly.*

So this research is for the benefit of many people as well as myself.

As my fieldwork progressed I reflected on my feelings as a researcher, this enabled me to recognise that I was gradually "fitting in" to the field. I was clearly also developing skills in participant observation:

28th July 2005
I do feel a bit like an enormous cuckoo in the nest and am hugely aware that I am unsettling the field at the moment – perhaps I am being too ambitious thinking that I will become accepted so quickly.

21st September 2005
My persona, or the way that other people think of me, is gradually changing. They seem to be thinking of me as more of a team member, they are starting to come and find me when there is a meeting that may be of interest. They also have started to come and talk to me about incidents that have happened when I am not around or to talk about things I have observed.

Over time my diary tended to be used more as a vehicle to review progress and plan future action. My lack of enthusiasm for writing about my own thoughts sometimes showed:

19th February 2006
I'm gradually getting worse and worse at writing this diary, all that self stuff does not really appeal, it detracts from my real purpose.

As I have reflected on the research I have concluded that my years of being a nurse undoubtedly influenced the whole research process. It was pivotal to the selection of the research question. I am aware that I have been selective in what I have observed and what I have chosen to report. To portray as fair a picture as possible I focused my observations on patients and essentially recorded all the data available whilst I was with them. This depth and intensity of recording was only possible because of the long periods of time that they spent alone and the brief, functional nature of most interactions. This approach allowed me to present an authentic account of what was happening in practice.

As I observed practice I reflected on my own performance as a registered nurse caring for people with dementia. One of my supervisors challenged the "harshness and critical perspective" that I offered in my research. I found this a difficult concept as I believe I have presented a fair account although I am sure that the care I observed was measured against my own standards. Some of the practice I saw appalled me, a few incidents were inhumane and I felt that staff delivering "care" in this way should not be allowed to continue in practice. However the majority of care was delivered in an automatic way, not unkind, but with no respect for the personhood of individuals. I questioned why I found this so difficult and painful to observe; had I too been drawn into the habitus and become unthinking in my practice? This thought stayed with me throughout the research process. Eventually I concluded that I had not worked in such an unthinking way although my departure from direct care had allowed me to step back and view practice from a new perspective.

Although I have not entirely reconciled myself with reflexivity it is something that I have achieved. It is suggested by Cutcliffe (2003:139) that to be truly reflexive there is a requirement for "temet nosce", a need to know myself. I would argue that perhaps we never fully know ourselves as we are in a state of constant change. My aim has been to disclose my value base, do justice to my personal stance (Savin-Baden 2004) and provide a clear audit trail (Koch and Harrington 1998) whilst not allowing this to dominate the work.

The Nature of the Doctor of Professional Practice Programme

As I began the doctoral programme my predominant feeling was one of excitement. I wondered what I had taken on as the course leader told us more about the programme. One of the features of this doctorate is that it is punctuated by various hurdles including the submission of a research proposal, a transfer report, a transfer viva and the production of annual reports. At times these just seemed like more work. In retrospect they have been hugely helpful in terms of forcing me to stop and take stock of what I had achieved and plan the next steps. At times the enormity of the work became daunting, achieving the milestones throughout the course was a useful way of stopping me degenerating into complete panic.

Supervision and the Peer Group

Throughout the course I have had regular meetings with my two supervisors who have been unerringly supportive. I often left supervision sessions feeling quite overwhelmed by the sheer breadth and depth of the feedback on current work and new ideas that we had discussed. I learnt to note key words during the session and accept that it would take me several days to really think through what had been said and the implications of this for my work. My supervisors have been enormously constructive in their critique of my work. Looking back at some of the work they reviewed in the early stages this must have been challenging, however it has been invaluable in adding to my inherent motivation. The seeming confidence of my supervisors over the four years has been much appreciated.

I have found working with a small peer group throughout the course a very positive experience. Within the cohort there has been a high level of support and a notable absence of competition. It is suggested by Ellis (2005) that the support network is one of the major strengths of these programmes, particularly when the group is multi-professional.

Whilst I have always believed that the professional doctorate is the right path for me to follow doubts began to emerge as I discussed my work with others. I found that I had to work particularly hard to explain my thesis to those who view this qualification as a second class doctorate; this experience seems relatively common to others on this journey (Yam 2005, Galvin and Carr 2003). I have been aware of the scepticism of others towards professional doctorates (Ellis 2005). I have become particularly frustrated by those who insist that this is a “taught” programme, perhaps a sign of my own academic elitism. Limitations of the professional doctorate are summarised by Ellis (2005) as a lack of academic equivalence, status and currency compared with a traditional doctorate. Despite the negativity of some, and at times my own personal doubts, I am convinced that this has been the right course for me. It has embraced creativity and autonomous learning (Ellis 2005), it has been situated in the “real world” (Lee et al 2000), it has contributed to the body of knowledge and has made a tangible difference in practice. The thesis as a whole represents more than its component parts; the final work is holistic. As professional doctorates begin to flourish in the United Kingdom (Yam 2005) I believe that it will be the responsibility of those that have chosen this path to justify and defend their choice and ensure that the value of their work is acknowledged.

The Integrative Review

Chapter five has possibly been the most difficult for me to write. I have found myself experiencing some reluctance to engage with it as it signals that this work, which seemed impossibly vast at the beginning, has come to an end. This evokes feelings of both sadness and uncertainty. If asked about the process now I would immediately say that it is one I have totally enjoyed. I seem to have mentally set aside some of the emotions and difficulties I encountered during the four years. Reviewing my reflective diaries has reminded me that it has not all been plain sailing. Perhaps the most important achievement for me is the belief that I have made a genuine contribution to improving the care of people with dementia in acute hospitals. This was at the very core of my choice of subject and decision to undertake a professional doctorate. I am realistic in knowing that any change I have facilitated, whilst creditable, is a mere drop in the ocean at present. I am hopeful that I will be able to secure post doctoral funding to take this work forward and improve more widely the lot of this group. In some respects my timing with this study could not be better. I have piloted and evaluated a practice development project at a time when there is a huge increase in political interest in dementia care. This will be a great advantage for my future work.

Conclusion

Chapter five aims to draw together the elements of this study, the literature review, research study and practice development project to form an integrated whole. At the outset of the doctorate my aims were to enable the voices of people with dementia to be heard, to produce knowledge that would influence future practice and to set the work within the broader social and political context. Potential contributions to knowledge made by this work clearly demonstrate how these aims have been met. Limitations of the work and opportunities for further research and practice development have been identified. My personal and professional growth through the doctoral journey has been mapped. This illustrates the value of the professional doctorate as an approach that enables practitioners to engage in "real world" studies that are used to directly influence practice. The doctorate has enabled me to develop as a "scholarly professional" with skills in research that have been used to begin to improve the care of older people with dementia in the acute hospital setting.

BIBLIOGRAPHY

Adams, T. and Bartlett, R. (2003) Constructing dementia. In *Dementia Care* (eds, Adams, T. and Manthorpe, J.) Arnold, London, pp. 3-21.

Aggarwal, N., Vass, A., Minardi, H., Ward, R., Garfield, C. and Cybyk, B. (2003) People with dementia and their relatives: personal experiences of Alzheimer's and the provision of care. *Journal of Psychiatric and Mental Health Nursing,* **10**, 187 - 197.

Allan, K. (2002) A sense of possibility. *Mental Health Today,* **April**, 18 - 21.

Allen, D. (2000) Negotiating the role of expert carers on an adult hospital ward. *Sociology of Health and Illness,* **22**, 149-171.

—. (2004) Ethnomethodological insights into insider-outsider relationships in nursing ethnographies of healthcare settings. *Nursing Inquiry,* **11**, 14 - 24.

Althehide, D. and Johnson, J. (1998) Criteria for assessing interpretive validity in qualitative research. In *Collecting and Interpreting Qualitative Materials* (eds, Denzin, N. and Lincoln, Y.) Sage, Thousand Oaks, pp. 283-312.

Alzheimer's Society (2003) How is Dementia Diagnosed? http://alzheimers.org.uk/Howisdementiadiagnosed/Diagnosisprocess/info.diag (accessed 31.5.03)

—. (2006) http://www.alzheimers.org.uk/site/scripts/documents_info.php?categoryID=200120&documentID=341 (accessed 13.3.06)

—. (2007) Dementia UK: The Full Report. The Alzheimer's Society, London.

Andren, S. and Elmstahl, S. (2005) Family caregivers' subjective experiences of satisfaction in dementia care: aspects of burden, subjective health and sense of coherence. *Scandinavian Journal of Caring Sciences,* **19**, 157-168.

Appignanesi, J. (2006) Ex Memoria DVD. A Missing in Action Films Production. The Wellcome Trust.

Archibald, C. (2003) *People with Dementia in Acute Hospitals: A Practice Guide for Clinical Support Workers,* Dementia Services Development Centre, Stirling.

Arendt, H. (1973) *Men in Dark Times,* Penguin, New York.

Ashburner, C., Meyer, J., Johnson, B. and Smith, C. (2004) Using action research to address loss of personhood in a continuing care setting. *Illness, Crisis and Loss,* **12**(1), 23-37.

Ashworth, A. and Ashworth, P. (2003) The lifeworld as phenomenon and as research heuristic, exemplified by a study of lifeworld of a person suffering Alzheimer's disease. *Journal of Phenomenological Psychology,* **34**(2), 179 - 205.

Atkinson, P. (1992) *Understanding Ethnographic Texts,* Sage, Newbury Park CA.

Atkinson, P., Coffey, A. and Delamont, S. (1999) Ethnography post, past and present. *Journal of Contemporary Ethnography,* **28**(5), 460 - 471.

Audit Commission. (1997) The Coming of Age: Improving Care Services for Older People. The Audit Commission, London.

Aveyard, B. (2001) Education and person-centred approaches to dementia care. *Nursing Older People,* **12**(10), 17 - 19.

Ayers, L. and Poirier, S. (1996) Virtual text and the growth of meaning in qualitative analysis. *Research in Nursing and Health,* **19**, 163-169.

Azar, B. (1997) Defining the trait that makes us most human. *APA Monitor,* **28**(11), 1-15.

Badley, G. (2004a) Does Ron Barnett have a problem with pragmatism? *Teaching in Higher Education,* **9**(1), 113 - 121.

—. (2004b) Reading an academic journal is like doing ethnography. In *Forum: qualitative Social Research.*

Bagshaw, M. and Adams, M. (1986) Nursing home nurses' attitudes, empathy and ideologic orientation. *International Journal of Aging and Human Development,* **22**, 235-246.

Bailey, P. (1996) Assuring quality in narrative analysis. *Western Journal of Nursing Research,* **2**, 186-194.

Bailey, P. and Tilley, S. (2002) Storytelling and the interpretation of meaning in qualitative research. *Journal of Advanced Nursing,* **38**(6), 574-583.

Ballard, C., O'Brien, J., James, I. and Swann, A. (2001) Training carers in behavioural management skills. In *Managing behavioural and psychological symptoms in people with dementia* (eds, Ballard, C., O'Brien, J., James, I. and Swann, A.) Oxford University Press, Oxford, pp. 169-193.

Bamford, C. and Bruce, E. (2000) Defining the outcomes of community care: the perspectives of older people with dementia and their carers. *Ageing and Society,* **20**, 543 - 570.

Bamford, C. and Bruce, E. (2002) Successes and challenges using focus groups with older people with dementia. In *The Perspectives of People with Dementia* (ed, Wilkinson, H.) Jessica Kingsley Publishers Ltd, London, pp. 139 - 164.

Banks, M. (2001) *Visual Methods in Social Research,* Sage, London.

Barnes, V., Clouder, D., Pritchard, J., Hughes, C. and Purkis, J. (2003) Deconstructing dissemination: dissemination as qualitative research. *Qualitative Research,* **3**(2), 147-164.

Barnett, E. (2000) *Including the Person with Dementia in Designing and Delivering Care,* Jessica Kingsley Publishers, London.

Barnett, R. (1997) *Higher Education: A Critical Business,* Society for Research into Higher Education and Open University Press, Buckingham.

—. (2000) *Realizing the University in an Age of Supercomplexity,* Society for Research into Higher Education and Open University Press, Buckingham.

Barnhart, R. (1988) *The Barnhart Dictionary of Etymology,* H.W. Wilson Company, New York.

Bartlett, R. (2000) Dementia as a disability: can we learn from disability studies and theory? *Journal of Dementia Care,* **8**(5), 33 - 36.

—. (2007) 'You can get in alright but you can't get out': social exclusion and men with dementia in nursing homes: insights from a single case study. *Quality in Ageing - Policy, Practice and Research,* **8**(2), 16-26.

Bartlett, H. and Martin, W. (2002) Ethical issues in dementia care research. In *The Perspectives of People with Dementia* (ed, Wilkinson, H.) Jessica Kingsley Publishers Ltd, London, pp. 47 - 61.

Beach, M., Roter, D., Larson, S., Levinson, W., Ford, D. and Frankel, R. (2004) What do physicians tell patients about themselves? A qualitative analysis of physician self-disclosure. *Journal of General Internal Medicine,* **19**, 911-916.

Beauchamp, T. and Childress, J. (1989) *Principles of Biomedical Ethics,* Oxford University Press, Oxford.

Beavis, D. (2007) Specialist Dementia Nurse in an Acute Trust. personal email.

Beck, J. and Young, M. (2005) The assault on professions and the restructuring of academic and professional identities: a Bernsteinian analysis. *British Journal of Sociology of Education,* **26**, 183-197.

Becker, R. (1998) Taking the misery out of experiential learning. *Training,* **35**, 78-81.

Beckett, D. (2001) Workplace learning as post-modernist enactment: a model for dementia. *Journal of Vocational Education and Training,* **53**, 141-159.

Bell, M. and Proctor, S. (1998) Developing nurse practitoners to develop practice: the experiences of nurses working on a nursing development unit. *Journal of Nursing Management,* **6**(2), 61-69.

Bell, V. and Troxel, D. (2003a) Javier, Jane and Mary at Happy Valley. a new day for staff training in a dementia care facility. *Alzheimer's Care Quarterly,* **4**(1), 69-72.

Bell, V. and Troxel, D. (2003b) Javier, Jane and Mary at happy Valley. A look at dementia care training today part 3. *Alzheimer's Care Quarterly,* **4**(2), 153-157.

Bellini, L., Balme, M. and Shea, J. (2002) Variation of mood and empathy during internship. *Journal of the American Medical Association,* **287**, 3143-3146.

Bellini, L. and Shea, J. (2005) Mood change and empathy decline persist during three years internal medicine training. *Academic Medicine,* **80**, 164-167.

Bennett, A. (2005) *Untold Stories,* Faber, London.

Berg, B. (1998) *Qualitative Research Methods for the Social Sciences,* Allyn and Bacon, Boston.

Berman, M. (2000) *Wandering God. A Study in Nomadi Spirituality,* New York Press, Albany, New York.

Bernard, M. and Phillips, J. (2000) The challenge of ageing in tomorrow's Britain. *Ageing and Society,* **20**, 33-54.

Bertakis, K., Roter, D. and Putman, S. (1991) The relationship of physician medical interview style to patient satisfaction. *Journal of Family Practice,* **32**(175-181).

Biddle, J. (1996) The stories of adolescent mothers: hearing their voices in context and community. *Dissertation Abstracts International: The Humanities and Social Sciences,* **56**(8), 3329 - 30.

Binnie, A. and Titchen, A. (1999) *Freedom to Practice: the Development of Patient-Centred Nursing,* Butterworth-Heinemann, Oxford.

Bleakley, A. (2005) Stories as data, data as stories: making sense of narrative inquiry in clinical education. *Medical Education,* **39**, 534-540.

Boettcher, I., Kemeny, B. and Boerman, R. (2004a) Training for and sustaining person-centered dementia care. *Annals of Long-Term Care,* **12**(12), 26-28.

Boettcher, I., Kenmeny, B., DeShon, R. and Stevens, A. (2004b) A system to develop staff behaviours for person-centered care. *Alzheimer's Care Quarterly,* **5**(3), 188-196.

Bogdan, R. and Biklen, S. (1982) *Qualitative Research for Education: An Introduction to Theory and Methods,* Allyn and Bacon, Boston.

Bond, J. and Corner, L. (2001) Researching dementia: are there unique methodological challenges for health services research? *Ageing and Society,* **21**, 95 - 116.

Booth, A. (2001) Cochrane or cock-eyed? how should we conduct systematic reviews of qualitative research? http://www.leeds.ac.uk/educol/documents/00001724.htm (accessed 11.7.04)

Bourdieu, P. (1977) *Outline of a Theory of Practice,* Cambridge University Press, Cambridge.

—. (1984) *Distinction: A Social Critique of the Judgement of Taste,* Routledge and Kegan Paul, London.

Bourdieu, P. and Wacquant, L. (1992) *A Invitation to Reflexive Sociology,* Polity Press, Cambridge.

Bourgeois, M., Dijkstra, K., Burgio, L. and Allen, R. (2004) Communication skills training for nursing aides of residents with dementia: the impact of measuring performance. *Clinical Gerontologist,* **27**(1/2), 119-138.

Bova, B. and Kroth, M. (2001) Workplace learning and generation X. *Journal of Workplace Learning,* **13**(2), 57-65.

Brindle, N. and Holmes, J. (2005) Capacity and coercion: dilemmas in the discharge of older people with dementia from general hospital settings. *Age and Ageing,* **34**, 16-20.

Britten, N., Campbell, R., Pope, C., Donovan, J. and Morgan, M. (2002) Using meta ethnography to synthesise qualitative research: a worked example. *Journal of Health Services Research and Policy,* **7**(4), 209 - 215.

Brody, E. (1971) Excess disabilities of mentally impaired aged: impact of individualised treatment. *The Gerontologist,* **25**, 124-133.

Broe, G., Jorm, A., Creasey, H., Casey, B., Bennett, H., Cullen, J., Edelbrock, D., Waite, L. and Grayson, D. (1999) Carer distress in the general population: results from Sydney Older Persons Study. *Age and Ageing,* **28**, 307-311.

Brooker, D. (1995) Looking at them, looking at me: A review of observational studies into the quality of institutional care for elderly people with dementia. *Journal of Mental Health,* **4**, 145 - 156.

Brown, S. (1998) 'I don't want to go into a home': entering residential or nursing home care, care management and decision-making. In *British Society of Gerontology Annual Conference* Sheffield.

Brown, G. (1990) *Human Teaching for Human Learning An Introduction to Confluent Education,* Gestalt, New York.

Brown, J. and Hillam, J. (2004) *Dementia: your questions answered,* Churchill Livingstone, London.

Bruner, J. (1986) *Actual Minds, Possible Worlds,* Harvard University Press, Cambridge.

Buber, M. (1937) *I and Thou,* Continuum, London.

Burgener, S., Jirovec, M., Murrell, L. and Barton, D. (1992) Caregiver and environmental variables related to difficult behaviours in institutionalized demented elderly patients. *Journal of Gerontology,* **47**(4), 242-249.

Burgener, S. and Dickerson-Putman, J. (1999) Assessing patients in the early stages of irreversible dementia. *Journal of Gerontological Nursing,* **25**(2), 33 - 41.

Burgess, R. (1984) *In the Field: An Introduction to Field Research,* Routledge, London.

Burgess, L. and Page, S. (2003) Educating nursing staff involved in the provision of dementia care. *Nursing Times,* **99**(46), 34 - 37.

Burnard, P. (1991) A method of analysing interview transcripts in qualitative research. *Nurse Education Today,* **11**, 461 - 466.

Burnard, P. (2001) Writing skills. *Journal of Community Nursing,* **15**(4), 25-30.

Bytheway, B. (1995) *Ageism,* Open University Press, Buckingham.

Cabana, M., Rand, C. and Powe, N. (1999) Why don't physicians follow clinical practice guidelines. *Journal of the American Medical Association,* **282**, 1458-1465.

Carr, E., Galvin, K. and Todres, L. (in press) Facilitating nourished scholarship through a professional doctoral programme developing 'cohortness' as an emotional resource. *Studies in Continuing Education.*

Carradice, A. and Round, D. (2004) The reality of practice development for nurses working in an inpatient service for people with severe and enduring mental health problems. *Journal of Psychiatric and Mental Health Nursing,* **11**, 731-737.

Centre for Policy on Ageing. (1996) A Better Home Life: A Code of Good Practice for Residential and Nursing Home Care. Centre for Policy on Ageing, London.

Centre for Reviews and Dissemination (2001) Undertaking systematic reviews of research on effectiveness: CRD report Number 4 (2nd edition).

Chamberlayne, P., Bornat, J. and Wengraf, T. (2000) *The Turn to Biographical Methods in Social Science. Comparative Issues and Examples,* Routledge, New York.

Chase, S. (1996) Personal vulnerability and interpretive authority in narrative research. In *Ethics and Process in the Narrative Study of Lives* (ed, Josselson, R.) Sage, Thousand Oaks CA, pp. 45 - 59.

Chatterji, R. (1998) An ethnography of dementia. *Culture, Medicine and Psychiatry,* **22**, 355-382.
—. (2006) Ethnography. email personal communication.
Cheston, R. and Bender, M. (2003) *Understanding Dementia: The Man with the Worried Eyes,* Jessica Kingsley Publishers, London.
Clare, L. (2002) We'll fight it as long as we can: coping with the onset of Alzheimer's disease. *Aging and Mental Health,* **6**(2), 139-148.
—. (2003) Managing threats to self: awareness in early stage Alzheimer's disease. *Social Science and Medicine,* **57**(6), 1017-1029.
Clare, L., Roth, I. and Pratt, R. (2005) Perceptions of change over time in early-stage Alzheimer's disease. *Dementia: The International Journal of Social Research and Practice,* **4**(4), 487-520.
Clarke, C. and Keady, J. (1996) Researching dementia care and family caregiving: extending ethical responsibilities. *Health Care in Later Life,* **1**(2), 85 - 95.
Clarke, C. and Keady, J. (2002) Getting down to brass tacks: a discussion of data collection with people with dementia. In *The Perspectives of People with Dementia* (ed, Wilkinson, H.) Jessica Kingsley Publishers Ltd, London, pp. 25 - 46.
Clarke, C. and Proctor, S. (1999) Practice development: ambiguity in research and practice. *Journal of Advanced Nursing,* **30**, 975-982.
Clarke, C. and Wilcockson, J. (2001) Professional and organizational learning: analysing the relationship with the development of practice. *Journal of Advanced Nursing,* **34**(2), 264-272.
Clarke, L. (1992) Qualitative research: meaning and language. *Journal of Advanced Nursing,* **17**(2), 243 - 252.
Cleary, M. and Walter, G. (2004) Apportioning out time and energy: oral presentation, poster, journal article or other? *International Journal of Mental Health Nursing,* **13**, 204-207.
Clifford, J. (1986) Introduction: Partial Truths. In *Writing Culture: the Poetics and Politics of Ethnography* (eds, Clifford, J. and Marcus, G.) University of California Press, Berkeley CA, pp. 1 - 26.
—. (1997) *Routes: Travel and Translation in the Late Twentieth Century,* Harvard University Press, Cambridge MA.
Coffey, A. (1999) *The Ethnographic Self: Fieldwork and the Representation of Identity,* Sage Publications, London.
Coffey, A. and Atkinson, P. (1996) *Making Sense of Qualitative Data,* Sage, London.
Cohen, D. and Eisdorfer, C. (1986) *The Loss of Self,* Norton, New York
Cohen, S., Dove, D. and Bachelder, E. (2001) Time to treat learners as consumers. *Training and Development,* **55**(1), 54-57.

Cohen-Mansfield, J. and Werner, P. (1995) Environmental influences on agitation: an integrative summary of an observational study. *The American Journal of Alzheimer's Care and Related Disorders and Research,* **10**(1), 32-39.

Collopy, B., Boyle, P. and Jennings, B. (1991) New directions in nursing home ethics. *Hastings Center Report,* **21**, 1-15.

Cook, A. (2002) Using video observation to include the experiences of people with dementia in research. In *The Perspectives of People with Dementia* (ed, Wilkinson, H.) Jessica Kingsley Publishers Ltd, London, pp. 209 - 222.

—. (2003) Using video to include the experiences of people with dementia in research. *Research Policy and Planning,* **21**(2), 23 - 32.

Coombs, M. and Ersser, S. (2004) Medical hegemony in decision-making - a barrier to interdisciplinary working in intensive care. *Journal of Advanced Nursing,* **46**(3), 245 - 252.

Cornwall County Council. (2007) Time for Action: The Report of the Health and Adult Social Care Overview and Scrutiny Committee's Care Pathways Steering Group., accessed 14.6.07 available from: www.cornwall.gov.uk/media/pdf/r/3/dementia_report.pdf.

Costello, J. (2002) Do not resuscitate orders and older patients: findings from an ethnographic study of hospital wards for older people. *Journal of Advanced Nursing,* **39**(5), 491 - 499.

Cotrell, V. and Schulz, R. (1993) The perspective of the patient with Alzheimer's disease: a neglected dimension of dementia research. *The Gerontologist,* **33**(2), 205 211.

Coyne, I. (1997) Sampling in Qualitative Research: Purposeful and Theoretical Sampling: Merging or Clear Boundaries. *Journal of Advanced Nursing,* **26**, 623 - 630.

Creswell, J. (1998) *Qualitative Inquiry and Research Design: Choosing Among Five Traditions,* Sage Publications, Thousand Oaks.

CSIP (2005) Everybody's Business. www.everybodysbusiness.org.uk (accessed 21.7.06)

Cutcliffe, J. (2003) Reconsidering reflexivity: introducing the case for intellectual entrepreneurship. *Qualitative Health Research,* **13**(1), 136 - 148.

Dahlberg, K. (2006) The publication of qualitative findings. *Qualitative Health Research,* **16**(3), 444-446.

Daily Mail (2006) http://www.dailymail.co.uk/pages/you/article.html?in_article_id=384603&in_page_id=1909 accessed 6.9.06.

Daniels, K., Lamson, A. and Hodgson, J. (2007) An exploration of the marital relationship and Alzheimer's disease: one couple's story. *Families, Systems and Health,* **25**(2), 162-177.

Davidson, D. (2001) *Subjective, Intersubjective, Objective,* Oxford University Press, Oxford.

Davies, H., Nutley, S. and Walter, I. (2005) Approaches to assessing the non-academic impact of social science research. School of Management, University of St Andrews, St Andrews.

Dean, R. (1995) Stories of AIDS: the use of narrative as an approach to understanding AIDS support groups. *Clinical Social Work Journal,* **23**(3), 287-384.

Dellasega, C. and Nolan, M. (1997) Admission to care: facilitating role transition amongst family carers. *Journal of Clinical Nursing,* **6**, 443-451.

Dementia Advocacy Support Network International (2008) http://www.dasninternational.org/ accessed 30.05.2008.

Denzin, N. (1983) Interpretive interactionism. In *Beyond Method: Strategies for Social Research* (ed, Morgan, G.) Sage, Beverly Hills, pp. 129 - 146.

—. (1995) *The Cinematic Society,* Sage, Thousand Oaks.

—. (1997) *Interpretive Ethnography,* Sage, Thousand Oaks.

Denzin, N. and Lincoln, Y. (1994) Handbook of Qualitative Research, Sage, Thousand Oaks.

Denzin, N. (2000) Aesthetics and the practices of qualitative inquiry. *Qualitative Inquiry,* **6**(2), 256-265.

—. (2001) The reflexive interview and a performative social science. *Qualitative research,* **1**, 23-46.

Department of Health (1992) *The Health of the Nation*. Department of Health. London

—. (1999a) Better Government for Older People: Strategem Bulletin 1. Department of Health. London

—. (1999b) *Patient and Public Involvement in the New NHS.* Department of Health. London

—. (2000) *The NHS Plan*. Department of Health. London

—. (2001a) *Seeking consent: working with older people,* Department of Health, London.

—. (2001b) *National Service Framework for Older People.* Department of Health. London

Desjarlais, R. (1994) Struggling along: the possibilities for experience among the homeless mentally ill. *American Anthropologist,* **96**(4), 886-901.

Dewing, J. (1999) Dementia part 1: person-centred care. *Professional Nurse,* **14**(8), 585 - 588.

—. (2001) Care for older people with dementia in acute hospital settings. *Nursing Older People,* **13**(3), 18 - 20.

—. (2002) From ritual to relationship. *Dementia: The International Journal of Social Research and Practice,* **1**(2), 157-171.

—. (2003) Rehabilitation for people with dementia. *Nursing Standard,* **18**(6), 42 - 48.

—. (2004) Concerns relating to the application of frameworks to promote person-centredness in nursing with older people. *International Journal of Older People Nursing,* **13**(3a), 39-44.

Dick, J., Guiloff, R., Stewart, A., Blackstock, J., Bielawska, C., Paul, E. and Marsden, C. (1984) Mini-mental state examination in neurological patients. *Journal of Neurology, Neurosurgery and Psychiatry,* **47**, 496 - 499.

Dingwall, R. (1992) Don't mind him - he's from Barcelona: qualitative methods in health studies. In *Researching Health Care* (eds, Daly, J., McDonald, I. and Willis, E.) Tavistock / Routledge, London, pp. 161 - 175.

Diseker, R. and Michielutte, R. (1981) An analysis of empathy in medical students before and following clinical experience. *Journal of Medical Education,* **56**, 1004-1010.

Doane, G. (2005) Towards Compassionate Action: Pragmatism and the Inseparability of Theory / Practice. *Advances in Nursing Science,* **28**(1), 81 - 90.

Downs, M. (1997) The emergence of the person in dementia research. *Ageing and Society,* **17**, 597 - 607.

Downs, M. and Rae, C. (1997) General Practitioners reasons for withholding and sharing a diagnosis of dementia. In *50th Annual Meeting of the Gerontological Society of America* Washington.

Edwards, A., Elwyn, G., Hood, K. and Rollnick, S. (2000) Judging the 'weight of evidence' in systematic reviews: introducing rigour into the qualitative overview stage by assessing Signal and Noise. *Journal of Evaluation in Clinical Practice,* **6**(2), 177 - 184.

Edwards, A., Russell, I. and Stott, C. (1998) Signal versus noise in the evidence base for medicine: an alternative to hierarchies of evidence? *Family Practice,* **15**(4), 319-322.

Ekman, I. and Skott, C. (2005) Developing clinical knowledge through narrative-based method of interpretation. *European Journal of Cardiovascular Nursing,* **4**, 251-256.

Elderworld (2006) www.elderworld.com (in production).

Elliott, J. (2005) *Using Narrative in Social Research,* Sage Publications, London.

Ellis, L. (2005) Professional doctorates for nurses: mapping provision and perceptions. *Journal of Advanced Nursing,* **50**(4), 440-448.

Ellis, C. and Bochner, A. (2006) Analyzing analytic authoethnography an autopsy. *Journal of Contemporary Ethnography,* **35**(4), 429-449.

Emden, C. (1998) Conducting a narrative analysis. *Collegian,* **5**(3), 34-37.

Emerson, R., Fretz, R. and Shaw, L. (2001) Participant Observation and Fieldnotes. In *Handbook of Ethnography* (eds, Atkinson, P., Coffey, A., Delamont, S., Lofland, J. and Lofland, L.) Sage Publications, London, pp. 352 - 368.

Engestrom, Y. (2001) Expansive learning at work: toward an actively theoretical conceptualisation. *Journal of Education and Work,* **14**(133-156).

Eriksson, C. and Saveman, B.-I. (2002) Nurses' experiences of abusive / non-abusive caring for demented patients in acute care settings. *Scandinavian Journal of Caring Sciences,* **16**, 79 - 85.

European Agency for the Evaluation of Medicinal Products (1997) Notes for *Guidance on Medicinal Products in the Symptomatic Treatment of AD.* Committee for Proprietary Medicinal Products Working Party, London.

Evans, R. (2003) Patient centred medicine: reason, emotion, and human spirit? Some philosophical reflections on being with patients. *Journal of Medical Ethics: Medical Humanities,* **29**, 8-15.

Fagermoen, M. (1997) Professional identity: values embedded in meaningful nursing practice. *Journal of Advanced Nursing,* **25**, 434-441.

Farsides, C. (2003) The Ethics of Clinical Research. In *Manual for Research Ethics Committees* (ed, Eckstein, S.) Cambridge University Press, Cambridge, pp. 5 - 14.

Faulkner, M. (2001) Empowerment, disempowerment and the care of older people. *Nursing Older People,* **13**(5), 18 - 20.

Fetterman, D. (1998) *Ethnography,* Sage, Thousand Oaks CA.

Finfgeld, D. (2003) Metasynthesis: The State of the Art - So Far. *Qualitative Health Research,* **13**(7), 893 - 904.

Finlay, L. (2002a) Negotiating the swamp: the opportunity and challenge of reflexivity in research practice. *Qualitative Research,* **2**(2), 209 - 230.

—. (2002b) 'Outing' the researcher: the provenance, process and practice of reflexivity. *Qualitative Health Research,* **12**(4), 531 - 545.

Finlay, L. and Gough, B. (2003) Prologue. In *Reflexivity: a Practical Guide for Researchers in Health and Social Sciences* (eds, Finlay, L. and Gough, B.) Blackwell Science, Oxford, pp. ix-xi.

Flood, G. (1999) *Beyond Phenomenology: Rethinking the Study of Religion,* Cassell, London.

Folstein, M., Folstein, S. and McHugh, P. (1975) 'Mini-mental state': a practical method for grading the cognitive state of patients for the clinician. *Journal of Psychiatric Research,* **12**, 189-198.

Francke, A. and Erkens, T. (1994) Confluent education: an integrative method for nursing (continuing) education. *Journal of Advanced Nursing,* **19**, 354-361.

Freshwater, D. and Avis, M. (2004) Analysing interpretation and reinterpreting analysis: exploring the logic of critical reflection. *Nursing Philosophy,* **5**, 4 - 11.

Fretwell, J. (1982) *Freedom to Change,* Royal College of Nursing, London.

Frid, I., Ohlen, J. and Bergbom, I. (2000) On the use of narratives in nursing research. *Journal of Advanced Nursing,* **32**(3), 695-703.

Gabriel, Y. (1995) The unmanaged organization: stories, fantasies and subjectivity. *Organization Studies,* **16**(3), 477 - 501.

Galvin, K. and Carr, E. (2003) The emergence of professional doctorates in nursing in the UK: where are we now? *Nursing Times Research,* **8**(4), 293-307.

Garbett, R. and McCormack, B. (2001) The experience of practice development: an exploratory telephone interview study. *Journal of Clinical Nursing,* **10**(94-102).

Garner, J. and Ardern, M. (1998) Reflection on old age. *Aging and Mental Health,* **2**(2), 923.

Gee, J. (1986) Units in the production of narrative discourse. *Discourse Processes,* **9**, 391-422.

—. (1991) A linguistic approach to narrative. *Journal of Narrative and Life History,* **1**(1), 15-39.

Geertz, C. (1973) *The Interpretation of Cultures,* Fontana, New York.

Gehring, F. (1973) Anthropology and Education. In *Handbook of Social and Cultural Anthroplogy*(Ed, Honigman, J.) Rand McNally, Chicago.

George, L., Landerman, R. and Blazer, D. (1991) Cognitive Impairment. In *Psychiatric Disorders in America* (eds, Robbins, R. and Reiger, L.) Free Press, New York, pp. 291 - 327.

Gerdner, L. and Buckwater, K. (1994) A nursing challenge: assessment and management of agitation in Alzheimer's patients. *Journal of Gerontological nursing,* **20**(4), 11-20.

Germain, C. (1993) Ethnography: The Method. In *Nursing Research: a Qualitative Perspective* (eds, Munhall, P. and Oiler Boyd, C.) National League for Nursing Press, New York, pp. 237 - 268.

Gibson, G., Timlin, A., Curran, S. and Watts, J. (2004) The scope for qualitative methods in research and clinical trials in dementia. *Age and Ageing,* **33**(4), 422 - 426.

Gilgun, J. (2005) Lighten up: the citation dilemma in qualitative research. *Qualitative Health Research,* **15**(5), 721-724.

Gillies, B. (2000) A memory like clockwork: accounts of living through dementia. *Aging and Mental Health,* **4**(4), 366 - 374.

Gilmour, J. (2002) Dis/integrated care: family caregivers and in-hospital respite care. *Journal of Advanced Nursing,* **39**(6), 546-553.

Gilmour, J. and Huntington, A. (2005) Finding the balance: living with memory loss. *International Journal of Nursing Practice,* **11**, 118-124.

Goffman, E. (1961) *Asylums,* Penguin, London.

—. (1974) *Stigma: Notes on the Management of Spoiled Identity,* Penguin, Harmondsworth.

Gold, R. (1958) Roles in Sociological Field Observations. *Social Forces,* **36**(3), 217 - 223.

Goldstein, A. and Goedhart, A. (1973) The use of structured learning for empathy enhancement in paraprofessional psychotherapists. *Journal of Community Psychology,* **1**, 168-173.

Goldsmith, M. (2002) *Hearing the Voice of People with Dementia,* Jessica Kingsley, London.

Gould, D., Kelly, D., Goldstone, L. and Maidwell, A. (2001) The changing training needs of clinical nurse managers: exploring issues fro continuing professional development. *Journal of Advanced Nursing,* **34**(1), 7-17.

Graneheim, U. and Jansson, L. (2006) The meaning of living with dementia and disturbing behaviour as narrated by three persons admitted to a residential home. *Journal of Clinical Nursing,* **15**, 1397-1403.

Gray, R. (2003) Performing on and off the stage: the place(s) of performance arts-based approaches to qualitative inquiry. *Qualitative Inquiry,* **9**(2), 254-267.

Gray, R., Sinding, M., Ivonoffski, V., Fitch, M., Hampson, A. and Greenberg, M. (2000) The use of research-based theatre in a project related to metastatic breast cancer. *Health Expectations,* **3**, 137-144.

Gray, R., Sinding, M. and Fitch, M. (2001) Navigating the social context of metastatic breast cancer: reflections on a project linking research to drama. *Health,* **5**(2), 233-248.

Gray, R., Fitch, M., Labrecque, M. and Greenberg, M. (2003) Reactions of health professionals to a research-based theatre production. *Journal of Cancer Education,* **18**(4), 223-229.

Grout, G. (2004) Using negotiated consent in research and practice. *Nursing Older People,* **16**(4), 18-20.

Guardian (1999) http://www.guardian.co.uk/health/story/00,282056,00.html#article_continue accessed 6.9.06.

—. (2006) http://www.guardian.co/family/story/0,1680652,00.html|#article-continue accessed 6.9.06.

Gubrium, J. (1975) *Living and Dying at Murray Manor,* St Martin's, New York.

Gwyther, L. (1997) The perceptions of the person with Alzheimer's disease. What outcomes matter most in early to middle stage dementia? *Alzheimer's Disease and Related Disorders,* **11**(supplement 6), 18-24.

Hallberg, L. (1990) *Vocally Disruptive Behaviour in Severely Demented Patients in Relation to Institutional Care Provided,* University of Umeai, Department of Advanced Nursing.

Halpern, J. (2003) What is clinical empathy? *Journal of General Internal Medicine,* **18**, 670-674.

Halse, K. and Hage, A. (2006) An acute hospital ward, densely populated with students during a 12-week clinical study period. *Journal of Nursing Education,* **45**(4), 133-136.

Hammersley, M. (1991) *What's Wrong with Ethnography?* Routledge, London.

Hammersley, M. and Atkinson, P. (1983) *Ethnography Principles in Practice,* Routledge, London.

Hammersley, M. and Atkinson, P. (1995) *Ethnography: Principles in Practice 2nd ed,* Routledge, London.

Hansebo, G. and Kihlgren, M. (2001) Carers; reflections about their video-recorded interactions with patients suffering from severe dementia. *Journal of Clinical Nursing,* **10**, 737 - 747.

Hanson, E., Magnusson, L., Arvidsson, H., Claesson, A., Keady, J. and Nolan, M. (2007) Working together with persons with early stage dementia and their family members to design a user-friendly technology-based support service. *Dementia: The International Journal of Social Research and Practice,* **6**(3), 411-434.

Harborne, A. and Solly, A. (1996) Challenging behaviour in older people: nurses' attitudes. *Nursing Standard,* **11**(12), 39-43.

Harman, G. and Clare, L. (2006) Illness representations and lived experience in early-stage dementia. *Qualitative Health Research,* **16**(4), 484-502.

Harper, D. (1998) An Argument for Visual Sociology. In *Image Based Research: a Sourcebook for Qualitative Researchers* (ed, Prosser, J.) Falmer Press, London, pp. 113-126.

—. (2005) What's New Visually. In *The Sage Handbook of Qualitative Research 3rd ed* (eds, Denzin, N. and Lincoln, Y.) Sage, Thousand Oaks, pp. 747-762.

Harrington, B. (2003) The social psychology of access in ethnographic research. *Journal of Contemporary Ethnography,* **32**(5), 592 - 625.

Harris, P. and Durkin, C. (2002) Building resilience through coping and adapting. In *The Person with Alzheimer's Disease* (ed, Harris, P.) The Johns Hopkins University Press, Baltimore, pp. 165 - 184.

Hart, T. (1999) The refinement of empathy. *Journal of Humanistic Psychology,* **39**(4), 111-125.

Health Advisory Service (2000) Not Because They Are Old. London. HAS

Heiney, S. (1995) The healing power of story. *Oncology Nursing Forum,* **22**(6), 899-904.

Hellstrom, I., Nolan, M. and Lundh, U. (2005) 'We do things together'. *Dementia: The International Journal of Social Research and Practice,* **4**(1), 7-22.

Hellstrom, I., Nolan, M. and Lundh, U. (2007) Sustaining 'couplehood'. *Dementia: The International Journal of Social Research and Practice,* **6**(3), 383-409.

Hendricks, J., Mooney, D. and Berry, C. (1996) A practical strategy approach to use of reflective practice in critical care nursing. *Intensive and Critical Care Nursing,* **12**, 97 - 101.

Herskovits, E. (1995) Struggling over subjectivity: debates about the 'self' in Alzheimer's disease. *Medical Anthropology Quarterly,* **9**(2), 146-164.

Higginson, I., Finlay, I., Goodwin, D., Cook, A., Hood, K., Edwards, A., Douglas, H.-R. and Norman, C. (2002) Do hospital-based palliative care teams improve care for patients or families at the end of life? *Journal of Pain and Symptom Management,* **23**(2), 96 - 106.

Hirschhorn, L. (1997) *The Workplace Within: Psychodynamics of Organisational Life,* MIT Press, Cambridge, MA.

Hoffman, L. (1990) Empathy and justice motivation. *Motivation and Emotion,* **14**(2), 151-172.

Hubbard, G., Downs, M. and Tester, S. (2002) Including the perspectives of older people in institutional care in the consent process. In *The Perspectives of People with Dementia* (ed, Wilkinson, H.) Jessica Kingsley Publishers Ltd, London, pp. 63 - 81.

Hubbard, G., Downs, M. and Tester, S. (2003) Including older people with dementia: challenges and strategies. *Aging and Mental Health,* **7**(5), 351 - 362.

HMSO. (2005) The Mental Capacity Act. London. HM Government.

Hodkinson, B. (2004) Dealing with Dementia: a Carer's Perspective. unpublished paper.

Hoffman, L. (1990) Empathy and justice motivation. *Motivation and Emotion,* **14**(2), 151-172.

Hojat, M., Mangione, S., Nasca, T., Cohen, M., Gonnella, J., Erdmann, J., Veloski, J. and Magee, M. (2001) The Jefferson scale of empathy: development and preliminary data. *Educational and Psychological Measurement,* **61**, 349-365.

Hojat, M., Gonnella, J., Nasca, T., Mangione, S., M and Magee, M. (2002) Physician empathy: definition, components, measurement and relationship to gender and speciality. *American Journal of Psychiatry,* **159**, 1563-1569.

Holloway, I. and Todres, L. (2003) The status of methods: flexibility, consistency and coherence. *Qualitative Research,* **3**(3), 345 - 357.

Holloway, I. and Wheeler, S. (2002) *Qualitative Research in Nursing,* Blackwell Science Ltd, Oxford.

Holloway, W. and Jefferson, T. (2000) *Doing Qualitative Research Differently,* Sage, London.

Howie, J., Heaney, D., Maxwell, M., Walker, J., Freeman, G. and Rai, H. (1999) Quality at general practice consultations: cross sectional survey. *British Medical Journal,* **319**, 738-743.

Hubbard, G., Downs, M. and Tester, S. (2002) Including the perspectives of older people in institutional care in the consent process. In *The Perspectives of People with Dementia* (ed, Wilkinson, H.) Jessica Kingsley Publishers Ltd, London, pp. 63 - 81.

Hubbard, G., Downs, M. and Tester, S. (2003) Including older people with dementia: challenges and strategies. *Aging and Mental Health,* **7**(5), 351 - 362.

Hughes, C. (1992) 'Ethnography': what's in a word - process? product? promise? *Qualitative Health Research,* **2**(4), 439 - 450.

Hughes, E. (1984) *The Sociological Eye,* Transaction Books, London.

Im, E.-O. and Chee, W. (2003) Fuzzy Logic and Nursing. *Nursing Philosophy,* **4**, 53 - 60.

Innes, A. (2000) *Training and Development for Dementia Care Workers,* Jessica Kingsley, London.

—. (2002) The social and political context of formal dementia care provision. *Ageing and Society,* **22**, 483-499.

James, I., Powell, I. and Kendell, K. (2003) The castle and the know-it-all access to the inner circle. *Journal of Dementia Care,* **11**(4), 24-26.

Jenkins, R. (2002) *Pierre Bourdieu,* Routledge, Abingdon.

Jeon, Y.-H., Brodaty, H. and Chesterton, J. (2005) Respite care for caregivers and people with severe mental illness: literature review. *Journal of Advanced Nursing,* **49**(3), 297-306.

Jones, K. (2003) The turn to a narrative knowing of persons: one method explored. *NT Research,* **8**(1), 60-71.

—. (2004a) Mission drift in qualitative research, or moving toward a systematic review of qualitative studies, moving back to a more systematic narrative review. *The Qualitative Report,* **9**(1), 95 - 112.

—. (2004b) The turn to narrative knowing of persons. In *New Qualitative Methodologies in Health and Social Care Research* (ed, Rapport, F.) Routledge, London, pp. 35-54.

—. (2006) Informal care as relationship: the case of the Magnificent Seven. *Journal of Psychiatric and Mental Health Nursing,* **13**, 214-220.

Jones, P. and Martinson, I. (1992) The experience of bereavement in caregivers of family members with Alzheimer's disease. *Journal of Nursing Scholarship,* **24**(3), 172-176.

Josselson, R. (1996a) Introduction. In *Ethics and Process in the Narrative Study of Lives* (ed, Josselson, R.) Sage, Thousand Oaks CA, pp. xi - xviii.

—. (1996b) On writing other people's lives: self-analytic reflections of a narrative researcher. In *Ethics and Process in the Narrative study of Lives* (ed, Josselson, R.) Sage, Thousand Oaks CA, pp. 60 -71.

Junker, B. (1960) *An Introduction to the Social Sciences,* University of Chicago Press, Chicago.

Kanuha, V. (2000) 'Being' native versus 'going native': conducting social work research as an insider. *Social Work,* **45**(5), 439 - 447.

Katsuno, T. (2003) Personal spirituality of persons with early-stage dementia. *Dementia: The International Journal of Social Research and Practice,* **2**(3), 315 - 335.

Katz, J. (1997) Ethnography's warrants. *Sociological Methods and Research,* **25**(4), 391 - 423.

—. (2001) 'From how to why: on luminous description and causal inference in ethnography' (part 1). *Ethnography,* **2**(4), 443-473.

Katzenbach, J. and Smith, D. (1998) *The Wisdom of Teams: Creating the High Performance Team,* Harvard Business School Press, Boston.

Keady, J. (1996) The experience of dementia: a review of the literature and implications for nursing practice. *Journal of Clinical Nursing,* **5**, 275 - 288.

Keady, J. and Gilliard, J. (2002) The experience of neuropsychological assessment for people with suspected Alzheimer's disease. In *The Person with Alzheimer's Disease* (ed, Harris, P.) The Johns Hopkins University Press, Baltimore, pp. 3 - 28.

Keady, J. and Williams, S. (2007) Co-constructed inquiry: a new approach to generating, disseminating and discovering knowledge in qualitative research. *Quality in Ageing,* **8**(2), 27-36.

Keady, J., Williams, S. and Hughes-Roberts, J. (2005) Emancipatory practice development through life-story work: changing care in a memory clinic in North Wales. *Practice Development in Health Care,* **4**(4), 203-212.

Keady, J., Williams, S. and Hughes-Roberts, J. (2007) 'Making mistakes' Using Co-Constructed Inquiry to illuminate meaning and relationships in the early adjustment to Alzheimer's disease - a single case study approach. *Dementia: The International Journal of Social Research and Practice,* **6**(3), 343-364.

Keane, W. (1994) The patient's perspective: The Alzheimer's Association. *Alzheimer Disease and Associated Disorders,* **8 (Suppl 3)**, 151-155.

Keen, S. and Todres, L. (2006) Communicating Qualitative Research Findings; An Annotated Bibliographic Review of Non-Traditional Dissemination Strategies. Institute of Health and Community Studies, Bournemouth University, Bournemouth.

Keating, E. (2001) The Ethnography of Communication. In *Handbook of Ethnography* (eds, Atkinson, P., Coffey, A., Delamont, S., Lofland, J. and Lofland, L.) Sage, London, pp. 285 - 301.

Kemeny, B., Boettcher, I., DeShon, R. and Stevens, A. (2006) Using experiential techniques for staff development. *Journal of Gerontological Nursing,* **August**, 9-14.

Killick, J. (2001) 'The best way to improve this place': gathering views informally. In *Hearing the User's Voice: Encouraging People with Dementia to Reflect on their Experiences of Services* (eds, Murphy, C., Killick, J. and Allan, K.) University of Stirling, Stirling, pp. 6 - 9.

—. (2002) 'I can't take this place at all': the nursing home experience. In *The Person with Alzheimer's Disease* (ed, Harris, P.) The Johns Hopkins University Press, Baltimore, pp. 270 - 281.

—. (2004) Dementia, identity and spirituality. *Journal of Religious Gerontology,* **16**(3-4), 59-74.

Kim, S., Cox, C. and Caine, E. (2002a) Impaired decision making ability in subjects with Alzheimer's disease and willingness to participate in research. *American Journal of Psychiatry,* **159**(5), 797 - 802.
Kim, S., Karlawish, J. and Caine, E. (2002b) Current state of research on decision-making competence of cognitively impaired elderly persons. *American Journal of Geriatric Psychiatry,* **10**(2), 151-165.
Kirk, W. and Thomas, A. (1982) A brief in-service training strategy to increase levels of empathy of psychiatric nursing personnel. *Journal of Psychiatric Treatment and Evaluation,* **4**, 177-179.
Kitwood, T. (1997a) *Dementia Reconsidered: The Person Comes First,* Open University Press, Buckingham.
—. (1997b) The experience of dementia. *Aging and Mental Health,* **1**(1), 13 - 22.
Kitwood, T. and Benson, S. (1995) *The New Culture of Dementia Care,* Hawker Publications, London.
Kitwood, T. and Bredin, K. (1992) A new approach to the evaluation of dementia care. *Journal of Advances in Health and Nursing Care,* **1**(5), 41 - 60.
Kitson, A. (1994) Clinical Nursing Practice Development and Research Activity in the Oxford Region. National Institute for Nursing, Oxford.
Koch, T. (1994) Establishing rigour in qualitative research: the decision trail. *Journal of Advanced Nursing,* **19**, 976 - 986.
—. (1998) Story telling: is it really research? *Journal of Advanced Nursing,* **28**(6), 1182 - 1190.
Koch, T. and Harrington, A. (1998) Reconceptualizing rigour: the case for reflexivity. *Journal of Advanced Nursing,* **28**(4), 882 - 890.
Koch, T., Webb, C. and Williams, A. (1995) Listening to the voices of older patients: an existential-phenomenological approach to quality assurance. *Journal of Clinical Nursing,* **4**(3), 185 - 193.
Kontos, P. and Naglic, G. (2006) Expressions of personhood in Alzheimer's: moving from ethnographic text to performing ethnography. *Qualitative Research,* **6**(3), 301-317.
Kuang-Hsu Chiang, I. (2003) Learning experiences of doctoral students in UK universities. *International Journal of Sociology and Social Policy,* **23**(1/2), 4-32.
Kvale, S. (1996) *InterViews An Introduction to Qualitative Research Interviewing,* Sage Publications, Thousand Oaks.
LaMonica, E., Carew, D., Winder, A., Bernazza-Hasse, A. and Blanchard, K. (1976) Empathy training as the major thrust of a staff development program. *Nursing Research,* **25**, 447-451.

LaMonica, E., Wolf, R., Madea, A. and Oberst, M. (1987) Empathy and nursing care outcomes. *Scholarly Inquiry for Nursing Practice,* **1**, 197-213.

Landreville, P., Dicaire, L., Verreault, R. and Levesque, L. (2005) A training program for managing agitation of residents in long-term care facilities. *Journal of Gerontological Nursing,* **31**(3), 34-42.

Lane, J. (2000) *Pierre Bourdieu,* Pluto Press, London.

Langdon, S., Eagle, A. and Warner, J. (2007) Making sense of dementia in the social world: a qualitative study. *Social Science and Medicine,* **64**, 989-1000.

Larson, E. and Yao, X. (2005) Clinical empathy as emotional labor in patient physician relationships. *Journal of the American Medical Association,* **293**, 1100-1106.

Lave, J. and Wenger, E. (1991) *Situated Learning: Legitimate Peripheral Participation,* Cambridge University Press, Cambridge.

Lawler, J. (1991) *Behind the Screens: Nursing, Somology and the Problem of the Body,* Churchill Livingstone, Edinburgh.

Lee, A., Green, B. and Brennan, M. (2000) Organisational knowldge, professional practice and the professional doctorate at work. In *Research and Knowledge at Work: Perspectives, Case-Studies and Innovative Strategies* (eds, Garrick, J. and Rhodes, C.) Routledge, London, pp. 117-136.

Lerum, K. (2001) Subjects of desire: academic armor, intimate ethnography, and the production of critical knowledge. *Qualitative Inquiry,* **7**(4), 466-483.

Lett, J. (1987) *The Human Enterprise: a Critical Introduction to Anthropological Theory,* Westview Press, Boulder CO.

Lewycka, M. (1998) *Finding and Paying for Residential and Nursing Home Care,* Age Concern, London.

Li, R. and Orleans, M. (2002) Personhood in a world of forgetfulness: an ethnography of the self-process among Alzheimer's patients. *Journal of Aging and Identity,* **7**(4), 227-244.

Lieblich, A., Tuval-Mashiach, R. and Zilber, T. (1998) *Narrative Research: Reading, Analysis and Interpretation,* Sage, London.

Lincoln, Y. and Guba, E. (1985) *Naturalistic Inquiry,* Sage, Beverly Hills.

Lindstrom, H., Smyth, K., Sami, S., Dawson, N., Patterson, M., Bohinc, J., Post, S., Barber, M., Ollerton, S., Singer, M. and Whitehouse, P. (2006) Medication used to treat memory loss: perspectives of persons with dementia and their caregivers. *Dementia: The International Journal of Social Research and Practice,* **5**(1), 27-50.

Lintern, T., Woods, B. and Phair, L. (2000) Training is not enough to change care practice. *Journal of Dementia Care,* **8**(2), 15-17.

Livinson, W. and Roter, D. (1995) Physicians' psychosocial beliefs correlate wit their patient communication skills. *Journal of General Internal Medicine,* **10**, 375-379.

Lockyer, J., Fidler, H., Hogan, D., Pereles, L., Wright, B., Lebeuf, C. and Gerritsen, C. (2005) Assessing outcomes through congruence of course objectives and reflective work. *The Journal of Continuing Education in the Health Professions,* **25**, 76-86.

Lomas, J. (1997) Improving research dissemination and uptake in the health sector: beyond the sound of one hand clapping. McMaster University Centre for Health Economics and Policy Analysis, Ontario.

Lomborg, K. and Kirkevold, M. (2003) Truth and validity in grounded theory - a reconsidered realist interpretation of the criteria: fit, work, relevance and modifiability. *Nursing Philosophy,* **4**, 189 - 200.

Lumme-Sandt, K. and Virtanen, P. (2002) Older people in the field of medication. *Sociology of Health and Illness,* **24**(3), 285-304.

Lundh, U., Sandberg, J. and Nolan, M. (2000) 'I don't have any other choice': spouses' experiences of placing a partner in a care home for older people in Sweden. *Journal of Advanced Nursing,* **32**(5), 1178-1186.

Lyman, K. (1998) Living with AD: the creation of meaning among persons with dementia. *Journal of Clinical Ethics,* **9**(1), 49-57.

MacLeod, R. (2000) Learning to care: a medical perspective. *Palliative Medicine,* **14**(209-216).

Macquarrie, C. (2005) Experiences in early stage Alzheimer's disease: understanding the paradox of acceptance and denial. *Aging and Mental Health,* **9**(5), 430-441.

Maggs-Rapport, F. (2001) 'Best research practice': in pursuit of methodological rigour. *Journal of Advanced Nursing,* **35**(3), 373 - 383.

Malacrida, C. (2005) Discipline and dehumanization in a total institution: institutional survivors' descriptions of time-out rooms. *Disability and Society,* **20**(5), 523-537.

Mallet, J. (1997) Forging new roles. *Nursing Times,* **93**, 38-39.

Malloy, D. and Hadjistavropoulos, T. (2004) The problem of pain management among persons with dementia, personhood, and the ontology of relationships. *Nursing Philosophy,* **5**, 147-159.

Manley, K. (2001) Consultant Nurse: Concept, Processes, Outcome. Manchester University / RCN Institute, London.

Manley, K. and McCormack, B. (2003) Practice development: purpose, methodology, facilitation and evaluation. *Nursing in Critical Care,* **8**(1), 22-29.

Marcus, G. (1998) What comes (just) after "post"? The case of ethnography. In *The Landscape of Qualitative Research: Theories and Issues* (eds, Denzin, N. and Lincoln, Y.) Sage, Thousand Oaks CA, pp. 383 - 406.

Marshall, M. (1999) 'They should not really be here': people with dementia in the acute sector. *Age and Ageing,* **28**, 9 - 11.

Marson, D., Hawkins, L., McInturff, B. and Harrell, L. (1997) Cognitive models that predict physician judgments of capacity to consent in mild Alzheimer's disease. *Journal of the American Geriatrics Society,* **45**, 458 - 464.

Martin, L., Rozon, L., McDowell, S., Cetinski, G. and Kemp, K. (2004) Evaluation of a training programme for long-term care staff on bathing techniques for persons with dementia. *Alzheimer's Care Quarterly,* **5**(3), 217-229.

Marzanski, M. (2000) Would you like to know what is wrong with you? on telling the truth to patients with dementia. *Journal of Medical Ethics,* **26**(2), 108 - 113.

Mason, E., Clare, L. and Pistrang, N. (2005) Processes and experiences of mutual support in professionally-led support groups for people with early-stage dementia. *Dementia: The International Journal of Social Research and Practice,* **4**(1), 87-112.

McAuley, W., Travis, S. and Safewright, M. (1997) Personal accounts of the nursing home search and selection process. *Qualitative Health Research,* **7**, 236-254.

McCormack, B. (2001a) Autonomy and the relationship between nurses and older people. *Ageing and Society,* **21**(4), 417 - 446.

—. (2001b) Clinical effectiveness and clinical teams: effective practice with older people. *Nursing Older People,* **13**(5), 14 - 17.

—. (2002) The person of the voice: narrative identities in informed consent. *Nursing Philosophy,* **3**, 114 - 119.

—. (2003) Knowing and acting - a strategic practitioner-focused approach to nursing research and practice development. *NT Research,* **8**(2), 86-100.

—. (2004) Person-centredness in gerontological nursing: an overview of the literature. *International Journal of Older People Nursing,* **13**(3a), 31-38.

McCormack, B. and Garbett, R. (2003) The characteristics, qualities and skills of practice developers. *Journal of Clinical Nursing,* **12**, 317-325.

McCormack, B., Manley, K., Kitson, A., Titchen, A. and Harvey, G. (1999) Towards practice development - a vision in reality or a reality without vision? *Journal of Nursing Management,* **7**(5), 255 - 264.

McDaniel, S., Hepworth, J. and Doherty, W. (1995) Medical family therapy with somaticizing patients: the co-creation of therapeutic stories. *Family Process,* **34**, 349 - 361.

McLean, S. (1987) Assessing dementia part 1: difficulties, definitions and differential diagnosis. *The Australian and New Zealand Journal of Psychology,* **21**, 142 - 174.

McLeod, J. and Balamoutsou, S. (2000) A method for qualitative narrative analysis of psychotherapy transcripts. In *Qualitative Psychotherapy Research: Methods and Methodology* (eds, Frommer, J. and Rennie, D.) Pabst, Berlin.

McSherry, R. and Driscoll, J. (2004) Practice development: promoting quality improvement in orthopaedic care. as well as one's self. *Journal of Orthopaedic Nursing,* **8**(3), 171-178.

McSherry, R. and Warr, J. (2006) Practice development: confirming the existence of a knowledge and evidence base. *Practice Development in Health Care,* **5**(2), 55-79.

Means, R., Morbey, H. and Smith, R. (2002) *From Community Care to Market Care? The Developments of Welfare Services for Older People,* The Policy Press, Bristol.

Meleis, A. (1999) *Theoretical Nursing: Development and Progress,* Lippincott, Philadelphia.

Menne, H., Kinney, J. and Morhardt, D. (2002) Trying to continue to do as much as they can. *Dementia: The International Journal of Social Research and Practice,* **1**(3), 367 - 382.

Menzies Lyth, I. (1988) *Containing Anxiety in Institutions vol 1 Selected Essays,* Free Association Books, London.

Meyer, J., Bridges, J. and Spilsbury, K. (1999) Caring for people in acute settings: lessons learned from an action research study in accident and emergency. *NT Research,* **4**(5), 327-339.

Mickus, M., Wagenaar, D., Averill, M., Colenda, C., Gardiner, J. and Luo, A. (2002) Developing effective bathing strategies for reducing problematic behavior for residents with dementia: the PRIDE approach. *Journal of Mental Health and Aging,* **8**, 37-4.

Mienczakowski, J. (1995) The theatre of ethnography: the reconstruction of ethnography into theatre with emancipatory potential. *Qualitative Inquiry,* **1**(3), 360-375.

—. (1997) Theatre of change. *Research in Drama Education,* **2**(2), 159-172.

—. (2000) Applied Ethnography: Performance Texts, Research and Classroom Dilemmas. In http://www.leeds.ac.uk/educol/documents/00001578.htm accessed 13.2.07.

—. (2001) Ethnodrama: performed research - limitations and potential. In *Handbook of Ethnography* (eds, Atkinson, P., Coffey, A., Delamont, S., Lofland, J. and Lofland, L.) Sage, London, pp. 468-476.

Mienczakowski, J. and Morgan, S. (1993) *Busting: The Challenge of the Drought Spirit,* Griffith University Reprographics, Brisbane.

Mienczakowski, J., Smith, R. and Sinclair, M. (1996) On the road to catharsis: a theoretical framework for change. *Qualitative Inquiry,* **2**(4), 439-462.

Mills, M. (1997) Narrative Identity and Dementia: a study of Emotion and Narrative in Older People with Dementia. *Ageing and Society,* **17**, 673 - 698.

—. (2003) A meeting of minds: allowing older people with dementia to share their thoughts and experiences about health and social care, using counselling skills. *Research Policy and Planning,* **21**(2), 33 - 42.

Milton, C. (2000) Informed consent: process or outcome? *Nursing Science Quarterly,* **13**(4), 291 - 298.

Misch, D. and Peloquin, S. (2005) Developing empathy through confluent education. *Journal of Physical Therapy Education,* **19**(3), 41-51.

Monaghan, C. and Begley, A. (2004) Dementia diagnosis and disclosure: a dilemma in practice. *International Journal of Older People Nursing,* **13**(3a), 22 - 29.

Moniz-Cooke, E., Agar, S., Woods, R., Waang, M. and Elston, C. (1998) Can staff training reduce carer stress and behavioural disturbance in the elderly mentally ill? *International Journal of Geriatric Psychiatry,* **13**(1), 149-158.

Moon, G. (2000) Risk and protection: the discourse of confinement in contemporary mental health policy. *Health and Place,* **6**, 239-250.

Moore, T. and Hollett, J. (2003) Giving voice to persons living with dementia: the researchers opportunities and challenges. *Nursing Science Quarterly,* **16**(2), 163-167.

Moore, T., Hollett, J., Pilkington, B. and Jonas-Simpson, C. (2003) A pilot study of the lived experience for persons with dementia residing on a locked unit. *Perspectives,* **27**(2), 5 - 14.

Morgan, G. (1983) Exploring choice reframing the process of evaluation. In *Beyond Method: Strategies for Social Research*(Ed, Morgan, G.) Sage, Beverley Hills, pp. 392 - 404.

Morgan, D. (1999) Risk and Family Practices: Accounting for Change and Fluidity in Family Life. In *The New Family* (eds, Silva, E. and Smart, C.) Sage, London.

Moriarty, J. and Webb, S. (1997) How do older people feel about assessment. *Journal of Dementia Care,* **Sept / Oct**, 20 - 22.

Mounce, H. (2000) Pragmatism. *Nursing Philosophy,* **1**, 80 - 81.

Mueller-Hergl, C. (2003) Focus on the change agent. *Journal of Dementia Care,* **Nov/Dec**, 8-10.

Mulhall, A. (2003) In the field: notes on observation in qualitative research. *Journal of Advanced Nursing,* **41**(3), 306 - 313.

Mullen, C. (2003) Guest editors introduction: 'A self fashioned gallery of aesthetic practice'. *Qualitative Inquiry,* **9**(2), 165-181.

Mulrow, C. and Cook, D. (1998) *Systematic Reviews,* American College of Physicians, Philadelphia.

Murphy, J., Tester, S., Hubbard, G., Downs, M. and MacDonald, C. (2005) Enabling frail older people with a communication difficulty to express their views: the use of Talking Mats as an interview tool. *Health and Social Care in the Community,* **13**(2), 95-107.

Murphy, E. and Dingwall, R. (2001a) The Ethics of Ethnography. In *Handbook of Ethnography* (eds, Atkinson, P., Coffey, A., Delamont, S., Lofland, J. and Lofland, L.) Sage Publications, London, pp. 339 - 351.

Murphy, E. and Dingwall, R. (2001b) Qualitative methods in health technology assessment. In *The Advanced Handbook of Methods in Evidence Based Healthcare* (eds, Stevens, A., Abrams, K., Brazier, J., Fitzpatrick, R. and Lilford, R.) Sage, London, pp. 166 - 180.

Naidoo, M. and Bullock, R. (2001) *Integrated Care Pathway for Dementia,* Harcourt, New York.

National Audit Office. (2007) Improving Services and Support for People with Dementia. The Stationery Office, London.

Nelms, T. (1996) Living a caring presence in nursing: a Heideggerian hermeneutical analysis. *Journal of Advanced Nursing,* **24**(2), 368 - 374.

Nelson-Jones, R. (1993) *Practical counselling and helping skills: how to use the lifeskills helping model,* Cassell, London.

Neuman, R. (2005) Doctoral differences: professional doctorates and PhDs compared. *Journal of Higher Education and Management,* **27**(2), 173-188.

NICE (2006) *Dementia: Supporting People with Dementia and their Carers in Health and Social Care,* National Institute for Health and Clinical Excellence, London.

Nolan, L. (2007) Caring for people with dementia in the acute setting: a study of nurses' views. *British Journal of Nursing,* **16**(7), 419-422.

Nolan, M. (2003) Ageism: what's in a word? *Journal of Advanced Nursing,* **41**(1), 8 - 9.

Nolan, M., Ryan, T., Enderby, P. and Reid, D. (2002) Towards a more inclusive vision of dementia care and practice. *Dementia: The International Journal of Social Research and Practice,* **1**(2), 193-211.

Nolan, M. and Tolson, D. (2000) Gerontological nursing 1: challenges of nursing older people in acute care. *British Journal of Nursing,* **9**(1), 39 - 43.

Norman, R. (2003a) Acute nursing care for people with dementia. What happens when a person with dementia is admitted to hospital for acute care. University of the West of England, Bristol.

—. (2003b) Acute Nursing Care for People with Dementia. Developing practice guidance - dementia care in acute hospital settings. University of the West of England, Bristol.

—. (2006) Observations of the experiences of people with dementia on general hospital wards. *Journal of Research in Nursing,* **11**(5), 453-465.

Normann, H., Apslund, K. and Norberg, A. (1999) Attitude of Registered Nurses towards patients with severe dementia. *Journal of Clinical Nursing,* **8**, 353 - 359.

Northway, R. (2000) Disability, nursing research and the importance of reflexivity. *Journal of Advanced Nursing,* **32**(2), 391 - 397.

Nutley, S., Walter, I. and Davies, H. (2002) From knowing to doing: a framework for understanding the evidence into practice agenda. available from www.st-andrews.ac.uk/%7Eruru/publications.htm. University of St Andrews, St Andrews.

Nygard, L. and Starkhammar, S. (2007) The use of everyday technology by people with dementia living alone: mapping out the difficulties. *Aging and Mental Health,* **11**(2), 144-155.

O'Connor, S. (2007) Developing professional habitus: a Bernsteinian analysis of the modern nurse apprenticeship. *Nurse Education Today,* **27**, 748-754.

Ogg, J., Grimley Evans, J., Jefferys, M. and MacMahon, D. (1998) Professional responses to the challenge of old age. In *The Social Policy of Old Age - Moving into the 21st Century* (eds, Bernard, M. and Phillips, J.) Centre for Policy on Ageing, London.

Ogier, M. (1982) *An Ideal Sister?* Royal College of Nursing, London.

—. (1986) An ideal sister - seventy years on? *Nursing Times,* **82**, 54-57.

—. (1989) *Working and Learning,* Scutari Press, London.

Olofsson, B. and Norberg, A. (2001) Experiences of coercion in psychiatric care as narrated by patients, nurses and physicians. *Journal of Advanced Nursing,* **33**(1), 89-97.

Olsen, D. (1997) Development of an instrument to measure the cognitive structure to understand personhood in patients. *Nursing Research,* **46**, 78-84.

O'Neill, A. and Duffey, M. (2000) Communication of Research and Practice Knowledge in Nursing Literature. *Nursing Research,* **49**, 224-230.

O'Reilly, K. (2005) *Ethnographic Methods,* Routledge, Oxon.

Ortigara, A. and Rapp, C. (2004) Caregiver education for excellence in dementia care. *Alzheimer's Care Quarterly,* **5**(3), 179-180.

Packer, T. (2000a) A person-centred approach to the people who care. *Journal of Dementia Care,* **Nov / Dec**, 28 - 30.

—. (2000b) Does person-centred care exist? *Journal of Dementia Care,* **May / June**, 19 - 21.

—. (2001c) Acute sector care for people with dementia: time to get our heads out of the sand! *Signpost,* **5**(4), 33 - 36.

Page, S. (1998) Narrowing the gap between practice development and service management. In *The Practice Development Unit: an Experiment in Multidisciplinary Innovation* (eds, Page, S., Allsopp, D. and Casley, S.) Wharr, London.

Page, S. and Hamer, S. (2002) Practice development - time to realize the potential. *Practice Development in Health Care,* **1**(1), 2-17.

Parker, J. (2005) Constructing dementia and dementia care. *Journal of Social Work,* **5**(3), 261-278.

Patton, M. (1990) *Qualitative Evaluation and Research Methods,* Sage, Newbury Park.

Pearce, A., Clare, L. and Pistrang, N. (2002) Managing sense of self: coping in the early stages of Alzheimer's disease. *Dementia: The International Journal of Social Research and Practice,* **1**(2), 173 - 192.

Pellatt, G. (2003) Ethnography and reflexivity: emotions and feelings in fieldwork. *Nurse Researcher,* **10**(3), 28 - 37.

Phinney, A. (1998) Living with Dementia from the Patient's Perspective. *Journal of Gerontological Nursing,* **24** (6), 8 - 15.

—. (2002a) Fluctuating awareness and the breakdown of the illness narrative in dementia. *Dementia: The International Journal of Social Research and Practice,* **1**(3), 329 - 344.

—. (2002b) Living with the symptoms of Alzheimer's disease. In *The Person with Alzheimer's Disease* (ed, Harris, P.) The Johns Hopkins University Press, Baltimore, pp. 49 - 74.

Phinney, A., Wallhagen, M. and Sands, L. (2002) Exploring the meaning of symptom awareness and unawareness in dementia. *Journal of Neuroscience Nursing,* **34**(2), 79 - 90.

Phinney, A. (2006) Family strategies for supporting involvement in meaningful activity by persons with dementia. *Journal of Family Nursing,* **12**(1), 80-101.

Pickard, S., Shaw, S. and Glendinning, C. (2000) Health care professionals' support for older carers. *Ageing and Society,* **20**, 725 - 744.

Pillow, W. (2003) Confession, catharsis, or cure? Rethinking the uses of reflexivity as methodological power in qualitative research. *Qualitative Studies in Education,* **16**(2), 175 - 196.

Pink, S. (2003) Interdisciplinary agendas in visual research: re-situating visual anthropology. *Visual Studies,* **18**(2), 179-192.

Polkinghorne, D. (1988) *Narrative Knowing and the Human Sciences,* University of New York Press, Albany.

—. (1995) Narrative configuration in qualitative analysis. In *Life History and Analysis* (eds, Hatch, J. and Wisniewski, R.) The Falmer Press, London, pp. 5-23.

Popay, J., Rogers, A. and Williams, G. (1998) Rationale and standards for the systematic review of qualitative literature in health services research. *Qualitative Health Research,* **8**(3), 341 - 351.

Post, S. (1995) *The Moral Challenge of Alzheimer's Disease,* Johns Hopkins University Press, Baltimore.

Pratt, R. (2002) 'Nobody's ever asked how I felt'. In *The Perspectives of People with Dementia* (ed, Wilkinson, H.) Jessica Kingsley Publishers Ltd, London, pp. 165 - 182.

Pratt, R. and Wilkinson, H. (2001) *'Tell Me the Truth': the effect of being told the diagnosis of dementia from the perspective of the person with dementia,* The Mental Health Foundation, London.

Preston, R. (1997) Ethnography: studying the fate of health promotion in coronary families. *Journal of Advanced Nursing,* **25**(3), 554 - 561.

Preston, L., Marshall, A. and Bucks, R. (2007) Investigating the ways that older people cope with dementia: a qualitative study. *Aging and Mental Health,* **11**(2), 131-143.

Priest, H., Roberts, P. and Woods, L. (2002) An overview of three different approaches to the interpretation of qualitative data. Part 1: theoretical issues. *Nurse Researcher,* **10**(1), 30-42.

Pritchard, E. and Dewing, J. (2001) Older people with dementia in acute settings. *Nursing Older People,* **12**(10), 21 - 25.

Proctor, G. (2001) Listening to Older Women with Dementia: relationships, voices and power. *Disability and Society,* **16**(3), 361 - 376.

Prosser, J. (1998) the Status of Image Based Research. In *Image Based Research: a Sourcebook for Qualitative Research* (ed, Prosser, J.) Falmer Press, London, pp. 97-112.

—. (2006) Working Paper: Researching with Visual Images: Some Guidance Notes for Beginners. www.reallifemethods.ac.uk accessed 30.05.2008.

Pugh, J., Mitchell, M. and Brooks, F. (2000) Insider - outsider partnerships in an ethnographic study of shared governance. *Nursing Standard,* **14**, 43 - 44.

Qureshi, H., Bamford, C., Nicholas, E., Patmore, C. and Harris, J. (2000) *Outcomes in social care practice: developing an outcome focus in care management and use surveys,* Social Policy Research Unit, University of York.

Rapport, F., Wainwright, P. and Elwyn, G. (2004) The view from the edgelands. *Journal of Medical Ethics,* **30**, 5 - 6.

Rapport, F., Wainwright, P. and Elwyn, G. (2005) "Of the edgelands": broadening the scope of qualitative methodology. *Journal of Medical Ethics,* **31**, 37-42.

Redfern, S., Norman, I., Briggs, K. and Askham, J. (2002) Care at home for people with dementia: routines, control and care goals. *Quality in Ageing,* **3**(4), 12 - 23.

Redwood, R. (1999) Narrative and narrative analysis. *Journal of Clinical Nursing,* **8**, 674.

Reed, J. and Payton, V. (1996) Past the age of consent? A discussion of some ethical issues arising in a study involving older people. *Health Care in Later Life,* **1**(1), 52 - 61.

Reed, J. and Payton, V. (1998) Privileging the voices of older service users: a methodological challenge. *Social Sciences in Health,* **4**(4), 230 - 242.

Reid, D., Ryan, T. and Enderby, P. (2001) What does it mean to listen to the person with AD? *Disability and Society,* **16**(3), 377-392.

Rhynas, S. (2005) Bourdieu's theory of practice and its potential in nursing research. *Journal of Advanced Nursing,* **50**(2), 179-186.

Rice, K. and Warner, N. (1994) Breaking the bad news: what do psychiatrists tell patients with dementia about their illness? *International Journal of Geriatric Psychiatry,* **9**, 467-471.

Richardson, L. (1994) Writing: a Method of Inquiry. In *Handbook of Qualitative Research* (eds, Denzin, N. and Lincoln, Y.) Sage, Thousand Oaks, pp. 516-529.

Richardson, L. and St Pierre, E. (2005) Writing: a Method of Inquiry. In *The Sage Handbook of Qualitative Research 3rd ed* (eds, Denzin, N. and Lincoln, Y.) Sage, Thousand Oaks, pp. 959-978.

Riessman, C. (1993) *Narrative Analysis: Qualitative Research Methods Series 30,* Sage Publications, London.

Riddell, S., Wilkinson, H. and Baron, S. (1998) From emancipatory research to focus groups: people with learning difficulties and the research process. In *Articulating with difficulty: Research Voices in Inclusive Education* (eds, Clough, P. and Barton, L.) Paul Chapman Publishing Ltd, London, pp. 78 - 95.

Riley, R. and Manias, E. (2003) Snap-shots of live theatre: the use of photography to research governance in the operating room. *Nursing Inquiry,* **10**(2), 81-90.

Rittman, M., Rivera, J. and Goodwin, I. (1997) Phenomenological study of nurses caring for dying patients. *Cancer Nursing,* **20**, 115-119.

Roberts, K. and Turnbull, B. (2002-3) Scholarly productivity. *Australian Journal of Advanced Nursing,* **20**(2), 8-14.

Rock, P. (2001) Symbolic Interactionism and Ethnography. In *Handbook of Ethnography* (eds, Atkinson, P., Coffey, A., Delamont, S., Lofland, J. and Lofland, L.) Sage Publications, London, pp. 26 - 38.

Rodeheaver, D. and Datan, N. (1988) The challenge of double jeopardy - toward a mental health agenda for aging. *American Psychologist,* **43**(8), 648 - 654.

Rorty, R. (1979) *Philosophy and the Mirror of Nature,* Princeton University Press, New Jersey.

—. (1987) Science as Solidarity. In *The Rhetoric of Human Sciences: Language and Argument in Scholarship and Public Affairs* (eds, Nelson, J., Megill, A. and McCloskey, D.) University of Wisconsin Press, Madison, pp. 38 - 52.

Ross, C. (2005) Gaining insights into the realities of dementia. *Canadian Nursing Home,* **16**(1), 41-50.

Roter, D., Hall, J., Merisca, R., Nordstrom, B., Cretin, D. and Svarstad, B. (1998) Effectiveness of interventions to improve patient compliance: a meta analysis. *Medical Care,* **36**, 1138-1161.

Rubin, H. and Rubin, I. (1995) *Qualitative Interviewing: The Art of Hearing Data,* Sage, Thousand Oaks.

Rundqvist, E. and Severinsson, E. (1999) Caring relationships with patients suffering from dementia - an interview study. *Journal of Advanced Nursing,* **29**(4), 800 - 807.

Sabat, S. and Harre, R. (1992) The construction and deconstruction of self in Alzheimer's disease. *Ageing and Society,* **12**, 443 - 461.

Sabat, S. (1998) Voices of Alzheimer's disease sufferers: a call for treatment based on personhood. *The Journal of Clinical Ethics,* **9**(1), 35 - 48.

—. (2001) *The Experience of Alzheimer's Disease: Life Through a Tangled Veil,* Blackwell Publishers, Oxford.

—. (2002a) Surviving manifestations of selfhood in Alzheimer's disease. *Dementia: The International Journal of Social Research and Practice,* **1**(1), 25 - 36.

—. (2002b) Selfhood and Alzheimer's disease. In *The Person with Alzheimer's Disease* (ed, Harris, P.) The Johns Hopkins University Press, Baltimore, pp. 88 - 111.

—. (2006) Personal Communication. email.

Salinsky, J. and Sackin, P. (2000) What are you feeling, doctor? Identifying and avoiding defensive patterns in the consultation.

Sandelowski, M., Docherty, S. and Emden, C. (1997) Qualitative meta-synthesis: issues and techniques. *Research in Nursing and Health,* **20**, 365 - 371.

Sapsford, R. and Abbott, P. (1992) *Research Methods for Nurses and the Caring Professions,* Open University Press, Buckingham.

Savage, J. (2000) Ethnography and health care. *British Medical Journal,* **321**(7273), 1400 - 1402.

Savin-Baden, M. (2004) Achieving reflexivity: moving researchers from analysis to interpretation in collaborative inquiry. *Journal of Social Work Practice,* **18**(3), 365 - 378.

Scheff, T. (1997) *Emotions, the social bond and human reality part/whole analysis,* University Press, Cambridge MA.

Schofield, I. (1986) Patient centred care in the management of postoperative orthopaedic patients with an acute confusional state. *Journal of Orthopaedic Nursing,* **1**, 71-75.

Schofield, J. (1993) Increasing the generalizability of qualitative research. In *Social Research: Philosophy, Politics and Practice*(Ed, Hammersley, M.) Sage, London, pp. 200 - 225.

Schofield, H., Block, S., Herman, H., Murphy, B., Nankervis, J. and Singh, B. (1998) *Family Caregivers: Disability, Illness and Ageing,* Allen and Unwin, Sydney.

Schwandt, T. and Halpern, E. (1988) *Linking Auditing and Meta-Evaluation,* Sage, Newbury Park CA.

Scott, D. (1997) The researcher's personal responses as a source of insight in the research process. *Nursing Inquiry,* **4**, 130 - 134.

Scottish Dementia Working Group (2008) http://www.alzscot.org/pages/sdwg/aimsobjectives.htm accessed 30.05.2008.

Sedney, M., Baker, J. and Gross, E. (1994) The story of a death: therapeutic considerations with bereaved families. *Journal of Marital and Family Therapy,* **20**(3), 287-296.

Seely Brown, J. and Duguid, P. (1991) Organisational learning and communities of practice: toward a unified view of working, learning and innovation. *Organisation Science,* **2**(1), 40-57.

Sells, D., Topor, A. and Davidson, L. (2004) Generating coherence out of chaos: examples of the utility of empathic bridges in phenomenological research. *Journal of Phenomenological Psychology,* **35**(2), 253-271.

Serrant-Green, L. (2006) Narrative methods offer a valuable opportunity to us all. *Nurse Researcher,* **3**(3), 3.

Shah, A. and Dickenson, D. (1999) The capacity to make decisions in dementia: some contemporary issues. *International Journal of Geriatric Psychiatry,* **14**, 803 - 806.

Sherwood, G. (1999) Meta-synthesis: merging qualitative studies to develop nursing knowledge. *International Journal of Human Caring,* **3**(1), 37-42.

Sidenvall, B. (1999) Meal procedures in institutions for elderly people: a theoretical interpretation. *Journal of Advanced Nursing,* **30**(2), 319-328.

Silverman, D. (1997) Towards an aesthetics of research. In *Qualitative Research: Theory, Method and Practice* (ed, Silverman, D.) Sage, London, pp. 239 - 253.

Simpson, R., Scothern, G. and Vincent, M. (1995) Survey of carer satisfaction with the quality of care delivered to in-patients suffering from dementia. *Journal of Advanced Nursing,* **22**, 517-527.

Sinding, M., Gray, R., Fitch, M. and Greenberg, M. (2002) Staging breast cancer, rehearsing metastatic disease. *Qualitative Health Research,* **12**(1), 61-73.

Snow, D., Morrill, C. and Anderson, L. (2003) Elaborating analytic ethnography: linking fieldwork and theory. *Ethnography,* **4**, 181-200.

Snyder, L. (2003) Satisfactions and challenges in spiritual faith and practice for persons with dementia. *Dementia: The International Journal of Social Research and Practice,* **2**(3), 299 - 313.

Spradley, J. (1980) *Participant Observation,* Holt, Rinehart and Winston, New York.

Springwood, C. and King, C. (2001) Unsettling engagements: on the ends of rapport in critical ethnography. *Qualitative Inquiry,* **7**(4), 403 - 417.

Stake, R. (1995) *The Art of Case Study Research,* Sage, Thousand Oaks CA.

Stanford (2005a) The Correspondence Theory of Truth

http://plato.stanford.edu/entries/truth-correspondence (accessed 17.10.2005).

—. (2005b) The Coherence Theory of Truth http://plato.stanford.edu/entires/truth-coherence (accessed 17.10.2005).

Stanley, L. and Wise, S. (1983) Breaking Out: Feminist Consciousness and Feminist Research.

Steeman, E., Godderis, J., Grypdonck, M., de Bal, N. and Dierckx de Casterle, B. (2007) Living with dementia from the perspective of older people: is it a positive story? *Aging and Mental Health,* **11**(2), 119-130.

Steplen, K. and Baernstein, A. (2006) Educating for empathy: a review. *Journal of General Internal Medicine,* **21**, 524-530.

Stokes, G. (2000) *Challenging Behaviour in Dementia,* Winslow, Bicester.

Streubert Speziale, H. and Carpenter, D. (2003) *Qualitative Research in Nursing: Advancing the Humanistic Imperative,* Lippincott Williams and Wilkins, Philadelphia.

Suchman, A., Roter, D., Green, M. and Lipkin, M. (1993) Physician satisfaction with primary care office visits. *Medical Care,* **31**, 1083-1092.

Svanstrom, R. and Dahlberg, K. (2004) Living with dementia yields a heteronomous and lost existence. *Western Journal of Nursing Research,* **26**(6), 671 - 687.

Thomas, J. (1993) *Doing Critical Ethnography,* Sage, Newbury Park.

Thorne, S., Jensen, L., Kearney, M., Noblit, G. and Sandelowski, M. (2004) Qualitative Metasynthesis: Reflections on methodological orientation and ideological agenda. *Qualitative Health Research,* **14**(10), 1342 - 1365.

Thornton, P. (2000) *Older People Speaking Out,* Joseph Rowntree Foundation, York.

Tobin, S. (1999) *Preservation of self in the oldest years,* Springer, New York.

Todres, L. (2004) The meaning of understanding and the open body: some implications for qualitative research. *Existential Analysis,* **15**(1), 38-54.

Todres, L. and Holloway, I. (2004) Descriptive phenomenology: life-world as evidence. In *New Qualitative Methodologies in Health and Social Care Research* (ed, Rapport, F.) Routledge, London, pp. 79-98.

Tolson, D., Smith, M. and Knight, P. (1999) An investigation of the components of best nursing practice in the care of acutely ill hospitalized older patients with coincidental dementia: a multi-method design. *Journal of Advanced Nursing,* **30**(5), 1127 - 1136.

Tolson, D., McAloon, M., Hotchkiss, R. and Schofield, I. (2005) Progressing evidence-based practice: an effective nursing model? *Journal of Advanced Nursing,* **50**(2), 124-133.

Torode, B. (1998) Narrative analysis using Code-A-Text. *Qualitative Health Research,* **8**(3), 414-432.

Train, G., Nurock, S., Manela, M., Kitchen, G. and Livingston, G. (2005) A qualitative study of the experiences of long-tern care for residents with dementia, their relatives and staff. *Aging and Mental Health,* **9**(2), 119-128.

Traynor, V., Pritchard, E. and Dewing, J. (2004) Illustrating the importance of views and experiences of users and carers in evaluating the effectiveness of drug treatments for dementia. *Dementia: The International Journal of Social Research and Practice,* **3**(2), 145-159.

Troman, G. (2001) *Tales from the Interface: Disseminating Ethnography for Policy Making,* JAI, London.

Trotman, D. (2006) Evaluating the imaginative: situated practice and the conditions for professional judgment in imaginative education. *http://www.leeds.ac.uk/educol/documents/143528.htm.*

Turner, V. (1986) *The Anthropology of Performance,* PAJ, New York.

Turton, C. (1997) Ways of knowing about health: an Aboriginal perspective. *Advances in Nursing Science,* **19**(3), 28 - 36.

Tutton, E. and Seers, K. (2004) Comfort on a ward for older people. *Journal of Advanced Nursing,* **46**(4), 380 - 389.

Unsworth, J. (2000) Practice development: a concept analysis. *Journal of Nursing Management,* **8**(6), 317-326.

Van der Staay, S. (1994) Stories of (social) distress: applied narrative analysis and public policy for the homeless. *Journal of Social Distress and the Homeless,* **3**(4), 299 - 319.

Van Dijkhuizen, M., Clare, L. and Pearce, A. (2006) Striving for connection. *Dementia: The International Journal of Social Research and Practice,* **5**(1), 73-94.

Van Maanen, J. (1988) *Tales of the Field: on Writing Ethnography,* University of Chicago Press, Chicago.

Van Manen, M. (1997) *Researching Lived Experience: Human Science for an Action Sensitive Pedagogy (2nd edition),* Althouse Press, Ontario.

—. (2006) Writing qualitatively, or the demands of writing. *Qualitative Health Research,* **16**(5), 713-722.

Van Teijlingen, E. and Hundley, V. (2002) Getting your paper in the right journal: a case study of an academic paper. *Journal of Advanced Nursing,* **37**(6), 506-511.

Vassilas, C. (1999) How often do GPs tell people with dementia the truth about their diagnosis? *Alzheimer's Disease Society,* **Feb** 12-14.

Vermeire, E., Hearnshaw, H., Van Royen, P. and Denekens, J. (2001) Patient adherence to treatment: three decades of research. A comprehensive review. *Journal of Clinical Pharmacolgical Therapy,* **26**, 331-342.

Vernooij - Dassen, M., Derksen, E., Scheltens, P. and Moniz-Cooke, E. (2006) Receiving a diagnosis of dementia: the experience over time. *Dementia: The International Journal of Social Research and Practice,* **5**(3), 397-410.

Vescio, T., Sechrist, G. and Paolucci, M. (2003) Perspective taking and prejudice reduction: the mediational role of empathy arousal and situational attributions. *European Journal of Social Psychology,* **33**(455-472).

Victor, C. (1992) Do we need institutional care? In *Social Policy and Elderly People* (eds, Laczko, F. and Victor, C.) Gower, Aldershot, pp. 161-172.

Viney, L. and Bousfield, L. (1991) Narrative analysis: a method of psychosocial research for aids-affected people. *Social Science and Medicine,* **32**, 757-765.

Vittoria, A. (1998) Preserving selves, identity work and dementia. *Research on Aging,* **20**(1), 91-136.

Volicer, L. and Ganzini, L. (2003) Health professionals' views on standards for decision-making capacity regarding refusal of medical treatment in mild Alzheimer's disease. *Journal of the American Geriatrics Society,* **51**, 1270 - 1274.

Waddell, C. (2002) So much research evidence, so little dissemination and uptake; mixing the useful with the pleasing. *Evidence Based Nursing,* **5**, 38-40.

Walker, E. and Dewar, B. (2001) How do we facilitate carers' involvement in decision making. *Journal of Advanced Nursing,* **34**(3), 329-337.

Walsh, D. and Downe, S. (2005) Meta-synthesis method for qualitative research: a literature review. *Journal of Advanced Nursing,* **50**(2), 204 - 211.

Walsh, M. (2000) *Nursing Frontiers: Accountability and the Boundaries of Care,* Butterworth-Heinemann, Oxford.

Walter, I., Nutley, S. and Davies, H. (2003) Research impact: a cross sector review [on line] St Andrews University of St Andrews. available from www.st-andrews.ac.uk/%7Eruru/publications.htm accessed 3.1.07.

Ward-Griffin, C., Bol, N. and Oudshoorn, A. (2006) Perspectives of women with dementia receiving care from their adult daughters. *Canadian Journal of Nursing Research,* **38**(1), 120-146.

Ward-Griffin, C., Oudshoorn, A., Clark, K. and Bol, N. (2007) Mother-adult daughter relationships within dementia care. *Journal of Family Nursing,* **13**(1), 13-32.

Warms, C. and Schroeder, C. (1999) Bridging the Gulf between Science and action: The "New Fuzzies" of Neopragmatism. *Advances in Nursing Science,* **22**(2), 1 - 10.

Warner, L. and Wexler, S. (1998) Eight hours a day and taken for granted? The Princess Royal Trust for Carers, London.

Webb, C. (2003) Introduction to guidelines on reporting qualitative research. *Journal of Advanced Nursing,* **42**(6), 544 - 545.

Wells, D. and Dawson, P. (2000) Description of retained abilities in older persons with dementia. *Research in Nursing and Health,* **23**, 158 - 166.

Wenger, E. (1998) *Communities of Practice: Learning Meaning and Identity,* Cambridge University Press, Edinburgh.

—. (2000) Communities of practice and social learning systems. *Organization,* **7**, 225-246.

—. (2003) *Communities of Practice: Learning, Meaning and Identity 2nd ed,* Cambridge University Press, Cambridge.

Wenger, E., McDermott, R. and Snyder, W. (2002) *Cultivating Communities of Practice,* Harvard Business School Press, Boston MA.

Wengraf, T. (2001) *Qualitative Research Interviewing Biographic Narrative and Semi-Structured Methods,* Sage, London.

Werezak, L. and Stewart, N. (2002) Learning to live with early dementia. *Canadian Journal of Nursing Research,* **34**(1), 67 - 85.

Wheeler, S. (2006) Ethical Principles and Research Ethics Review. unpublished report.

White, H. (1981) The value of narrativity in the representation of reality. In *On Narrative* (ed, Mitchell, W.) Chicago University Press, Chicago.

WHO (1992) ICD 10 - Classification of Mental and Behavioral Disorders. Clinical Descriptions and Diagnostic Guidelines. World Health Organisation, Geneva.

Wilkinson, H. (2002) Including people with dementia in research: methods and motivations. In *The Perspectives of People with Dementia* (ed, Wilkinson, H.) Jessica Kingsley Publishers Ltd, London, pp. 9 - 24.

Wilkinson, H. and Milne, A. (2003) Sharing a diagnosis of dementia - learning from the patient perspective. *Aging and Mental Health,* **7**(4), 300 - 307.

Williams, R. (1988) *Key Words: a Vocabulary of Culture and Society (revised edition),* Fontana, London.

Willis, P. (2004) From 'the things themselves' to a 'feeling of understanding': finding different voices in phenomenological research [on line] available from www.ipip.org/august2004/willis4e1.pdf accessed 23.12.06. *Indo-Pacific Journal of Phenomenology,* **4**(1), 1-13.

Wolcott, H. (1994) *Transforming Qualitative Data: Description, Analysis and Interpretation,* Sage, Thousand Oaks.

Wong, J., Clare, I., Holland, A., Watson, P. and Gunn, M. (2000) The capacity of people with 'mental disability' to make a health care decision. *Psychological Medicine,* **30**, 295 - 306.

Wood, M. (2002) Experiential learning for undergraduates: a simulation about functional change and aging. *Gerontology and Geriatrics Education,* **23**, 37-48.

Wooding, S., Hanney, S., Buxton, M. and Grant, J. (2004) The returns from arthritis research: vol 1 approach, analysis and recommendations. In *A report prepared for the Arthritis Research Campaign* RAND, Europe.

Woods, L., Priest, H. and Roberts, P. (2002) An overview of three different approaches to the interpretation of qualitative data. Part 2: practical illustrations. *Nurse Researcher,* **10**(1), 43-51.

Wright, F. (1998) *Continuing to Care. The Effect on Spouses and Children of an Older Person's Admission to a Care Home,* York Publishing Services Ltd, York.

Yam, B. (2005) Professional doctorate and professional nursing practice. *Nurse Education Today,* **25**, 564-572.

Yanow, D. (1995) Writing organizational tales: four authors and their stories about culture. Introduction. *Organization Science,* **6**, 225 - 226.

Young, R. (2002) Medical experiences and concerns of people with Alzheimer's disease. In *The Person with Alzheimer's Disease* (ed, Harris, P.) The Johns Hopkins University Press, Baltimore, pp. 29 - 46.

Zarit, S., Gaugler, J. and Jarrott, S. (1999) Useful services for families: research findings and directions. *International Journal of Geriatric Psychiatry,* **14**, 165-177.

INDEX